T0344436

Geriatric Rehabilitation

Geriatric Rehabilitation

DAVID X. CIFU, MD

Associate Dean of Innovation and System
   Integration
Virginia Commonwealth University
   School of Medicine
Richmond, VA, United States
Herman J. Flax, MD Professor and Chair
Department of PM&R
Virginia Commonwealth University
   School of Medicine
Richmond, VA, United States
Senior TBI Specialist
Principal Investigator, Chronic Effects of
   Neurotrauma Consortium
U.S. Department of Veterans Affairs
Richmond, VA, United States
Director, Sports Sciences
NHL Florida Panthers
Richmond, VA, United States

HENRY L. LEW, MD

Tenured Professor and Chair
University of Hawai'i School of Medicine
Department of Communication Sciences
   and Disorders
Honolulu, HI, United States
Adjunct Professor
Virginia Commonwealth University
   School of Medicine
Department of Physical Medicine and
   Rehabilitation
Richmond, VA, United States

MOOYEON OH-PARK, MD

Director of Geriatric Rehabilitation
Kessler Institute for Rehabilitation
Research Scientist
Kessler Foundation
West Orange, NJ, United States
Professor
Vice Chair of Education
Department of Physical Medicine and
   Rehabilitation
Rutgers New Jersey Medical School
Newark, NJ, United States

ELSEVIER

ELSEVIER

3251 Riverport Lane
St. Louis, Missouri 63043

GERIATRIC REHABILITATION

ISBN: 978-0-323-54454-2

Notices

Content Strategist: Kayla Wolfe
Content Development Manager: Taylor Ball
Content Development Specialist: Kristen Helm
Publishing Services Manager: Deepthi Unni
Project Manager: Janish Ashwin Paul
Designer: Gopalakrishnan Venkatraman

Printed in United States of America

Last digit is the print number: 9   8   7   6   5   4   3   2   1

Working together to grow libraries in developing countries

www.elsevier.com • www.bookaid.org

List of Contributors

Editors

David X. Cifu, MD
Associate Dean of Innovation and System Integration
Virginia Commonwealth University School of
    Medicine
Richmond, VA, United States
Herman J. Flax, MD Professor and Chair
Department of PM&R
Virginia Commonwealth University School of
    Medicine
Richmond, VA, United States
Senior TBI Specialist
Principal Investigator, Chronic Effects of Neurotrauma
    Consortium
U.S. Department of Veterans Affairs
Richmond, VA, United States
Director, Sports Sciences
NHL Florida Panthers
Richmond, VA, United States

Blessen C. Eapen, MD
Section Chief, Polytrauma Rehabilitation Center
TBI/Polytrauma Fellowship Program Director
Site Director, Defense and Veterans Brain Injury
    Center (DVBIC)
South Texas Veterans Health Care System
San Antonio, TX, United States
Associate Professor
Department of Rehabilitation Medicine
UT Health San Antonio
San Antonio, TX, United States

Henry L. Lew, MD
Tenured Professor and Chair
University of Hawai'i School of Medicine
Department of Communication Sciences and
    Disorders
Honolulu, HI, United States
Adjunct Professor
Virginia Commonwealth University School of
    Medicine
Department of Physical Medicine and Rehabilitation
Richmond, VA, United States

Mooyeon Oh-Park, MD
Director of Geriatric Rehabilitation
Kessler Institute for Rehabilitation
Research Scientist
Kessler Foundation
West Orange, NJ, United States
Professor
Vice Chair of Education
Department of Physical Medicine and Rehabilitation
Rutgers New Jersey Medical School
Newark, NJ, United States

Authors

Venu Akuthota, MD
Professor and Chair
Department of Physical Medicine and Rehabilitation
School of Medicine, University of Colorado
Aurora, CO, United States

Matthew N. Bartels, MD, MPH
Professor and Chairman of the Physical Medicine and
    Rehabilitation
Albert Einstein College of Medicine
Bronx, NY, United States
Chairman
Department of Rehabilitation Medicine
Montefiore Medical Center
Bronx, NY, United States

Christina L. Bell, MD, PhD
Hawaii Permanente Medical Group
Clinical Associate Professor
Department of Geriatric Medicine
University of Hawaii John A. Burns School of
    Medicine
Honolulu, HI, United States

Jaewon Beom, MD, PhD
Assistant Professor
Department of Physical Medicine and Rehabilitation
Chung-Ang University Hospital
Seoul, South Korea

Shih-Ching Chen, MD, PhD
Professor
Dean
College of Medicine
Taipei Medical University
Taipei, Taiwan, Republic of China

Michelle Didesch, MD
Traumatic Brain Injury Service
Department of Physical Medicine and Rehabilitation
University of Pittsburgh Medical Center
Pittsburgh, PA, United States

Walter R. Frontera, MD, PhD
Professor
Department of Physical Medicine, Rehabilitation, and
  Sports Medicine
Department of Physiology
University of Puerto Rico School of Medicine
San Juan, PR, United States

Shari Goo-Yoshino, MS, CCC-SLP
Department of Communication Sciences and
  Disorders
John A. Burns School of MedicineUniversity of
  Hawai'i at Mānoa
Honolulu, HI, United States
Kaiser Permanente Moanalua Medical Center
Honolulu, HI, United States

Der-Sheng Han, MD, PhD
Medical Director
National Taiwan University Hospital Beihu Branch,
Taipei, Taiwan, Republic of China
Assistant Professor
College of Medicine
National Taiwan University
Taipei, Taiwan, Republic of China

Eric K. Holder, MD
Hospital for Special Surgery
Department of Physiatry
New York, NY, United States

Carlos A. Jaramillo, MD, PhD
Staff Physician/Clinical Investigator
Polytrauma Rehabilitation Center
South Texas Veterans Health Care System
San Antonio, TX, United States
Assistant Professor
UT Health San Antonio
San Antonio, TX, United States

Dennis D.J. Kim, MD
Associate Professor,
Department of Rehabilitation Medicine
Montefiore Medical Center
Albert Einstein College of Medicine
Bronx, NY, United States

Jongmin Lee, MD, PhD
Professor
Chair
Department of Rehabilitation of Medicine
Konkuk University School of Medicine and Konkuk
  University Medical Center
Seoul, Republic of Korea

Sang Y. Lee, MD, PhD
Assistant Professor
Department of Rehabilitation Medicine
Seoul National University Boramae Medical Center
Seoul, Republic of Korea

Sewon Lee, MD
Associate Professor
Department of Rehabilitation Medicine
Montefiore Medical Center
Albert Einstein College of Medicine
Bronx, NY, United States

Carol Li, MD
Department of Rehabilitation Medicine
University of Texas Health Science Center San Antonio
San Antonio, TX, United States

Jae-Young Lim, MD, PhD
Professor and Chair
Department of Rehabilitation Medicine
Seoul National University College of Medicine
Seoul National University Bundang Hospital
Seongnam-si, Republic of Korea

Adele Meron, MD
Physical Medicine and Rehabilitation
University of Colorado
Aurora, CO, United States

William Micheo, MD
Professor and Chair
Sports Medicine Fellowship Director
Physical Medicine, Rehabilitation and Sports
  Medicine Department
University of Puerto Rico, School of Medicine
San Juan, PR, United States

Peter J. Moley, MD
Assistant Attending Physiatrist,
Hospital for Special Surgery
Assistant Professor of Clinical Rehabilitation Medicine
Weill Cornell Medical College
New York, NY, United States

Yeonsil Moon, MD, PhD
Clinical Assistant Professor
Department of Neurology
Konkuk University Medical Center
Seoul, Republic of Korea

Jean Oh, PhD
Systems Scientist
Robotics Institute
Carnegie Mellon University
Pittsburgh, PA, United States

Manisha S. Parulekar, MD, FACP, CMD
Program Director
Geriatrics fellowship
Assistant Professor
Rutgers New Jersey Medical School
West Orange, NJ, United States
Associate Professor
St. George's Medical School, St. George's, Grenada
Interim Chief
Division of Geriatrics
Hackensack University Medical Center
Hackensack Meridian Health
Hackensack, NJ, United States

Kanakadurga R. Poduri, MD, FAAPMR
Professor and Chair of PM&R and Professor of
    Neurology
Department of Physical Medicine and Rehabilitation
University of Rochester School of Medicine and
    Dentistry and Medical Center
Rochester, NY, United States

David Z. Prince, MD
Assistant Professor
Albert Einstein College of Medicine
Bronx, NY, United States
Director
Cardiopulmonary Rehabilitation
Montefiore Medical Center
Bronx, NY, United States

Christopher K. Rogers, MPH
Research Associate
Division of Geriatrics
Hackensack University Medical Center
Hackensack Meridian Health
Hackensack, NJ, United States

Luis A. Sánchez, MD
Sports Medicine Fellow
Physical Medicine, Rehabilitation and Sports
    Medicine Department
University of Puerto Rico, School of Medicine
San Juan, PR, United States

Chiemi Tanaka, PhD CCC-A
Audiology Specialist
Audmet KK (Oticon Japan, DiaTec Company)
Kawasaki-shi, Kanagawa, Japan
Adjunct Assistant Professor
Department of Communication Sciences & Disorders
University of Hawai'i at Mānoa, John A. Burns School
    of Medicine
Honolulu, HI, United States

Lisa D. Taniguchi, AuD
Department of Communication Sciences and
    Disorders
John A. Burns School of Medicine
University of Hawai'i at Mānoa
Honolulu, HI, United States

Maria Vanushkina, MD
Department of Physical Medicine and Rehabilitation
University of Rochester School of Medicine and
    Dentistry and Medical Center
Rochester, NY, United States

Foreword

Currently, the total number of people aged 60 years and older in the world is 900 million strong, and by 2050, it is expected to exceed 2 billion. With improvements in public health and medical care, people are expected to live longer lives, but it does not mean that the geriatric population will automatically maintain functional independence and high quality of life. It is essential that health professionals work together to achieve this goal. Although geriatric rehabilitation is an important topic, there has not been a single, easy-to-read clinical handbook to guide practitioners in the care of their elderly patients. This *Geriatric Rehabilitation Handbook* provides the fundamental knowledge that is required to design and implement a practical rehabilitation program for elderly individuals over a wide functional range. Exemplary chapters discuss the most common issues in the elderly population, such as nutritional and swallowing problems, hearing impairment, osteoporosis, sarcopenia, polypharmacy, deconditioning, as well as cognitive impairment and psychiatric disorders. It is our hope that this handbook will serve as a practical resource for rehabilitation specialists, geriatricians, and other healthcare professionals who care for the elderly population. We applaud the efforts of the editors (Dr. David Cifu, Dr. Henry Lew, and Dr. Mooyeon Oh-Park) and authors for publication of this handbook.

Jerris Hedges, MD, MS
Professor and Dean, John A. Burns School of Medicine, University of Hawaii at Manoa

Kamal Masaki, MD
Professor and Chair, Department of Geriatric Medicine
John A. Burns School of Medicine, University of Hawaii at Manoa

Preface

The world's older population continues to grow at an unprecedented rate. Longitudinal studies have revealed the presence of multiple risk factors for disability, including behavioral and individual characteristics (e.g., low physical activity, alcohol consumption, increased age, reduced social contacts) and chronic conditions (e.g., cardiovascular disease, osteoarthritis, cancer, diabetes mellitus). Although this is hardly surprising, what is interesting and particularly pertinent to this *Geriatric Rehabilitation* handbook is that a substantial proportion of individuals who are disabled *report improvement on subsequent assessments*. In effect, disability is a product of the disease or diseases, a sedentary lifestyle, and physiologic declines from normal aging or pathologic processes that are not specific diseases but instead result from factors such as inflammation or endocrine changes. As these predisposing conditions change, they have an impact on the initiation of disability and on changes in the status of already established disability. These findings have especially significant implications on the role of rehabilitation efforts for older adults; concerted efforts to optimize baseline and postdisability physical, cognitive, and behavioral functioning can effectively "reverse the effects of time." Disability and aging are not inexorably linked. Although the impact of degenerative and inflammatory processes on the body's systems will often be expressed in physical and cognitive limitations, there are a wide range of physical medicine and rehabilitation interventions that can be applied to both bolster the functional reserve of elders and reverse many of the acute and even chronic disabilities seen. The geriatric population is diverse in its level of functional independence, ranging from elite athletes to those totally dependent. The wide range of topics and conditions covered in this *Geriatric Rehabilitation* issue provide the reader with the age-specific impacts commonly experienced, scientific background supporting the management strategies, and practical approaches to the assessments and interventions for this growing population. The authors have identified the key topics, delivered the information in a user-friendly style, and highlighted the vital rehabilitation principles necessary to affect older adults with disability. In the fast-paced 21st century, awash in high technology and precision medicine, the core principles of rehabilitation medicine offer proven treatments that are universal in their efficacy and that can provide durable and meaningful outcomes. We hope that the readers of this important work will find it an easy-to-use and practical resource that will augment their skills and enable their patients. Many thanks to all who contributed and supported the development and execution of this work.

David X. Cifu, MD
Henry L. Lew, MD, PhD
Mooyeon Oh-Park, MD

Contents

CHAPTER 1

Epidemiology of Aging, Disability, Frailty and Overall Role of Physiatry

KANAKADURGA R. PODURI, MD, FAAPMR • MARIA VANUSHKINA, MD

INTRODUCTION

There is no agreement in the literature, practice, or policymaking for considering an individual to be truly "old." Although not the most clinically relevant, chronologic age is the commonly accepted criterion for categorization, with most Western societies arbitrarily choosing 65 years as the cutoff to consider a person as a member of the geriatric population.[1] Terms frequently used to describe this population are young old (60+), old old (75+), and oldest old (85+).[1] When demographers mention "aging," they are referring to the increase in the proportion of the population in the older age ranges.[2] When life sciences experts discuss "aging," they are referring to the progressive changes in functional properties at the cellular and tissue level leading to decreased adaptability to stressors and an overall vulnerability to morbidity and mortality.[3] These changes are not linear or consistent, are sometimes reversible, and correlate only loosely with chronologic age. Some mechanisms of aging are random, whereas others are strongly associated with biological, social, environmental, and behavioral factors intrinsic to the individual.[4]

As we age our health is the predominant characteristic that affects the available opportunities and the ability to engage in meaningful activities. Individuals with good health in their later years have very few limitations. However, if the extra years in later life are dominated by consequences of deteriorating physical and mental capacities, the implications for both the society and the older individual are more detrimental. Although it is often assumed that the trend of increased longevity is accompanied by an extended period of good health and preserved function, the evidence that older people today are "healthier" than their parents is not encouraging, especially for the American population. Both demographic and biological "aging" have tremendous implications for local and global health and healthcare, public policy, and economy.[4] Unlike most societal level changes that may occur over the next 50 years, the trends associated with aging are largely predictable and amenable to interventions. The future framework for global action should focus on strengthening and preparing older adults to thrive in a turbulent and evolving environment.[4] This chapter provides an overview of aging demographics and physiology, reviews emerging concepts and terminology in geriatric medical practice, and addresses current practice models designed to compress morbidity and mortality in this complex population.

EPIDEMIOLOGY OF AGING: DEMOGRAPHICS AND WHAT IS "NORMAL"

Demographics

For the first time in recorded history, most individuals are expected to live beyond 60 years. Accordingly, all current research predicts a steep increase in the aging population over the next 4 decades. In some countries such as Brazil or Myanmar, a child born in 2015 can expect to live 20 years longer than one born 50 years earlier.[4] When combined with globally decreasing fertility trends, the increasing life expectancy is expected to have dramatic impacts on the structure of global populations.[4] Worldwide, the 65+ years sector is projected to grow from 524 to 1.5 billion between 2010 and 2050.[5] In the United States the population of adults over the age of 65 years is expected to double between 2012 and 2050, reaching a projected maximum of 83.7 million. By 2030, more than 20.3% of US residents are projected to be over 65 years old, compared with 13.7% in 2010 and 9.8% in 1970.[2] This population is expected to become more racially and ethnically diverse with a shift toward more equal gender distribution during this time.[2] This accelerated growth is attributed to improvements in life expectancy over the past century.[2,5] In the United States, life expectancy at age 65 years was 15.2 years in 1972 and rose to 19.1 years in 2010.[2] For those turning 85 years in 1972, the average length of life was 5.5 years, which increased to 6.5 years in 2010.[2]

This oldest old population is expected to grow by 351% by 2050.[5] Similar trends have been observed in almost all developed nations.[2,5]

Changes Associated With "Normal" Aging

Aging affects the physiologic function of multiple organ systems as summarized in Table 1.1.

CHRONIC CONDITIONS IN OLDER ADULTS
Chronic Conditions at a Glance

The life expectancy improvements discussed earlier are reflections of multiple public health efforts in the 20th century, such as advances in living conditions, sanitation, and introduction of vaccination protocols. In fact, the global burden of morbidity and mortality has shifted from infectious illnesses to chronic noncommunicable conditions, such as heart disease, stroke, diabetes, cancer, arthritis, obesity, and respiratory disease.[2,5,6] In 2008 chronic conditions accounted for an estimated 86% of the burden of disease in developed countries.[5] The prevalence of chronic conditions will continue to increase in the future decades. In the United States, almost half the general population is projected to have at least one chronic condition by 2020.[7] It has been estimated that 20% of the Medicare beneficiaries have five or more chronic conditions.[8] It is important to note that chronic conditions affect all age groups and the majority of persons with chronic conditions are not disabled or "old."[9]

Only about one-fourth of individuals with chronic conditions have one or more daily activity limitations.[10] Such individuals often require family or professional caregiver presence in the house. Caregivers are currently present in only one of five US households.[11] Most caregiving in United States is informal, provided by women (usually wives or daughters) on a daily basis, averaging between 4 and 8 hours and lasting from weeks to multiple decades. This type of informal care accounts for about 75% of all the care provided to the older population in the United States.[1] Access to and quantity of social supports is positively correlated with happiness, life satisfaction, physical health, lower mortality, and rates of institutionalization in the geriatric population.[12,13] Unfortunately, not everyone has equal access to social supports. Social dependency is more common in women who are more likely to be widowed than age-matched men. Older adult men are more likely to have the support of a spouse who is typically younger and in better health.[1] The toll on caregivers' health and well-being is tremendous and accounts for significant costs to families, employers, and communities.[11]

Chronic diseases are among the most common and costly of all the health problems but also the most preventable. Chronic disease prevention, to be most effective, must occur in multiple sectors and across individuals' entire life spans. Prevention encompasses health promotion activities that encourage healthy living. Current research consistently associates many adult-onset health problems and later-onset disability to early life, or even in utero, socioeconomic conditions, and associated health complications. Ensuring adequate living conditions, healthcare access, and health literacy in childhood will reduce the future health burden of older populations.[5] Studies repeatedly demonstrate that the onset of multimorbidity and its associated complications occurred between 10 and 15 years earlier in people living in the most deprived areas compared with the most affluent, and socioeconomic deprivation is particularly associated with multimorbidity.[14] It is noteworthy that the scope and severity of the chronic disease problem in the United States has not escaped the attention of the public. More than two-thirds of the adults believe that the healthcare system should place more emphasis on chronic disease preventive care, and more than eighty percent Americans favor public funding for such prevention programs.[15]

DISABILITY IN OLDER ADULTS
Comorbidity

The term "comorbidity" was introduced in 1970 by Feinstein and refers to the combination of diseases beyond an index condition that may affect prognosis.[16] Many current inpatient and outpatient clinical practice models continue to focus on an index condition and address comorbid conditions only as part of the risk factor modification for the index problem. "Comorbidity" is also an important determinant in the formula used for the rehabilitation prospective payment system implemented in 2002 by the Centers for Medicare and Medicaid services. It further defines and characterizes the burden of care.

Multimorbidity

The term "multimorbidity" was introduced in 2002 by Bastra and colleagues and denotes the complex interplay between multiple conditions in an individual.[6,17] This concept is slowly shifting the clinical practice models for providers caring for these individuals (see section on complex care teams for further discussion). Multimorbidity is most often defined as the coexistence of at least three chronic conditions over a span of at least 1 year.[6,18] Although the absolute number of

TABLE 1.1
Physiologic Changes of Aging

Body System	Change	Consequences
Nervous	↓ Number of neurons ↓ Action potential speed ↓ Axon/dendrite branches	↓ Muscle innervation ↓ Fine motor control
Muscle	Fibers shrink ↓ Type II (fast twitch) fibers ↑ Lipofuscin and fat deposits	Tissue atrophies ↓ Tone and contractility ↓ Strength
Skin	↓ Thickness ↑ Collagen cross-links	Loss of elasticity
Skeletal	↓ Bone density Joints become stiffer, less flexible	Movement slows and may become limited
Cardiovascular		
Heart	↑ Left ventricular wall thickness ↑ Lipofuscin and fat deposits	Stressed heart is less able to respond
Vasculature	↑ Stiffness ↓ Responsiveness to agents	
Pulmonary	↓ Elastin fibers ↑ Collagen cross-links ↓ Elastic recoil of the lung ↑ Residual volume ↓ Vital capacity, forced expiratory volume, and forced vital capacity	↓ Effort-dependent and effort-independent respiration (quiet and forced breathing) ↓ Exercise tolerance and pulmonary reserve
Eyes	↑ Lipid infiltrates/deposits ↑ Thickening of the lens ↓ Pupil diameter	↓ Transparency of the cornea Difficulty in focusing on near objects ↓ Accommodation and dark adaptation
Ears	↑ Thickening of tympanic membrane ↓ Elasticity and efficiency of ossicular articulation ↑ Organ atrophy ↓ Cochlear neurons ↓ Number of neurons in the utricle, saccule, and ampullae ↓ Size and number of otoliths	↑ Conductive deafness (low-frequency range) ↑ Sensorineural hearing loss (high-frequency sounds) ↓ Detection of gravity, changes in speed, and rotation
Digestive	↑ Dysphagia ↑ Achlorhydria Altered intestinal absorption ↑ Lipofuscin and fat deposition in pancreas ↑ Mucosal cell atrophy	↓ Iron absorption ↓ B_{12} and calcium absorption ↑ Incidence of diverticula, transit time, and constipation
Urinary	↓ Kidney size, weight, and number of functional glomeruli ↓ Number and length of functional renal tubules ↓ Glomerular filtration rate ↓ Renal blood flow	↓ Ability to resorb glucose ↓ Concentrating ability of kidney

Continued

TABLE 1.1
Physiologic Changes of Aging—cont'd

Body System	Change	Consequences
Immune	↓ Primary and secondary response	↓ Immune functioning
	↑ Autoimmune antibodies	
	↓ T-cell function, fewer naive and more memory T cells	↓ Response to new pathogens
	Atrophy of thymus	↓ T lymphocytes, natural killer cells, cytokines needed for growth and maturation of B cells
Endocrine	↑ Atrophy of certain glands (e.g., pituitary, thyroid, thymus)	Changes in target organ response, organ system homeostasis, response to stress, functional capacity
	↓ Growth hormone, dehydroepiandrosterone, testosterone, estrogen	
	↑ Parathyroid hormone, atrial natriuretic peptide, norepinephrine, baseline cortisol, erythropoietin	

From Fedarko NS, McNabney MK. Biology. In: Medina-Walpole A, Pacala JT, Potter JF, eds. *Geriatrics Review Syllabus: A Core Curriculum in Geriatric Medicine*. 9th ed. New York: American Geriatrics Society; 2016; with permission.

people with multimorbidity is higher for the below 65-year age ranges, the prevalence of multimorbidity increases substantially with age.[6,14] Coexistence of multiple chronic conditions is becoming the "normal" in geriatric patients rather than the exception.[6,14,18] The reported prevalence of multimorbidity in older persons ranges from 55% to 98%.[6,9,14,19] Chronic neuropsychiatric disorders, such as mental health disorders or dementia, and lower socioeconomic status are strongly associated with increased physical morbidities[14] and long-term care dependency.[5,18] Chronic diseases can exacerbate symptoms of depression, and depressive disorders can themselves lead to chronic diseases. The correlation between multimorbidity and mortality is still a controversial topic in the literature. There is strong evidence to suggest that multimorbid individuals die earlier,[18,20,21] are 99 times more likely to be admitted to the hospital for ambulatory care sensitive conditions,[19] have higher rates of functional decline and disability,[6,18] are more likely to be dependent for long-term care at an younger age,[18] report poorer quality of life,[6,18,22] and have higher healthcare costs.[6,9,18,19] Persons with chronic conditions have greater health needs at any age and, not surprisingly, their costs are disproportionately higher.[9] The direct healthcare costs of US adults with more than one chronic condition is estimated to account for greater than three-fourth of total annual healthcare expenditures, with 1990 costs exceeding $659 billion per year.[9] The per capita Medicare expenditures are more than 66 times higher for beneficiaries with multiple chronic conditions compared with their "healthy" counterparts.[19]

GERIATRIC SYNDROMES

One of the main challenges to traditional clinical care and research models for the geriatric population is the presence of multiple chronic conditions and geriatric syndromes that cross organ systems and discipline-based boundaries.[14,18,23] The term "geriatric syndrome" is used to capture a clinical condition affecting the geriatric population that does not fit into a discrete disease category.[23] "Geriatric syndromes" are a valuable theoretical framework clinically as well as an educational tool for patients and medical providers alike.[24] The term "syndrome" may be a misnomer.[23,24] A syndrome is classically defined as the "aggregate of symptoms and signs associated with any morbid process, and it constitutes together the picture of the disease."[25] Geriatric syndromes are more accurately conceptualized as "multifactorial health conditions that occur when the accumulated effects of impairments in multiple systems render an older person vulnerable to situation challenges."[26] This definition emphasizes the nonlinear contribution of multiple etiologic factors and their varying degrees of synergism to the observable characteristics of a manifestation[23] (Fig. 1.1). Many of the most common conditions treated in geriatric patients across all the care settings are classified as geriatric syndromes, including delirium, dizziness, syncope, urinary incontinence, pressure ulcers, falls, and frailty.[23] There are four shared risk factors consistently identified across all the geriatric syndromes suggesting a shared pathophysiologic mechanism: older age, functional impairment, cognitive impairment, and impaired mobility.

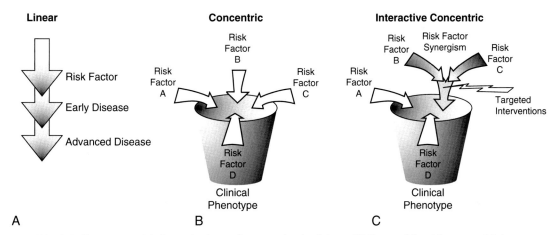

FIG. 1.1 Concept models for geriatric syndrome pathophysiology. **(A)** The traditional linear model does not adequately capture the multifactorial nature of geriatric syndromes. **(B)** The concentric model may also not be suitable for geriatric syndromes because interventions targeting only one risk factor would address only a small portion of the overall risk for such conditions, whereas multicomponent pharmaceutical interventions risk being unfocussed and could lead to adverse effects typically associated with geriatric polypharmacy. **(C)** The interactive concentric model is a means of reconciling the need for mechanistic research with the condition's multifactorial complexity, by focusing on pathways associated with risk factor synergisms, thus offering a locus for the design of targeted interventions. (From Inouye SK, Studenski S, Tinetti ME, et al. Geriatric syndromes: clinical, research, and policy implications of a core geriatric concept. *J Am Geriatr Soc.* 2007;55(5):780–791; with permission.)

Excluding older age, the remaining risk factors (functional impairment, cognitive impairment, and impaired mobility) are amenable to interventions, preventative strategies to provide reorientation for cognitive impairment, exercise, balance training, and mobilization.[23]

There has been substantial progress in clarifying risk factors and intervention strategies for some common geriatric syndromes such as delirium and falls. Unfortunately, these advances have failed to widely translate into the clinical implementation.[23] Delirium is a very common life-threatening geriatric syndrome for hospitalized older patients, occurring in 14%–56% and associated with in-hospital mortality of 22%–76%.[27] Unfortunately, delirium is unrecognized in 66%–77% of these patients and documented in only 3% of the patients when it is present clinically. These factors preclude effective interventions.[28,29] Up to 30%–40% of delirium may be preventable with appropriate interventions, such as the Hospital Elder Life Program (HELP), which may also reduce delirium duration when it does occur, prevent functional decline and falls, and lead to higher rates of home discharge post hospitalization.[30-32]

Unintentional injury is the sixth most common cause of death among older individuals. Falls are the leading cause of unintentional injury and occur at very high rates (30%–40%) in the geriatric population.[33] Gait instability accounts for approximately 20% of falls in older adults.[34] Although some physicians may worry about falls, gait instability is in itself an indication for initiating an exercise program and can be improved significantly through strength and balance training.[35] Falls are associated with functional decline, hospitalization, institutionalization, and increased healthcare costs. However, only 37% of primary care providers document screening their older patients for falls.[33,36] Based on 2008 data, over 60 fall-reduction interventional trials have been conducted, with an approximated 30% relative risk reduction noted post intervention.[33,37] The Connecticut Collaboration for Fall Prevention (CCFP) program is an example of a local effort to translate research into practice by providing targeted providers in emergency departments, primary care offices, home care agencies, and rehabilitation centers with the fall risk evaluation and management resources and education.[38]

There are many challenges to the successful implementation and sustainability of HELP, CCFP, and similar programs, including the need for clinician leadership and limited funding.[39] The data collected as part of the CCFP project showed multiple barriers to dissemination, including lack of knowledge regarding the importance and preventability of falls in providers and patients alike, false perception that fall risk evaluation and management were not allowed by Medicare, poor Medicare reimbursement for fall-related services, ongoing healthcare focus on diseases rather than multifactorial geriatric syndromes, and competing demands for frequent clinical visits.[38] As with most interventions, a national-level shift of focus to prevention will be required for the geriatric population for optimal results.

FRAILTY

The Concept of Frailty

"Frailty" can be thought of as one more example of a geriatric syndrome that overlaps with but is distinct from disability, multimorbidity, and "normal" aging (Fig. 1.2).[40,41] Frailty as defined or rather described by Walston et al. is "[Frailty is] a state of increased vulnerability to stressors due to age-related declines in physiologic reserve across neuromuscular, metabolic and immune systems."[43] It is a clinical syndrome presenting the following symptoms:
- Self-reported exhaustion
- Low physical activity
- Unintentional weight loss (10 lbs or more than 5% of body weight in past year)
- Weakness (grip strength in lowest 20th percentile)
- Slow walking speed (15 ft; lowest 20th percentile)

Multimorbidity is an etiologic risk for disability and is a potential outcome of frailty.[41] Although frailty is poorly defined in the literature,[40,42] broadly agreed upon manifestations include accumulation of multidimensional loss of reserves across neuromuscular, metabolic, cognitive, and immune systems that give rise to vulnerability.[40,43,44] It is sometimes referred to as a loss of "functional homeostasis."[45] Frailty is associated with aging and increases in prevalence in older age groups, although exact estimates vary based on the population studied. For example, among community-dwelling adults in Canada 65–102 years old, 22.7% were frail. Of the subgroup of individuals aged 85 years and older, frailty was noted in 40%.[46] Other studies mentioned rates as low as 6.9% in community-dwelling American geriatric populations.[41] Independent of age, frailty is thought to be predictive of mortality, hospitalization, institutionalization, falls, and worsening health status.[40,41,44,46–50] Frailty is also thought of as bidirectional and can be reversed with appropriate interventions.[51]

Both the high rates of associated morbidity and availability of "reversal" modalities for frailty make it a high-yield clinical construct for screening in the aging population. There are many operational definitions and screening tools. These tools tend to be based on a predefined set of rules, a summation of impairments, or reliant on clinical judgment.[44] Each assessment has associated drawbacks to clinical implementation, such

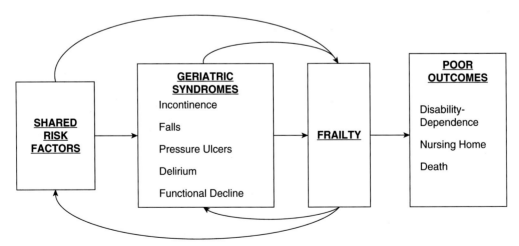

FIG. 1.2 Conceptual model of shared risks leading to geriatric syndromes. Conceptual model demonstrating the interconnected nature with multiple feedback mechanisms of risk factors, geriatric syndromes, frailty, and poor outcomes. These self-sustaining pathways hold important implications for elucidating pathophysiologic mechanisms and designing effective intervention strategies for this patient population. (From Inouye SK, Studenski S, Tinetti ME, et al. Geriatric syndromes: clinical, research, and policy implications of a core geriatric concept. *J Am Geriatr Soc.* 2007;55(5):780–791; with permission.)

as the need to consider a list of no fewer than 70 possible disorders for models based on summation of impairments.[44] Examples of validated assessment tools used to determine frailty status include the Cardiovascular Health Study Frailty Phenotype (CHSFP),[41] the Frailty Index,[48,49] and the Clinical Frailty Score (CFS).[44] The CHSFP is an example of a rules-based approach that diagnoses frailty based on the presence of at least three of the criteria listed below:

- Unintentional weight loss of 10 or more pounds over a period of 1 year
- Self-reported exhaustion
- Grip strength weakness
- Slow walking speed
- Low physical activity.[41]

The CFS is a seven-point system that may be the easiest to administer in clinical practice than the other tools. It mixes items such as comorbidity, cognitive impairment, and disability that some other groups separate by focusing on physical manifestations of frailty. Scores range from 1 (patient is in robust health) to 7 (patient has complete functional dependence on others).[44] The utilization of one of the many available tools should be incorporated into clinical practice by all providers dealing with this population.

Brief Note on Polypharmacy and Deprescribing

Although not a true "geriatric syndrome," polypharmacy is a rampant problem in the older adults. Optimizing pharmacotherapy is a critical aspect of geriatric care, as this population is at high risk for adverse drug events (ADEs). Polypharmacy is defined as the use of multiple medications by a patient, with 5–10 medications usually accepted as the cutoff.[52] In the United States, approximately 50% of Medicare beneficiaries take five or more medications at the same time.[8] Various criteria exist to help identify medications that should be avoided or used with caution in this patient population, although compliance with these medication lists is suboptimal. A widely used example of such lists in the United States is Beers Criteria, which was revised in 2015.[53] ADEs are associated with high rates of hospitalization in older adults. Prescribing cascades (when providers confuse ADEs with a new disease process), drug-drug interactions, and inappropriate drug doses are some of the most common causes of preventable ADEs in this population. Evidence suggests that clinicians are consistently avoiding overprescribing of inappropriate drug therapies but are more likely to underprescribe indicated drug therapies (e.g., statins).

DISABILITY IN OLDER ADULTS

It is important to differentiate disability from frailty, as patients may have one or both.[54] Among disabled older patients only 28% are frail; nearly 75% of frail older patients can complete all their activities of daily living (ADLs), and 40% do not have difficulty performing all instrumental activities of daily living (IADLs).[41] Disability may be physical, emotional, or social or due to disease-related changes. However, disability does not typically occur across multiple organ systems as does frailty.[55] The most common definition of disability focuses on physical limitations and is thought of as impairments in performance of ADLs and/or IADLs or difficulty with independent mobility.

Disability is often used in research as a measure of health and function in the aging population.[5] The increase in overall lifespan has raised an interesting question: are individuals living healthier and longer, or are the additional years spent in poor health and/or chronic disability? Currently, there is a significant controversy surrounding the relationship between increased life expectancy and overall health status in part because this topic is difficult to research. Some researchers think there will be a decrease in the prevalence of disability as life expectancy increases, termed "compression of morbidity," whereas others foretell an "expansion of morbidity" as life expectancy increases. Several studies of the US population have noted positive trends suggesting that the healthcare system can affect not only the duration but also the quality of life in the aging population. Between 1982 and 2001, severe disability decreased about 25% among those aged 65 years or older, and life expectancy increased.[5] Unfortunately, this positive trend may not persist because of alarmingly increasing rates of obesity among pediatric, adult, and geriatric populations alike. Several population-based studies from the late 2000s found stark health differences between non-Hispanic white older adults in the United States and the adults in England and 10 other European countries.[5] Significantly higher rates of chronic diseases and disability were reported for American adults aged 50–75 years compared with their European counterparts. These discrepancies in health status were at all levels of wealth, educational levels and behavioral risk factors.

THE CRITICAL IMPORTANCE OF PHYSICAL ACTIVITY

There are numerous benefits to physical activity. It is often believed that the development and worsening of chronic disease is part of normal aging. As discussed earlier, this is not a valid conclusion. Regular physical activity has been shown to reduce both the development and worsening of chronic diseases.[56] In addition, physiologic changes associated with age should not preclude an individual from engaging in exercises, even though the absolute gains are noted to be less in older adults.[57]

With very few exceptions, physical activity is recommended and should be promoted for everyone by healthcare providers. Lack of advice to exercise is often interpreted by patients as condoning a sedentary lifestyle.[58] The very few definitive contraindications to exercise, such as unstable cardiovascular conditions, are often transient.[59] The risks of sedentary behavior far outweigh the risks of a gentle exercise program.[58] Many physicians are hesitant to prescribe exercise for geriatric patients with cardiovascular disease and may order a preinitiation stress test.[35] There are several guidelines about stress testing in this setting. It is worth noting that more than 70% of patients over the age of 70 years will have abnormal stress tests with asymptomatic ischemia.[35] The American College of Sports Medicine recommends "exercise stress testing for all sedentary or minimally active older adults who plan to begin exercising at a vigorous intensity." However, most older adults can safely begin a moderate aerobic and resistance training exercises if they can begin slowly and gradually increase their level of activity without stress testing.[73] Older adults with coronary artery disease with unstable angina, uncontrolled hypertension, or dysrhythmia and a recent history of congestive heart failure must be evaluated with a stress test before starting any exercise program. Fortunately, evidence suggests that risk for a recurrent coronary event and associated disability in this population is actually reduced with exercise.[35] Patients with intermittent claudication frequently avoid exercise, and their physicians often hesitate to recommend physical activity given their symptoms of pain. Intermittent claudication is not a contraindication. These patients should be encouraged to exercise regularly, titrating the amount to pain tolerance with very gradual increase in duration and less emphasis on intensity.[60]

Benefits and Limitations

Despite the ample evidence supporting the critical role of physical activity for the reduction of morbidity and mortality at all ages, many individuals in the United States avoid physical exercise. Based on the data from 2015, up to 15% of adolescents did not participate in at least 60 min of physical activity for a minimum of 5 days per week if it produced signs of moderate effort such as increased heart rate or breathing difficulty.[61] Up to 65.3% of adolescent students do not

meet recommended levels of weekly physical activity.[62] For the adult population, more than one-third do not meet the recommendations for aerobic physical activity and 23% do not have leisure time physical activity for several months.[63] Only 51.7% of adults 18 years of age and over met the Physical Activity Guidelines for aerobic physical activity per the Centers for Disease Control and Prevention report (https://www.cdc.gov/nchs/fastats/exercise.htm). For the geriatric population, 45% of the 65- to 74-year-old group and 51% of the 75+ year-old group do not have any routine leisure time activity.[64] Fortunately, the greatest impact of exercise in improving functional status occurs in sedentary individuals who become active.[58]

Regular physical exercise has been shown to reverse some age-related decline in physiologic processes that occur with normal aging (such as improved body composition),[56,65] reduce or reverse frailty,[40] prevent onset of disability,[66,67] improve recovery from mobility loss,[68] prevent or mitigate physical dependency,[69] reduce institutional placement,[70] improve quality of life measures,[71] and, of particular importance to older adults, reduce the risk of falls and injuries from falls.[37,72] Research and clinical practice guidelines promote physical activity as a therapeutic modality for the management of hypertension,[73,74] coronary artery disease,[74-76] congestive heart failure,[77] hyperlipidemia,[74,78] peripheral vascular disease,[79] type 2 diabetes mellitus,[80,81] obesity,[82] osteoporosis,[83] osteoarthritis,[84-86] colon cancer,[87] breast cancer,[88] prostate cancer,[89] and many other common chronic conditions such as depression.[71] Cognitive function is closely linked with physical activity; increased participation is shown to prevent or delay cognitive decline and dementia.[90-92] Exercise improves bone health and reduces the risk of falling.[37]

The Geriatric Exercise Prescription

There is no consensus for the "optimal" exercise modality or frequency for geriatric patients. Innovative programs such as Exergames have not been shown to be superior to standardized or self-regulated programs.[70] Most evidence suggests that a multicomponent program inclusive of aerobic, resistance, balance, and flexibility training is preferred.[40] The key to success with any program is involving the patient in the plan and the endorsement of physical activity by physicians.[35] Participants should be counseled to view their training as a long-term commitment because frail adults can rapidly lose fitness gains upon exercise cessation.[93] Patients should directly be involved in creating an exercise plan because it seems to optimize safety and increase compliance.[35] When assisting patients with goal setting, focus on making choices that are SMART: specific, measurable, attainable, relevant, and time oriented.[58] As an example, "Get more active, do the best you can" is not SMART. Adding specifics, such as "Start by walking 5 min every day and add 1 min daily to achieve a 30 min daily walk time," is a more useful form of clinical endorsement and encouragement.[58]

In general, all programs should initially focus on the patients' current functional limitations and gradually implement a more generalized fitness plan as function improves.[35,94] The minimum suggested frequency for multicomponent training is two to three times per week at a moderate intensity (12–14 Rating of Perceived Exertion (RPE) or 3–4 on Borg CR10 point scale) for 30–45 min in frail adults and 45–60 min in prefrail adults.[40,93,95] For patients with severe clinical frailty, it is recommended that up to half of their training time should be spent on aerobic exercises.[40] Clinicians should actively work on progressing exercise prescriptions toward the upper end of the recommended range of intensity and frequency to facilitate longer-term exercise adherence and progression.[96] Resistance training exercise should include a variety of upper and lower body exercises that attempt to simulate functional tasks.[93] An emphasis should be placed on lower body muscles contributing to gross mobility (e.g., knee flexors and extensors, gluteal muscles), as these are necessary in maintaining physical independence and compensating for disproportional age-related loss of strength in the lower extremities compared with the upper body.[97] Intensity is initially established based on an individual's one repetition maximum weight, starting light at approximately 50%–60% and progressing to heavier loads.[40] Resistance exercise helps counteract neuromuscular changes associated with age-related weakness. With training, increases in voluntary muscle activation and antagonist muscle coactivation are noted. These changes are associated with overall strength gains in older adults.[98] Some evidence suggests that high-intensity progressive resistance strength training is safe and may improve lower-extremity strength more than lower-intensity programs but is not required to improve functional performance.[99] As in resistance training, the key focus of balance training is improvement of daily function. Tandem foot stance, line walking, and single leg stance should be performed after completion of resistance training as part of a cool down.[100] Patients should be instructed on proper technique before initiation of training and monitored carefully to reduce fall risk.

Group therapy programs have been shown to be effective for this population when combined with home therapy, allowing for peer interaction and some supervision for safety during the initial learning phase of an exercise routine.[100] Some group therapy classes focus on additional interventions, including nutritional education and psychosocial programs. These classes have been shown to have even greater success in the older population compared with exercise alone, improving functional status and reducing frailty.[101] Physical activity, however, is a crucial component, and educational programs alone are not sufficient to show benefits in physical function.[102]

Arthritis

Arthritis is the most common cause of disability in America, affecting one in every five adults.[103] By 60 years of age, 100% of individuals will have histologic changes consistent with degeneration. Data from the beginning of this century suggested that 40% of US adults reported having arthritis by age 60 years, and 10% had limitations in activity associated with arthritis symptoms.[104] As the US population ages, the number of adults with doctor-diagnosed arthritis is projected to increase from 46 to 67 million by 2030, and 25 million of these individuals will have limited activity as a result.[105] The disabling effects of arthritis are disproportionately prevalent in racial and ethnic minority populations. For example, compared with the white population, a higher proportion of African Americans reported severe pain as well as activity and work limitations attributable to arthritis.[106] Reducing the risk of functional dependency is the main focus of arthritis management.[35] The literature suggests that appropriate exercise programs can prevent and treat some arthritic disabilities and do not exacerbate pain or accelerate disease progression (which is contrary to popular belief).[94,107,108] Aerobic exercises, such as aquatics or walking, have been shown to increase the aerobic capacity and gait speed while improving symptoms of depression and anxiety in patients with osteoarthritis and rheumatoid arthritis when compared with simple range of motion exercises alone.[109] In addition to aerobics and resistance programs focusing on quadriceps training, a variety of nonpharmaceutical interventions have proven effective in managing osteoarthritis, including education, social support, well-cushioned customized shoes (e.g., extra depth, custom inserts to distribute plantar weight-bearing surfaces, toe box adjustments), canes, assistive devices, icing, and heating pads.[104] Proper footwear and skin care is especially critical in patients with diabetes. Obesity is one of the strongest risk factors for knee arthritis, second only to increasing age. Reducing body weight by 4.5 kg reduces the risk of developing symptomatic osteoarthritis by approximately 50%.[35] When specifically targeting weight loss in the geriatric population, calorie restriction combined with resistance training may have benefits over aerobic training by attenuating loss of hip and femoral neck bone mineral density.[110]

THE EMERGING ROLE OF MULTIDISCIPLINARY CARE TEAMS

The Problem

The growth of the aging population carries a special significance because of its implications for disability and its impact on those who provide preventative or restorative care. The geriatric patient can present with a complex set of issues and associated disability. They may have health, financial, and psychosocial issues resulting from one or more disabling conditions. On-going public interest in aging, multimorbidity, and geriatric syndromes has helped establish risk factors and effective intervention strategies for several age-related conditions. Unfortunately, much of this evidence has not been disseminated into clinical practice to date.[111] This can be attributed to:

1. Lack of commonly accepted definitions for the recognition, diagnosis, and coding of geriatric syndromes.
2. Lack of simple, measurable interventions for some geriatric syndromes.
3. Need for substantial provider time and longitudinal follow-up to intervene and assess effectiveness.
4. The fact that available interventions often require new behaviors or attitude shifts for patients and physicians. Examples include working as part of an interdisciplinary team and often requiring system-wide changes across extended systems of care with coordination across multiple disciplines.
5. Lack of champions for these interventions, particularly in the face of many other competing clinical demands and mandates.

The multifactorial nature of the geriatric syndromes requiring a coordinated, multifaceted approach does not adhere to the traditional disease model that drives most of the medical practice.[23] A more detailed assessment, such as an evaluation by a physiatry team or the Comprehensive Geriatric Assessment (CGA), can be most beneficial.

The Role of Physiatrists

Physiatrists play an important role in the care of older adults. They incorporate the biopsychosocial model of intervention with a goal-oriented team approach. Geriatric rehabilitation is an important emerging field, with a focus on evaluative, diagnostic, and therapeutic interventions with the purpose of restoring functional ability or enhancing residual functional capability in older people with disabling impairments and improving quality of life.[45,112] Frailty and other geriatric syndromes as well as multimorbidity make the medical management and rehabilitation of older adult care very complex.[45] Physiatrists receive targeted training and education to care for the many complex needs of this patient population, allowing them to provide improved care that addresses age-specific differences and manages multimorbidity in the context of disability.[1,113] Physiatrists are skilled in managing patients across multiple care settings, including acute inpatient rehab facilities; skilled nursing facilities, which are highly regulated by the Centers for Medicare and Medicaid Services; and in ambulatory clinics in the continuum of care of the growing geriatric population. Physiatrists may act as primary care physicians providing direct management of the medically complex conditions and their complications, coordinate the care, maximize function, lead interdisciplinary teams, or act as consultants. In the above-mentioned roles, physiatrists have been able to contribute to cost savings for the healthcare system by minimizing functional decline, reducing hospital length of stays and readmissions, and reducing functional dependency.[114]

Rehabilitation medicine has embraced the principles of "improving care of older patients" as set forth by the American Geriatrics Society.[115,116] Principles of rehabilitation practice emphasize a holistic assessment of patients, including the review of medical status, functional impairments, societal constraints, and the utility of adaptive equipment.[117] This comprehensive approach has been shown to improve outcomes in geriatric patients, and several practice models, such as the CGA, have been adapted to incorporate this holistic approach.[118] Interdisciplinary team work is the cornerstone of rehabilitation medicine. Many medical settings incorporate a variety of professionals; however, few are able to develop a truly interdisciplinary team process that often results in better outcomes than that provided by the traditional multidisciplinary methods.[117] For example, interdisciplinary treatment improves functional outcomes and decreases nursing home placement.[118] The interdisciplinary approach differs from the multidisciplinary approach by focusing on the common patient and team goals, compared with a discipline-specific focus. It emphasizes regular and effective communication, coordination, and integration of care.[117] The interdisciplinary model is ingrained in the Physical Medicine and Rehabilitation specialty as a fundamental component of their training. Learning to work with and leading a team are the core clinical competencies of physiatrists.[117]

Inevitably, rehabilitation services in the inpatient and/or outpatient setting are required for older adults to facilitate independent living in communities. Physiatrists may act as team leaders, primary care givers, or consultants to help provide the best available care for this complex population. Many questions arise in primary practices that are often difficult to manage or outside the providers' expertise, prompting referrals to physiatrists. For example, some key barriers to physical activity guideline implementation among primary care physicians include limitations in the knowledge of where to refer and what to recommend, access to pragmatic programs or resources, competing priorities for physician time, and/or lack of incentives.[119] These patients can be referred to physiatric practices to address their concerns.

Hospitalization is a risk for disability leading to decreased ability to live independently after discharge from the hospital. Physiatrists play a critical role in efficient and safe care transitions by determining the appropriate level of care required based on the intensity of services. Regardless of the setting, social integration is an important goal of a comprehensive rehabilitation program and requires in-depth knowledge of patient-related factors as well as available community resources.[120]

Successful integration in community living has measurable positive physical, cognitive, and psychosocial effects for older adults and disabled populations leading to increased awareness, new legislative efforts, and development of adaptive equipment and products.[120] However, this is often a complicated process that requires specific knowledge and training to navigate. Dwelling modifications that match functional needs are an important step in returning to the community. These often require significant out-of-pocket expense, as they are not routinely covered through Medicare.[120] Physiatrists and their interdisciplinary teams are often able to assist patients with these issues. Some information on housing resources can be found at the US Housing and Urban Development website. For the older adults, transportation is a vital link to "out of home" activities for work and pleasure. The US Division of Transportation is the designated agency with regulatory and enforcement responsibility for people with impairments. The risk of motor vehicle accidents increases significantly as individuals become older. Frequently, impaired older adult drivers voluntarily stop driving or adjust their driving to compensate for limitations.[121] Many physicians have poor knowledge on current licensing policies, the state-specific driving laws, and actions to be taken against potentially ineligible

drivers.[122] Physiatrists are an excellent resource for other physicians for this specific problem. A tactful but candid discussion with the patient and the family about the risks of driving is critical and may render reporting unnecessary, unless otherwise mandated by state regulations. The loss of driving privileges can be devastating to the patient and may place additional burden on their caregivers. Physiatrists are well equipped to reduce caregiver burden by providing psychological support, education, and resources for respite care. In turn, ongoing informal care can prolong a person's community living. Social supports are a complex network of programs, services, funding, and people that serve several needs of this population.[1]

Other common issues addressed by physiatrists include return to work issues as well as recommendations for recreational and leisure time activities. Physiatrists, and all healthcare providers, also play a critical role in patient advocacy. In the geriatric population, ageism is a major societal-level concern. Ageism is a negative societal belief that increasing chronologic age is synonymous with dementia, depression, dependence, isolation, and debility. Ageist views may lead to discrimination in the workplace, social settings, and medical care. Healthcare professionals must combat negative attitudes in providing care to older individuals, such as the common erroneous belief that decreased function is inevitable with aging.[1] Ageist's self-perception of some individuals can have a very negative impact on their own health and function. Modifying these negative stereotypes can have positive functional benefits; some common age-related gait changes were shown to be reversible with exposure of elders to positive images of aging.[123]

The Comprehensive Geriatric Assessment

The CGA is an interdisciplinary diagnostic and treatment protocol similar to physiatric assessments that is designed to identify biomedical, functional, environmental, and psychosocial limitations of older adults with the goal of developing a coordinated and personalized plan to maximize health and assist in clinical decision making.[124,125] In general, the interdisciplinary team consists of a physician (usually a geriatrician), nurse, social worker, and neuropsychologist and may draw on the expertise of physical and occupational therapists, nutritionists, pharmacists, podiatrists, opticians, and other medical personnel. It is imperative to consider the relevant social, spiritual, and economic domains when addressing geriatric syndromes in addition to the traditional biological framework for diseases.[23] There are six key steps in the assessment process, including data gathering, frequent team-based discussions with the patient and caregivers, development of treatment plan, implementation, monitoring for response, and revision of plan as needed. While gathering data, it is essential to evaluate the following components: frailty status, function, fall history and risk assessment, cognition, mood, polypharmacy, social support, finances, goals of care, advanced directives, and nutrition status.

Evidence from clinical trials and meta-analyses suggest that the healthcare setting may modify the effectiveness of CGA programs. Home and in-hospital programs have been consistently beneficial for multiple health outcomes.[126] Although there are conflicting and less consistent data, the majority of randomized trials have shown the efficacy of outpatient CGA in reducing functional decline, improving fatigue and depressive symptoms, and increasing social functioning.[127-130] The correlation between outpatient CGA and quality of life, risk of hospitalization, or institutionalization is still debatable.[131] So far, no benefit in overall survival has been reported in the literature for outpatient CGA models.[132]

CONCLUSIONS

Reducing severe disability from chronic health conditions will be the key for minimizing the social and economic burdens associated with aging. Extending mobility, functional independence, and independent community living in older adults will be crucial in minimizing costs.[5] Our current healthcare system is not designed to prevent chronic illnesses and must undergo changes to help reduce chronic diseases across the nation and globally. It is essential to have a coordinated, strategic prevention approach that promotes healthy behaviors, expands early detection and diagnosis of disease, supports people of every age, and eliminates health disparities. Clinically, this approach can be provided by multiple professionals in an interdisciplinary team to help address aging, geriatric syndromes, and multimorbidity in a holistic manner.

REFERENCES

1. Worsowicz GM, Stewart DG, Phillips EM, Cifu DX, Moreno L. Geriatric rehabilitation. 1. Social and economic implications of aging. *Arch Phys Med Rehabil.* 2004;85: 3–6. https://doi.org/10.1016/j.apmr.2004.03.005.
2. Ortman JM, Velkoff VA, Hogan H. *An Aging Nation: The Older Population in the United States Current Population Reports;* 2014. https://www.census.gov/prod/2014pubs/p25-1140.pdf.
3. Holliday R. The multiple and irreversible causes of aging. *J Gerontol A Biol Sci Med Sci.* 2004;59(6):B568–B572. http://www.ncbi.nlm.nih.gov/pubmed/15215266.
4. *World Report on Ageing and Health;* 2015. https://doi.org/10.1017/CBO9781107415324.004.
5. Suzman R, Beard J. Global health and aging. *NIH Publ No 117737.* 2011;1(4):273–277. https://doi.org/11-7737.
6. Marengoni A, Angleman S, Melis R, et al. Aging with multimorbidity: a systematic review of the literature. *Ageing Res Rev.* 2011;10(4):430–439. https://doi.org/10.1016/j.arr.2011.03.003.
7. Wu S, Green A. Projection of chronic illness prevalence and cost inflation. *RAND Heal.* 2000;18.
8. Tinetti ME, Bogardus ST, Agostini JV. Potential pitfalls of disease-specific guidelines for patients with multiple conditions. *N Engl J Med.* 2004;351(27):2870–2874. https://doi.org/10.1056/NEJMsb042458.
9. Hoffman C, Rice D, Sung HY. Persons with chronic conditions. Their prevalence and costs. *JAMA.* 1996;276 (18):1473–1479. http://www.ncbi.nlm.nih.gov/pubmed/8903258.
10. Anderson G. *Chronic Conditions: Making the Case for Ongoing Care;* 2004. Baltimore, MD.
11. *Caregiving in the U.S. Bethesda, MD and Washington, DC;* 2004. http://www.caregiving.org/data/04finalreport.pdf.
12. Koenig HG. Positive emotions, physical disability, and mortality in older adults. *J Am Geriatr Soc.* 2000;48(11):1525–1526. http://www.ncbi.nlm.nih.gov/pubmed/11083337.
13. Newsom JT, Schulz R. Social support as a mediator in the relation between functional status and quality of life in older adults. *Psychol Aging.* 1996;11(1):34–44. http://www.ncbi.nlm.nih.gov/pubmed/8726368.
14. Barnett K, Mercer SW, Norbury M, Watt G, Wyke S, Guthrie B. Epidemiology of multimorbidity and implications for health care, research, and medical education: a cross-sectional study. *Lancet.* 2012;380(9836):37–43. https://doi.org/10.1016/S0140-6736(12)60240-2.
15. [Press Release]. *Two-Thirds of Adult Americans Believe More Money Needs to Be Spent on Chronic Disease Prevention Programs, and They're Willing to Pay Higher Taxes to Fund Them, Survey Finds;* 2008.
16. Feinstein AR. The pre-therapeutic classification of co-morbidity in chronic disease. *J Chronic Dis.* 1970;23(7):455–468. http://www.ncbi.nlm.nih.gov/pubmed/26309916.
17. Batstra L, Bos EH, Neeleman J. Quantifying psychiatric comorbidity–lessons from chronic disease epidemiology. *Soc Psychiatry Psychiatr Epidemiol.* 2002;37(3):105–111. http://www.ncbi.nlm.nih.gov/pubmed/11995637.
18. Koller D, Schön G, Schäfer I, Glaeske G, van den Bussche H, Hansen H. Multimorbidity and long-term care dependency—a five-year follow-up. *BMC Geriatr.* 2014;14(1):70. https://doi.org/10.1186/1471-2318-14-70.
19. Wolff JL, Starfield B, Anderson G. Prevalence, expenditures, and complications of multiple chronic conditions in the elderly. *Arch Intern Med.* 2002;162(20):2269–2276. http://www.ncbi.nlm.nih.gov/pubmed/12418941.

20. Tooth L, Hockey R, Byles J, Dobson A. Weighted multi-morbidity indexes predicted mortality, health service use, and health-related quality of life in older women. *J Clin Epidemiol*. 2008;61(2):151–159. https://doi.org/10.1016/j.jclinepi.2007.05.015.

21. Menotti A, Mulder I, Nissinen A, Giampaoli S, Feskens EJ, Kromhout D. Prevalence of morbidity and multimorbidity in elderly male populations and their impact on 10-year all-cause mortality: the FINE study (Finland, Italy, Netherlands, Elderly). *J Clin Epidemiol*. 2001;54(7):680–686. http://www.ncbi.nlm.nih.gov/pubmed/11438408.

22. Byles JE, D'Este C, Parkinson L, O'Connell R, Treloar C. Single index of multimorbidity did not predict multiple outcomes. *J Clin Epidemiol*. 2005;58(10):997–1005. https://doi.org/10.1016/j.jclinepi.2005.02.025.

23. Inouye SK, Studenski S, Tinetti ME, Kuchel GA. Geriatric syndromes: clinical, research, and policy implications of a core geriatric concept. *J Am Geriatr Soc*. 2007;55(5):780–791. https://doi.org/10.1111/j.1532-5415.2007.01156.x.

24. Olde Rikkert MGM, Rigaud AS, van Hoeyweghen RJ, de Graaf J. Geriatric syndromes: medical misnomer or progress in geriatrics? *Neth J Med*. 2003;61(3):83–87. http://www.ncbi.nlm.nih.gov/pubmed/12765229.

25. Flacker JM. What is a geriatric syndrome anyway? *J Am Geriatr Soc*. 2003;51(4):574–576. http://www.ncbi.nlm.nih.gov/pubmed/12657087.

26. Tinetti ME, Inouye SK, Gill TM, Doucette JT. Shared risk factors for falls, incontinence, and functional dependence. Unifying the approach to geriatric syndromes. *JAMA*. 1995;273(17):1348–1353. http://www.ncbi.nlm.nih.gov/pubmed/7715059.

27. Inouye SK. Delirium in older persons. *N Engl J Med*. 2006;354(11):1157–1165. https://doi.org/10.1056/NEJMra052321.

28. Inouye SK, Foreman MD, Mion LC, Katz KH, Cooney LM. Nurses' recognition of delirium and its symptoms: comparison of nurse and researcher ratings. *Arch Intern Med*. 2001;161(20):2467–2473. http://www.ncbi.nlm.nih.gov/pubmed/11700159.

29. Inouye SK, Leo-Summers L, Zhang Y, Bogardus ST, Leslie DL, Agostini JV. A chart-based method for identification of delirium: validation compared with interviewer ratings using the confusion assessment method. *J Am Geriatr Soc*. 2005;53(2):312–318. https://doi.org/10.1111/j.1532-5415.2005.53120.x.

30. Inouye SK, Bogardus ST, Charpentier PA, et al. A multicomponent intervention to prevent delirium in hospitalized older patients. *N Engl J Med*. 1999;340(9):669–676. https://doi.org/10.1056/NEJM199903043400901.

31. Naughton BJ, Saltzman S, Ramadan F, Chadha N, Priore R, Mylotte JM. A multifactorial intervention to reduce prevalence of delirium and shorten hospital length of stay. *J Am Geriatr Soc*. 2005;53(1):18–23. https://doi.org/10.1111/j.1532-5415.2005.53005.x.

32. Marcantonio ER, Flacker JM, Wright RJ, Resnick NM. Reducing delirium after hip fracture: a randomized trial. *J Am Geriatr Soc*. 2001;49(5):516–522. http://www.ncbi.nlm.nih.gov/pubmed/11380742.

33. Tinetti ME, Baker DI, McAvay G, et al. A multifactorial intervention to reduce the risk of falling among elderly people living in the community. *N Engl J Med*. 1994;331(13):821–827. https://doi.org/10.1056/NEJM199409293311301.

34. Rubenstein LZ, Josephson KR. The epidemiology of falls and syncope. *Clin Geriatr Med*. 2002;18(2):141–158. http://www.ncbi.nlm.nih.gov/pubmed/12180240.

35. Roig RL, Worsowicz GM, Stewart DG, Cifu DX. Geriatric rehabilitation. 3. Physical medicine and rehabilitation interventions for common disabling disorders. *Arch Phys Med Rehabil*. 2004;85(7 suppl 3):S12-7-30. http://www.ncbi.nlm.nih.gov/pubmed/15221717.

36. Chou WC, Tinetti ME, King MB, Irwin K, Fortinsky RH. Perceptions of physicians on the barriers and facilitators to integrating fall risk evaluation and management into practice. *J Gen Intern Med*. 2006;21(2):117–122. https://doi.org/10.1111/j.1525-1497.2005.00298.x.

37. Lundebjerg N. Guideline for the prevention of falls in older persons. *J Am Geriatr Soc*. 2001;49(5):664–672. https://doi.org/10.1046/j.1532-5415.2001.49115.x.

38. Baker DI, King MB, Fortinsky RH, et al. Dissemination of an evidence-based multicomponent fall risk-assessment and -management strategy throughout a geographic area. *J Am Geriatr Soc*. 2005;53(4):675–680. https://doi.org/10.1111/j.1532-5415.2005.53218.x.

39. Bradley EH, Webster TR, Baker D, Schlesinger M, Inouye SK. After adoption: sustaining the innovation a case study of disseminating the hospital elder life program. *J Am Geriatr Soc*. 2005;53(9):1455–1461. https://doi.org/10.1111/j.1532-5415.2005.53451.x.

40. Bray NW, Smart RR, Jakobi JM, Jones GR. Exercise prescription to reverse frailty. *Appl Physiol Nutr Metab*. 2016;41(10):1112–1116. https://doi.org/10.1139/apnm-2016-0226.

41. Fried LP, Tangen CM, Walston J, et al. Frailty in older adults: evidence for a phenotype. *J Gerontol A Biol Sci Med Sci*. 2001;56(3):M146–M156. http://www.ncbi.nlm.nih.gov/pubmed/11253156.

42. Sternberg SA, Schwartz AW, Karunananthan S, Bergman H, Mark Clarfield A. The identification of frailty: a systematic literature review. *J Am Geriatr Soc*. 2011;59(11):2129–2138. https://doi.org/10.1111/j.1532-5415.2011.03597.x.

43. Walston J, Hadley EC, Ferrucci L, et al. Research agenda for frailty in older adults: toward a better understanding of physiology and etiology: summary from the American Geriatrics Society/National Institute on Aging Research Conference on Frailty in Older Adults. *J Am Geriatr Soc*. 2006;54(6):991–1001. https://doi.org/10.1111/j.1532-5415.2006.00745.x.

44. Rockwood K, Song X, McKnight C, et al. A global clinical measure of fitness and frailty in elderly people. *Can Med Assoc J*. 2005;173(5):489–495. https://doi.org/10.1503/cmaj.050051.

45. Wells JL, Seabrook JA, Stolee P, Borrie MJ, Knoefel F. State of the art in geriatric rehabilitation. Part I: review of frailty and comprehensive geriatric assessment. *Arch Phys Med Rehabil*. 2003;84(6):890–897. https://doi.org/10.1016/S0003-9993(02)04929-8.

46. Song X, Mitnitski A, Rockwood K. Prevalence and 10-year outcomes of frailty in older adults in relation to deficit accumulation. *J Am Geriatr Soc.* 2010;58(4):681–687. https://doi.org/10.1111/j.1532-5415.2010.02764.x.

47. Rockwood K, Mogilner A, Mitnitski A. Changes with age in the distribution of a frailty index. *Mech Ageing Dev.* 2004;125(7):517–519. https://doi.org/10.1016/j.mad.2004.05.003.

48. Song X, Mitnitski A, MacKnight C, Rockwood K. Assessment of individual risk of death using self-report data: an artificial neural network compared with a frailty index. *J Am Geriatr Soc.* 2004;52(7):1180–1184. https://doi.org/10.1111/j.1532-5415.2004.52319.x.

49. Jones DM, Song X, Rockwood K. Operationalizing a frailty index from a standardized comprehensive geriatric assessment. *J Am Geriatr Soc.* 2004;52(11):1929–1933. https://doi.org/10.1111/j.1532-5415.2004.52521.x.

50. Rockwood K, Stadnyk K, MacKnight C, McDowell I, Hébert R, Hogan DB. A brief clinical instrument to classify frailty in elderly people. *Lancet.* 1999;353(9148):205–206. https://doi.org/10.1016/S0140-6736(98)04402-X.

51. Roland KP, Theou O, Jakobi JM, Swan L, Jones GR. How do community physical and occupational therapists classify frailty? A pilot study. *J Frailty Aging.* 2014;3(4):247–250. https://doi.org/10.14283/jfa.2014.32.

52. Ferner RE, Aronson JK. Communicating information about drug safety. *BMJ.* 2006;333(7559):143–145. https://doi.org/10.1136/bmj.333.7559.143.

53. By the American Geriatrics Society 2015 Beers Criteria Update Expert Panel. American Geriatrics Society 2015 updated Beers criteria for potentially inappropriate medication use in older adults. *J Am Geriatr Soc.* 2015;63(11):2227–2246. https://doi.org/10.1111/jgs.13702.

54. Ahmed N, Mandel R, Fain MJ. Frailty: an emerging geriatric syndrome. *Am J Med.* 2007;120(9):748–753. https://doi.org/10.1016/j.amjmed.2006.10.018.

55. Fried LP, Ferrucci L, Darer J, Williamson JD, Anderson G. Untangling the concepts of disability, frailty, and comorbidity: implications for improved targeting and care. *J Gerontol A Biol Sci Med Sci.* 2004;59(3):255–263. http://www.ncbi.nlm.nih.gov/pubmed/15031310.

56. Haskell WL, Lee I-M, Pate RR, et al. Physical activity and public health. *Med Sci Sport Exerc.* 2007;39(8):1423–1434. https://doi.org/10.1249/mss.0b013e3180616b27.

57. Fahlman MM, Boardley D, Lambert CP, Flynn MG. Effects of endurance training and resistance training on plasma lipoprotein profiles in elderly women. *J Gerontol A Biol Sci Med Sci.* 2002;57(2):B54–B60. http://www.ncbi.nlm.nih.gov/pubmed/11818424.

58. Phillips EM, Bodenheimer CF, Roig RL, Cifu DX. Geriatric rehabilitation. 4. Physical medicine and rehabilitation interventions for common age-related disorders and geriatric syndromes. *Arch Phys Med Rehabil.* 2004;85(7 suppl 3):S18-22-30. http://www.ncbi.nlm.nih.gov/pubmed/15221718.

59. O'Grady M, Fletcher J, Ortiz S. Therapeutic and physical fitness exercise prescription for older adults with joint disease: an evidence-based approach. *Rheum Dis Clin North Am.* 2000;26(3):617–646. http://www.ncbi.nlm.nih.gov/pubmed/10989515.

60. Christmas C, Andersen RA. Exercise and older patients: guidelines for the clinician. *J Am Geriatr Soc.* 2000;48(3):318–324. http://www.ncbi.nlm.nih.gov/pubmed/10733061.

61. Kann L, McManus T, Harris WA, et al. Youth risk behavior surveillance United States, 2015. *MMWR Surveill Summ.* 2016;65(6):1–174. https://doi.org/10.15585/mmwr.ss6506a1.

62. Eaton DK, Kann L, Kinchen S, et al. Youth risk behavior surveillance–United States, 2007. *MMWR Surveill Summ.* 2008;57(4):1–131. http://www.ncbi.nlm.nih.gov/pubmed/18528314.

63. Centers for Disease Control and Prevention (CDC). Prevalence of self-reported physically active adults–United States, 2007. *MMWR Morb Mortal Wkly Rep.* 2008;57(48):1297–1300. http://www.ncbi.nlm.nih.gov/pubmed/19052527.

64. *Healthy People 2020.* 2011. Washington, D.C.

65. Nelson ME, Rejeski WJ, Blair SN, et al. Physical activity and public health in older adults: recommendation from the American College of Sports Medicine and the American Heart Association. *Circulation.* 2007;116(9):1094–1105. https://doi.org/10.1161/CIRCULATIONAHA.107.185650.

66. Tseng BS, Marsh DR, Hamilton MT, Booth FW. Strength and aerobic training attenuate muscle wasting and improve resistance to the development of disability with aging. *J Gerontol A Biol Sci Med Sci.* 1995;50 Spec No:113–119. http://www.ncbi.nlm.nih.gov/pubmed/7493203.

67. Keysor JJ. Does late-life physical activity or exercise prevent or minimize disablement? *A Crit Rev Sci Evid.* 2003;25:129–136. https://doi.org/10.1016/S0749-3797(03)00176-4.

68. Pahor M, Guralnik JM, Ambrosius WT, et al. Effect of structured physical activity on prevention of major mobility disability in older adults: the LIFE study randomized clinical trial. *JAMA.* 2014;311(23):2387–2396. https://doi.org/10.1001/jama.2014.5616.

69. Paterson DH, Jones GR, Rice CL. Ageing and physical activity: evidence to develop exercise recommendations for older adults. *Can J Public Health.* 2007;98(suppl 2):S69–S108. https://doi.org/10.1139/H07-111.

70. Oesch P, Kool J, Fernandez-Luque L, et al. Exergames versus self-regulated exercises with instruction leaflets to improve adherence during geriatric rehabilitation: a randomized controlled trial. *BMC Geriatr.* 2017;17(1):77. https://doi.org/10.1186/s12877-017-0467-7.

71. Bouaziz W, Vogel T, Schmitt E, Kaltenbach G, Geny B, Lang PO. Health benefits of aerobic training programs in adults aged 70 and over: a systematic review. *Arch Gerontol Geriatr.* 2017;69:110–127. https://doi.org/10.1016/j.archger.2016.10.012.

72. Chan WC, Fai Yeung JW, Man Wong CS, et al. Efficacy of physical exercise in preventing falls in older adults with cognitive impairment: a systematic review and meta-analysis. *J Am Med Dir Assoc.* 2015;16(2):149–154. https://doi.org/10.1016/j.jamda.2014.08.007.

73. Pescatello LS, Franklin BA, Fagard R, et al. American College of Sports Medicine position stand. Exercise and hypertension. *Med Sci Sports Exerc.* 2004;36(3):533–553. http://www.ncbi.nlm.nih.gov/pubmed/15076798.

74. Thompson PD, Buchner D, Pina IL, et al. Exercise and physical activity in the prevention and treatment of atherosclerotic cardiovascular disease: a statement from the Council on Clinical Cardiology (Subcommittee on Exercise, Rehabilitation, and Prevention) and the Council on Nutrition, Physical Activity, and Metabolism (Subcommittee on Physical Activity). *Circulation.* 2003;107(24):3109–3116. https://doi.org/10.1161/01.CIR.0000075572.40158.77.

75. Fletcher GF, Balady GJ, Amsterdam EA, et al. Exercise standards for testing and training: a statement for healthcare professionals from the American Heart Association. *Circulation.* 2001;104(14):1694–1740. http://www.ncbi.nlm.nih.gov/pubmed/11581152.

76. Williams MA, Haskell WL, Ades PA, et al. Resistance exercise in individuals with and without cardiovascular disease: 2007 update: a scientific statement from the American Heart Association Council on Clinical Cardiology and Council on Nutrition, Physical Activity, and Metabolism. *Circulation.* 2007;116(5):572–584. https://doi.org/10.1161/CIRCULATIONAHA.107.185214.

77. Chen YM, Li Y. Safety and efficacy of exercise training in elderly heart failure patients: a systematic review and meta-analysis. *Int J Clin Pract.* 2013;67(11):1192–1198. https://doi.org/10.1111/ijcp.12210.

78. Geliebter A, Maher MM, Gerace L, Gutin B, Heymsfield SB, Hashim SA. Effects of strength or aerobic training on body composition, resting metabolic rate, and peak oxygen consumption in obese dieting subjects. *Am J Clin Nutr.* 1997;66(3):557–563. http://www.ncbi.nlm.nih.gov/pubmed/9280173.

79. McDermott MM, Liu K, Ferrucci L, et al. Physical performance in peripheral arterial disease: a slower rate of decline in patients who walk more. *Ann Intern Med.* 2006;144(1):10–20. http://www.ncbi.nlm.nih.gov/pubmed/16389250.

80. Sigal RJ, Kenny GP, Wasserman DH, Castaneda-Sceppa C, White RD. Physical activity/exercise and type 2 diabetes: a consensus statement from the American Diabetes Association. *Diabetes Care.* 2006;29(6):1433–1438. https://doi.org/10.2337/dc06-9910.

81. Group DPPR. Reduction in the incidence of type 2 diabetes with lifestyle intervention or metformin. *N Engl J Med.* 2002;346(6):393–403. https://doi.org/10.1056/NEJMoa012512.

82. US Preventive Services Task Force. Screening for obesity in adults: recommendations and rationale. *Am J Nurs.* 2004;104(5):94-5, 97-8, 100, passim. http://www.ncbi.nlm.nih.gov/pubmed/15166736.

83. Going S, Lohman T, Houtkooper L, et al. Effects of exercise on bone mineral density in calcium-replete postmenopausal women with and without hormone replacement therapy. *Osteoporos Int.* 2003;14(8):637–643. https://doi.org/10.1007/s00198-003-1436-x.

84. Varela E, Oral A, Ilieva EM, et al. Osteoporosis. The role of physical and rehabilitation medicine physicians. The European perspective based on the best evidence. A paper by the UEMS-PRM Section Professional Practice Committee. *Eur J Phys Rehabil Med.* 2013;49(4):753–759. http://www.ncbi.nlm.nih.gov/pubmed/24084415.

85. Recommendations for the medical management of osteoarthritis of the hip and knee: 2000 update. *Arthritis Rheum.* 2000;43(9):1905–1915. https://doi.org/10.1002/1529-0131(200009)43:9<1905:: AID-ANR1>3.0.CO; 2-P.

86. Hochberg MC, Altman RD, April KT, et al. American College of Rheumatology 2012 recommendations for the use of nonpharmacologic and pharmacologic therapies in osteoarthritis of the hand, hip, and knee. *Arthritis Care Res (Hoboken).* 2012;64(4):465–474. http://www.ncbi.nlm.nih.gov/pubmed/22563589.

87. Meyerhardt JA, Giovannucci EL, Holmes MD, et al. Physical activity and survival after colorectal cancer diagnosis. *J Clin Oncol.* 2006;24(22):3527–3534. https://doi.org/10.1200/JCO.2006.06.0855.

88. Ibrahim EM, Al-Homaidh A. Physical activity and survival after breast cancer diagnosis: meta-analysis of published studies. *Med Oncol.* 2011;28(3):753–765. https://doi.org/10.1007/s12032-010-9536-x.

89. Friedenreich CM, Wang Q, Neilson HK, Kopciuk KA, McGregor SE, Courneya KS. Physical activity and survival after prostate cancer. *Eur Urol.* 2016;70(4):576–585. https://doi.org/10.1016/j.eururo.2015.12.032.

90. Larson EB, Wang L, Bowen JD, et al. Exercise is associated with reduced risk for incident dementia among persons 65 years of age and older. *Ann Intern Med.* 2006;144(2):73–81. http://www.ncbi.nlm.nih.gov/pubmed/16418406.

91. Tabbarah M, Crimmins EM, Seeman TE. The relationship between cognitive and physical performance: MacArthur studies of successful aging. *J Gerontol A Biol Sci Med Sci.* 2002;57(4):M228–M235. http://www.ncbi.nlm.nih.gov/pubmed/11909888.

92. Weuve J, Kang JH, Manson JE, Breteler MMB, Ware JH, Grodstein F. Physical activity, including walking, and cognitive function in older women. *JAMA.* 2004;292(12):1454. https://doi.org/10.1001/jama.292.12.1454.

93. Cadore EL, Moneo ABB, Mensat MM, et al. Positive effects of resistance training in frail elderly patients with dementia after long-term physical restraint. *Age (Omaha).* 2014;36(2):801–811. https://doi.org/10.1007/s11357-013-9599-7.

94. American Geriatrics Society Panel on Exercise and Osteoarthritis. Exercise prescription for older adults with osteoarthritis pain: consensus practice recommendations. A supplement to the AGS Clinical Practice Guidelines on the management of chronic pain in older adults. *J Am Geriatr Soc.* 2001;49(6):808–823. http://www.ncbi.nlm.nih.gov/pubmed/11480416.

95. Theou O, Stathokostas L, Roland KP, et al. The effectiveness of exercise interventions for the management of frailty: a systematic review. *J Aging Res.* 2011;2011:569194. https://doi.org/10.4061/2011/569194.

96. Liu CK, Fielding RA. Exercise as an intervention for frailty. *Clin Geriatr Med.* 2011;27(1):101–110. https://doi.org/10.1016/j.cger.2010.08.001.

97. Roos MR, Rice CL, Vandervoort AA. Age-related changes in motor unit function. *Muscle Nerve.* 1997;20(6):679–690.https://doi.org/10.1002/(SICI)1097-4598(199706)20:6<679:: AID-MUS4>3.0.CO; 2-5.

98. Arnold P, Bautmans I. The influence of strength training on muscle activation in elderly persons: a systematic review and meta-analysis. *Exp Gerontol.* 2014;58:58–68. https://doi.org/10.1016/j.exger.2014.07.012.

99. Raymond MJ, Bramley-Tzerefos RE, Jeffs KJ, Winter A, Holland AE. Systematic review of high-intensity progressive resistance strength training of the lower limb compared with other intensities of strength training in older adults. *Arch Phys Med Rehabil.* 2013;94(8):1458–1472. https://doi.org/10.1016/j.apmr.2013.02.022.

100. Barnett A, Smith B, Lord SR, Williams M, Baumand A. Community-based group exercise improves balance and reduces falls in at-risk older people: a randomized controlled trial. *Age Ageing.* 2003;32(4):407–414. https://doi.org/10.1093/ageing/32.4.407.

101. Seino S, Nishi M, Murayama H, et al. Effects of a multifactorial intervention comprising resistance exercise, nutritional and psychosocial programs on frailty and functional health in community-dwelling older adults: a randomized, controlled, cross-over trial. *Geriatr Gerontol Int.* 2017. https://doi.org/10.1111/ggi.13016.

102. Gill TM, Baker DI, Gottschalk M, Peduzzi PN, Allore H, Van Ness PH. A prehabilitation program for the prevention of functional decline: effect on higher-level physical function. *Arch Phys Med Rehabil.* 2004;85(7):1043–1049. http://www.ncbi.nlm.nih.gov/pubmed/15241748.

103. *Prevalence of Doctor-Diagnosed Arthritis and Arthritis-Attributable Activity limitation—United States, 2003–2005.* 2006. http://www.cdc.gov/mmwr/preview/mmwrhtml/mm5540a2.htm.

104. Loeser RF. Aging and the etiopathogenesis and treatment of osteoarthritis. *Rheum Dis Clin North Am.* 2000;26(3):547–567. http://www.ncbi.nlm.nih.gov/pubmed/10989512.

105. Hootman JM, Helmick CG. Projections of US prevalence of arthritis and associated activity limitations. *Arthritis Rheum.* 2006;54(1):226–229. https://doi.org/10.1002/art.21562.

106. Centers for Disease Control and Prevention (CDC). Racial/ethnic differences in the prevalence and impact of doctor-diagnosed arthritis–United States, 2002. *MMWR Morb Mortal Wkly Rep.* 2005;54(5):119–123. http://www.ncbi.nlm.nih.gov/pubmed/15703693.

107. Singh MAF. Exercise to prevent and treat functional disability. *Clin Geriatr Med.* 2002;18(3):431–462, vi–vii. http://www.ncbi.nlm.nih.gov/pubmed/12424867.

108. Penninx BW, Messier SP, Rejeski WJ, et al. Physical exercise and the prevention of disability in activities of daily living in older persons with osteoarthritis. *Arch Intern Med.* 2001;161(19):2309–2316. http://www.ncbi.nlm.nih.gov/pubmed/11606146.

109. Minor MA, Hewett JE, Webel RR, Anderson SK, Kay DR. Efficacy of physical conditioning exercise in patients with rheumatoid arthritis and osteoarthritis. *Arthritis Rheum.* 1989;32(11):1396–1405. http://www.ncbi.nlm.nih.gov/pubmed/2818656.

110. Beavers KM, Beavers DP, Martin SB, et al. Change in bone mineral density during weight loss with resistance versus aerobic exercise training in older adults. *J Gerontol A.* 2017. https://doi.org/10.1093/gerona/glx048.

111. Tinetti ME, Gordon C, Sogolow E, Lapin P, Bradley EH. Fall-risk evaluation and management: challenges in adopting geriatric care practices. *Gerontologist.* 2006;46(6):717–725. https://doi.org/10.1093/geront/46.6.717.

112. Boston Working Group on improving health care outcomes through geriatric rehabilitation. *Med Care.* 1997;35(6 suppl):JS4–20. http://www.ncbi.nlm.nih.gov/pubmed/9191710.

113. Strasser DC, Solomon DH, Burton JR. Geriatrics and physical medicine and rehabilitation: common principles, complementary approaches, and 21st century demographics. *Arch Phys Med Rehabil.* 2002;83(9):1323–1324. http://www.ncbi.nlm.nih.gov/pubmed/12235619.

114. Crosson FJ. *Report to the Congress: Medicare Payment Policy.* Washington, DC; 2017. http://www.medpac.gov/docs/default-source/reports/mar17_entirereport.pdf.

115. Landefeld CS, Palmer RM, Kresevic DM, Fortinsky RH, Kowal J. A randomized trial of care in a hospital medical unit especially designed to improve the functional outcomes of acutely ill older patients. *N Engl J Med.* 1995;332(20):1338–1344. https://doi.org/10.1056/NEJM199505183322006.

116. Nicholas JJ, Rybarczyk B, Meyer PM, Lacey RF, Haut A, Kemp PJ. Rehabilitation staff perceptions of characteristics of geriatric rehabilitation patients. *Arch Phys Med Rehabil.* 1998;79(10):1277–1284. http://www.ncbi.nlm.nih.gov/pubmed/9779684.

117. Stewart DG, Phillips EM, Bodenheimer CF, Cifu DX, Cretin D, Svarstad D. Geriatric rehabilitation. 2. Physiatric approach to the older adult. *Arch Phys Med Rehabil.* 2004;85:7–11. https://doi.org/10.1016/j.apmr.2004.03.006.

118. American Geriatrics Society, John A. Hartford Foundation. A statement of principles: toward improved care of older patients in surgical and medical specialties. *Arch Phys Med Rehabil.* 2002;83(9):1317–1319. http://www.ncbi.nlm.nih.gov/pubmed/12235617.

119. Clark RE, McArthur C, Papaioannou A, et al. "I do not have time. Is there a handout I can use?": combining physicians' needs and behavior change theory to put physical activity evidence into practice. *Osteoporos Int.* 2017. https://doi.org/10.1007/s00198-017-3975-6.

120. Bodenheimer CF, Roig RL, Worsowicz GM, Cifu DX. Geriatric rehabilitation. 5. The societal aspects of disability in the older adult. *Arch Phys Med Rehabil.* 2004;85(7 suppl 3):S23-6-30. http://www.ncbi.nlm.nih.gov/pubmed/15221719.

121. De Raedt R, Ponjaert-Kristoffersen I. The relationship between cognitive/neuropsychological factors and car driving performance in older adults. *J Am Geriatr Soc.* 2000;48(12):1664–1668. http://www.ncbi.nlm.nih.gov/pubmed/11129759.

122. Kelly R, Warke T, Steele I. Medical restrictions to driving: the awareness of patients and doctors. *Postgrad Med J.* 1999;75(887):537–539. http://www.ncbi.nlm.nih.gov/pubmed/10616686.

123. Hausdorff JM, Levy BR, Wei JY. The power of ageism on physical function of older persons: reversibility of age-related gait changes. *J Am Geriatr Soc.* 1999;47(11):1346–1349. http://www.ncbi.nlm.nih.gov/pubmed/10573445.

124. Stuck AE, Siu AL, Wieland GD, Adams J, Rubenstein LZ. Comprehensive geriatric assessment: a meta-analysis of controlled trials. *Lancet (London, England).* 1993;342(8878):1032–1036. http://www.ncbi.nlm.nih.gov/pubmed/8105269.

125. Devons CAJ. Comprehensive geriatric assessment: making the most of the aging years. *Curr Opin Clin Nutr Metab Care.* 2002;5(1):19–24. http://www.ncbi.nlm.nih.gov/pubmed/11790944.

126. Pilotto A, Cella A, Pilotto A, et al. Three decades of comprehensive geriatric assessment: evidence coming from different healthcare settings and specific clinical conditions. *J Am Med Dir Assoc.* 2017;18(2):192.e1–192.e11. https://doi.org/10.1016/j.jamda.2016.11.004.

127. Reuben DB, Frank JC, Hirsch SH, McGuigan KA, Maly RC. A randomized clinical trial of outpatient comprehensive geriatric assessment coupled with an intervention to increase adherence to recommendations. *J Am Geriatr Soc.* 1999;47(3):269–276. http://www.ncbi.nlm.nih.gov/pubmed/10078887.

128. Boult C, Boult LB, Morishita L, Dowd B, Kane RL, Urdangarin CF. A randomized clinical trial of outpatient geriatric evaluation and management. *J Am Geriatr Soc.* 2001;49(4):351–359. http://www.ncbi.nlm.nih.gov/pubmed/11347776.

129. Wenger NS, Roth CP, Shekelle PG, et al. A practice-based intervention to improve primary care for falls, urinary incontinence, and dementia. *J Am Geriatr Soc.* 2009;57(3):547–555. https://doi.org/10.1111/j.1532-5415.2008.02128.x.

130. Burns R, Nichols LO, Martindale-Adams J, Graney MJ. Interdisciplinary geriatric primary care evaluation and management: two-year outcomes. *J Am Geriatr Soc.* 2000;48(1):8–13. http://www.ncbi.nlm.nih.gov/pubmed/10642014.

131. Fletcher AE, Price GM, Ng ESW, et al. Population-based multidimensional assessment of older people in UK general practice: a cluster-randomised factorial trial. *Lancet (London, England).* 2004;364(9446):1667–1677. https://doi.org/10.1016/S0140-6736(04)17353-4.

132. Kuo H-K, Scandrett KG, Dave J, Mitchell SL. The influence of outpatient comprehensive geriatric assessment on survival: a meta-analysis. *Arch Gerontol Geriatr.* 2004;39(3):245–254. https://doi.org/10.1016/j.archger.2004.03.009.

CHAPTER 2

Sarcopenia

WALTER R. FRONTERA, MD, PHD

INTRODUCTION

The World Health Organization has recognized the aging of the population in countries around the world as one of the most significant challenges of the 21st century.[1] These demographic changes were discussed in more detail in Chapter 1 of this volume. In many countries, particularly in Asia and Europe, average life expectancy has already exceeded 80 years, especially among women, and aging of the population is happening very quickly. In 2015, Japan is the only country in the world, more than 30% of the population was aged 60 years or older. It has been projected that by the year 2050, this will be the case in more than 25 countries including nations in the Americas, Asia, and Europe.[1,2] It has been estimated that by the year 2025, the number of people above age 60 years in the planet will exceed 1 and 2 billion by the year 2050. Furthermore, a large proportion will be older than 80 years, some will be centenarians, and the majority will live in low- to middle-income countries. Not surprisingly, these changes in the age-group composition of the population have significant social, economic, political, and health implications. Thus, understanding age-related changes in human physiology and their functional consequences is of significant interest and relevance and has been identified as a research priority by the US National Institutes of Health.[3]

Aging is a continuum characterized by its significant variability. The source of this variability is multidimensional and includes a combination of factors such as individual genotype, environmental factors, health behaviors, and access to healthcare. Some of the most important contributors to the functional loss leading to impairment and disability are the multiple changes in the structure and function of the neuromuscular system. If not identified and addressed early, life-threatening complications, such as falls and bone fractures associated with muscle weakness, can occur. Many physiologic changes associated with advanced adult age contribute to a decline in skeletal muscle strength and mass, alterations in cellular and molecular processes within muscle fibers, impaired

motor performance, and the loss of the capacity of skeletal muscle to recover from injury. It is interesting that the qualitative nature of these changes is very similar to those experienced during the inactivity that follows injury or hospitalization, underlining the contribution of a sedentary life, inactivity, and immobilization to the age-associated loss of function and independence.

DEFINITION OF SARCOPENIA

The term sarcopenia was initially used by Rosenberg to describe the loss of lean body mass with aging.[4,5] For several years, it was used by scientists to refer only to the loss of skeletal muscle mass. More recently, in 2010, the European Working Group on Sarcopenia in Older People (EWGSOP) expanded the definition to include the presence of impaired performance measured by walking speed and/or muscle weakness in handgrip strength testing and proposed an algorithm (see Fig. 2.1) for a systematic evaluation of persons with possible sarcopenia.[6] This first consensus represented a significant development because it went beyond the static evaluation of muscle mass and underscored the physiologic and functional consequences of muscle atrophy with advanced adult age. In fact, from a functional and rehabilitative perspective, the addition of walking speed makes sense because this measurement correlates very well with the prevalence of limitations in activities of daily living, mobility, and survival.[7,8] It has been reported that in many countries around the world, the prevalence of limitations in activities of daily living is higher in older age-groups.[9]

The proposal by the EWGSOP was followed by similar efforts by the International Working Group on Sarcopenia,[10] the American Foundation for the National Institutes of Health,[11] and the Asian Working Group on Sarcopenia (AWGS).[12] The latter group updated their criteria in a more recent publication.[13] There are some differences among these proposals but many more similarities and agreement.

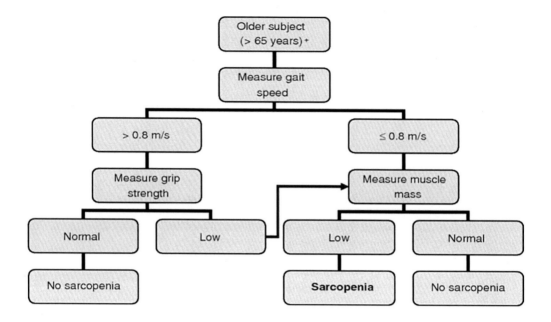

Comorbidity and individual circumstances that may explain each finding must be considered

+ This algorithm can also be applied to younger individuals at risk

FIG. 2.1 EWGSOP-suggested algorithm for sarcopenia case finding in older individuals. (From Cruz-Jentoft AJ, Baeyens JP, Bauer JM, et al. Sarcopenia: European consensus on definition and diagnosis: report of the European Working Group on Sarcopenia in older people. *Age Ageing*. 2010;39(4):420; with permission.)

MAKING THE DIAGNOSIS

In 2016, the 10th version of International Classification of Diseases (ICD-10-CM codes) added a code for the diagnosis of sarcopenia (M62.84) that could be used for reimbursement purposes under the general category of diseases of the musculoskeletal system and the specific group of disorders of muscle. Thus, an important question from a clinical practice point of view is who should be tested for sarcopenia. In general, the working groups mentioned above have recommended that community-dwelling individuals aged 65 years and older should be routinely screened. In addition, those who have experienced recent functional decline (i.e., repeated falls, unintentional weight loss, self-reported mobility difficulties, weakness, or self-reported slow walking speed) are good candidates for evaluation. It is likely that as we come to understand this condition better, indications for screening and testing will evolve and become more specific.

Since 2010, several groups have established criteria for the diagnosis of sarcopenia (see Table 2.1). This process requires the establishment of population-specific

normal values and the adjustment of measurements of muscle mass for differences in height. Several tests have been accepted for the testing of performance, muscle strength, and muscle mass. In the case of performance, most studies recommend the measurement of gait speed in a 6-m course. All study groups have recommended that a gait speed of ≤0.8 m/s be considered low and a justification for proceeding to testing muscle strength and mass. Static (isometric) strength is measured using a handgrip dynamometer. In general, normal values for men range between 26 and 30 kg and for women between 16 and 20 kg. It should be noted that handgrip strength by itself is associated with lower limb muscle power and mobility and is a good predictor of clinical outcomes.[14] In the case of muscle mass, both dual-energy X-ray absorptiometry and bioelectrical impedance (BIA) have been used. A skeletal muscle index is calculated as the sum of muscle mass of the four limbs divided by the square of the height. A measurement of 2 SD below the mean of a young reference group or in the lower quintile is considered abnormally low. In general, it is the

TABLE 2.1
Recommended Tests and Range of Normal Values for the Diagnosis of Sarcopenia

Variable	Specific Test	Recommended Value
Physical performance	6 m walking speed	≤0.8 m/s
Muscle strength	Handgrip	<30 and 20 kg for men and women, respectively
Muscle mass	Mass measured using DXA (absorptiometry) or BIA (bioelectrical impedance) and adjusted for height; 2 SD below the mean for a young control or the lowest quintile	7.2 and 5.6 kg/m^2 by DXA in men and women, respectively or 8.9 and 6.4 kg/m^2 using BIA in men and women, respectively

DXA, dual-energy X-ray absorptiometry.
Data from Cruz-Jentoft AJ, Baeyens JP, Bauer JM, et al. Sarcopenia: European consensus on definition and diagnosis. *Age Ageing*. 2010;39:412–423, Fielding RA, Vellas B, Evans WJ, et al. Sarcopenia: an undiagnosed condition in older adults. Current consensus definition: prevalence, etiology, and consequences. International Working Group on Sarcopenia. *J Am Med Dir Assoc*. 2011;12:249–256, Studenski SA, Peters KW, Alley DE, et al. The FNIH sarcopenia project: rationale, study description, conference recommendations, and final estimates. *J Gerontol A Biol Sci Med Sci*. 2014;69:547–558, Chen LK, Liu LK, Woo J, et al. Sarcopenia in Asia: consensus report of the Asian Working Group for Sarcopenia. *J Am Med Dir Assoc*. 2014;15:95–101, and Chen LK, Lee W-J, Peng L-N, et al. Recent advances in sarcopenia research in Asia: 2016 update from the Asian Working Group for Sarcopenia. *J Am Med Dir Assoc*. 2016;17:767.e1–767.e7.

combination of the three tests that helps make the diagnosis. According to the EWGSOP, if two measurements are abnormally low, sarcopenia is present, and if all measurements are below the criteria, the condition is severe sarcopenia. The recommendations of the different working groups are very similar, but there are some important differences. For example, according to the EWGSOP, if gait speed is normal (>0.8 m/s), handgrip strength is not measured and the next step is to measure muscle mass. In the case of the recommendations made by the AWGS, both gait speed and handgrip strength are measured at the beginning of the evaluation process. If one of these measurements is low, then muscle mass is measured.

It is interesting that at least two other approaches have been suggested to simplify the testing and screening process. A rapid questionnaire has been designed to diagnose sarcopenia quickly, including five questions about the difficulty of performing certain tasks as reported by the patient (difficulty in lifting and carrying 10 pounds, walking across the room, transferring from a chair or bed, and climbing a flight of 10 stairs) and the number of falls in the past year.[15] Each question is scored between 0 (no difficulty or no falls) and 2 (a lot or unable and 4 or more falls). The scores range from 0 to 10 and the authors suggested that a score equal or greater than 4 is predictive of sarcopenia and poor outcomes. This approach has obvious advantages in a clinical setting where more sophisticated resources may not be available. A second simplified approach

was proposed by Japanese investigators who found that an algorithm not including the measurement of gait speed, as proposed by the EWGSOP,[6] was equally useful in identifying sarcopenic individuals.[16] In other words, in this algorithm, a low measurement of handgrip strength is an indication to measure muscle mass, and only these two tests are the required measurements for the diagnosis of sarcopenia.

The importance of making the diagnosis early is that sarcopenia leads to many negative outcomes, such as reduced physical capacity, poorer quality of life, impaired cardiopulmonary performance, unfavorable metabolic effects, falls, disability, higher all-cause mortality, high healthcare expenditure, and poorer outcomes of medical or surgical treatment of cancer.[12,17] An early diagnosis may enhance the effectiveness of the interventions (see below).

PREVALENCE OF SARCOPENIA

The prevalence of sarcopenia varies significantly among countries.[13] It could be argued that biologic and cultural differences explain, at least partially, this variability. However, it is reasonable to conclude that variations in testing procedures and diagnostic criteria have also contributed to this. The prevalence of sarcopenia has been reported to vary between 4.0 and 27.1 and 2.5 and 22.1 in men and women of different nationalities, respectively. A high level of physical activity is associated with a lower prevalence of sarcopenia even in obese people.[18] It should be kept in mind that the prevalence of sarcopenia increases with age, and older groups may require more attention and careful evaluation. Finally, those living in long-term facilities have a higher prevalence probably due to a higher level of disability and the additional deleterious effect of inactivity.[19]

PHYSIOLOGICAL CHANGES ASSOCIATED WITH SARCOPENIA

Fig. 2.2 summarizes many of the physiologic changes with advanced adult age that may contribute to the development of sarcopenia.[20] It can be seen that dysfunction or negative adaptations in multiple organs and systems that under normal conditions favor an anabolic state contribute directly or indirectly to sarcopenia. Understanding sarcopenia is important because a reduction in skeletal muscle mass is associated with loss of functional capacity, many age-related diseases,

and an increase in mortality rate. Furthermore, muscles produce myokines (i.e., growth factors and cytokines secreted by muscle cells) that may improve metabolic homeostasis, increase stress resistance, and delay age-related functional decline in other tissues.[21] Thus, a loss of muscle mass that reduces the production and secretion of these myokines facilitates physiologic deterioration of tissues other than skeletal muscle. Many studies have been conducted in the last 10 years to understand the physiologic and cellular basis of the clinical manifestations of sarcopenia that can be measured in a clinical setting: impaired performance, weakness, and atrophy. In fact, the number of scientific manuscripts published and identifiable in PubMed on the topic of sarcopenia has increased by a factor of 9 (to almost 900 in 2016) in the same period. Several biomarkers of aging have been studied in detail. We will briefly summarize important observations regarding age-related alterations in muscle strength, muscle size, and muscle function or performance.

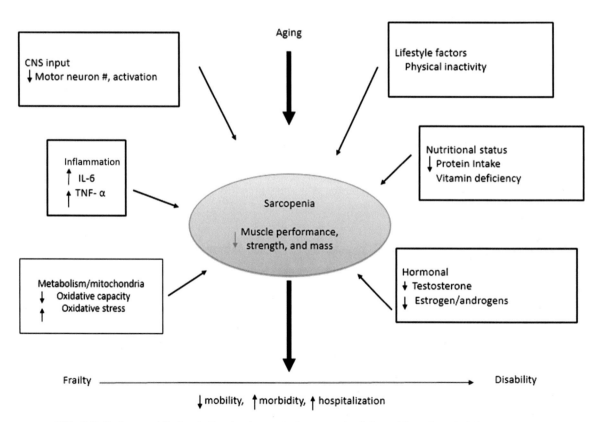

FIG. 2.2 Factors contributing to the development of sarcopenia. (Adapted from Joseph AM, Adhihetty PJ, Leeuwenburgh C. Beneficial effects of exercise on age-related mitochondrial dysfunction and oxidative stress in skeletal muscle. *J Physiol.* 2016;594(18):5107; with permission.)

Muscle Strength

The most important function of skeletal muscle is the production of force and generation of power. This is how movement and mobility become possible. The cellular elements that contribute to force generation change with advanced adult age, and this combination of changes results in muscle weakness. Both cross-sectional (comparison among age groups) and longitudinal (follow-up of the same population over the course of several years) studies show a decline in the strength of many muscle groups in both upper and lower limbs that ranges between 0.5% and 1.5% per year depending on the study design.[22,23] This reduction is less in the upper limbs (elbow flexors and extensors) particularly in women. The variability of this process is illustrated by the fact that approximately 10% of the older adults in one study showed no change or even an increase in the strength of the knee extensors and flexors over a 10-year follow-up.[24] This increase was even higher (32%) in the case of the elbow extensors and flexors in women. Differences in levels of physical activity, genetic influence, and hormonal factors may have contributed to the preservation of strength in some individuals. In another study, mobility-impaired older volunteers show a more significant decline in strength and muscle power over a 3-year period compared with healthy older adults.[25] The clinical importance of muscle strength is demonstrated by the fact that baseline muscle strength levels predict outcomes after falls with fractures and is associated with lower age-adjusted death rates from all causes and cancer in older patients. This loss of muscle strength makes the performance of activities of daily life more difficult and leads to the loss of independence.

Muscle Size

It has been repeatedly shown that the loss of muscle tissue explains, at least partially, the age-related loss of muscle strength. In one longitudinal study, the reduction in cross-sectional area over 12 years was 16.1% in the quadriceps and 14.9% in the knee flexor muscle group.[22] This loss of tissue is due to the loss of motor units and their muscle fibers, particularly type II (fast, glycolytic) fibers, in combination with atrophy of type I and II individual fibers. Muscle atrophy and accumulation of intermuscular fat are known to occur at the same time in many muscles of the body. Several studies using imaging techniques, such as magnetic resonance and ultrasonography, have shown that fat replacement increases with age and includes limb muscles as well as the paraspinal muscle group.[26]

Muscle Function and Performance

The loss of muscle function and performance typical of aging has been reported by many investigators. Tests of gait speed that correlate with leg muscle strength and power show a reduction in gait speed with age that predicts limitations in activities of daily living.[7,27] Other tests of functional performance, such as the Short Physical Performance Battery that not only includes gait speed but also tests for balance and muscle power,[23,28] also show a significant decline with age. Finally, muscle power (a parameter that combines muscle strength and speed or rate of force development) is lost at a faster rate than muscle strength.[23,25] This is important because power strongly correlates with functional performance, and its restoration may require a different rehabilitative approach (see below).

THE CELLULAR AND MOLECULAR BASIS OF MUSCLE WEAKNESS AND ATROPHY

Although activation of the neuromuscular system by central impulses contributes to muscle weakness in vivo, the ability of older muscle and muscle fibers to generate force is impaired even when maximal activation is achieved with maximal calcium concentrations in vitro. Furthermore, when force is adjusted for differences in muscle size (in vivo and in vitro), differences in strength between age-groups persist.[29–31] These two observations suggest that the intrinsic quality of muscle to generate force is impaired in the older muscle.

Like in many other cell types, several basic processes inside muscle fibers become dysfunctional with advanced adult age. Several general hallmarks underlying this dysfunction have been identified and include genomic instability, telomere shortening, epigenetic alterations, loss of proteostasis, and stem cell exhaustion.[32] Of note is a reduction in the number of satellite cells (stem cells of skeletal muscle), particularly those associated with type II fibers, and in the capacity of satellite cells to become activated in the presence of a stimulus that activates regenerating pathways.[33,34] This is relevant because it is an adaptation that reduces the regenerative capacity of older muscle at the same time that muscle fibers are being lost. With regard to telomeres, it is interesting to note that telomere shortening has been reported to be related more to physical inactivity than to chronological age.[35]

During the last 20 years, many studies have explored cellular and molecular alterations that may result in abnormal formation and function of the basic unit of force generation in muscle cells, the myosin-actin cross-bridge. For example, fragmentation of the excitation-contraction coupling system formed by t-tubules and the sarcoplasmic reticulum has been reported by Weisleder and collaborators.[36] This impairs the calcium homeostasis that is needed to activate cross-bridge formation. Changes in gene expression, including the upregulation of some genes and the downregulation of others, have been associated with an aging "signature."[37,38] It has been suggested that some of these alterations in gene transcription may be due to DNA methylation and may have an impact on the quantity and quality of proteins needed for muscle function, such as oxidative enzymes and contractile proteins.[39] Because physiological traits such as muscle strength and muscle size are partially regulated by genes, the possible contributions to sarcopenia of genotypes must be understood.[40]

Finally, several authors have reported chemical alterations, such as glycation and oxidation of the myosin molecule, that may interfere with cross-bridge kinetics.[41,42] Taken together, these studies strongly suggest that multiple alterations at the level of the cell itself contribute to muscle dysfunction in the elderly. The importance of changes in muscle quality at the level of the muscle cells was demonstrated in a very comprehensive study by Brocca and collaborators.[43] These investigators combined the assessment of in vivo muscle function with in vitro analysis of isolated single muscle fibers with proteomic analysis. They concluded that qualitative adaptations in muscle proteins due to phosphorylation and/or oxidation contribute significantly to muscle aging. It is important to note that their subjects were healthy volunteers with the same level of physical activity.

EXERCISE AND NUTRITIONAL SUPPLEMENTATION AS COUNTERMEASURES

A comprehensive discussion of the effects of exercise training on sarcopenia is beyond the scope of this chapter, and the exercise recommendations for older adults are discussed in Chapter 14 in this volume. However, it is appropriate to make some comments about the role of exercise in preventing and slowing down the development of sarcopenia.

One of the main goals of a geriatric rehabilitation program is to correct the impairments in the musculoskeletal system associated with advanced adult age. Although aging cannot be completely reversed or

stopped, some of the changes in skeletal muscle discussed above may be due to the presence of factors such as the lack of physical activity or exercise and inappropriate nutritional practices and not to inevitable consequences of the aging process.[35,44] This idea has stimulated many investigators to examine the beneficial effects of exercise on muscle strength and mass in older men and women. Cross-sectional studies have shown that the prevalence of sarcopenia is lower in older men and women with a higher level of habitual physical activity.[18] In addition, many exercise training studies have shown that strength training (i.e., resistance training, weightlifting) results in significant gains in strength and muscle mass in older people. In general, based on multiple studies, it can be concluded that the use of free weights or strength training devices (type of exercise), to perform three to four sets of 8–10 repetitions each (duration of training), two to three times per week (frequency of training), at 60%–80% of the one repetition maximum (intensity), results in significant physiologic and functional gains.[19,45] Considering that many activities of daily living do not require maximal force (strength) but rather the development of submaximal level of force quickly, several investigators have developed exercise training programs that include a high-velocity component, particularly during the concentric actions of the exercise.[46,47] These exercise programs have resulted in significant gains in strength, increases in muscle power, and functional improvements.

Another important question relates to the use of additional interventions that, in combination with exercise, may optimize the benefits of exercise training. Although anabolic agents such as testosterone and human growth hormone have been shown to be effective in short-duration studies, its long-term use in the older population cannot be recommended because it is not clear that prolonged administration of these agents is safe. On the other hand, many studies have demonstrated that nutritional interventions, such as amino acid and protein supplementation, effectively increases muscle protein synthesis and can act synergistically to enhance the benefits of exercise training.[48] In fact, these beneficial effects on strength and mobility can persist even several years after the intervention has been stopped.[49]

CONCLUDING STATEMENT

Aging and associated processes such as the development of sarcopenia represent important challenges for rehabilitation professionals. Our understanding of the underlying mechanisms has improved significantly and our diagnostic approach has been enhanced considerably. It is important to educate health professionals working with older populations on the benefits of exercise training in this population.

REFERENCES

1. World Health Organization. *World Report on Ageing and Health*; 2015.
2. www.who.org.
3. Frontera WR, Bean JF, Damiano D, et al. Rehabilitation research at the National Institutes of Health: moving the field forward (executive summary). *Am J Phys Med Rehabil.* 2017;96:211–220.
4. Rosenberg IH. Summary comments. *Am J Clin Nutr.* 1989;50:1231–1233.
5. Rosenberg IH. Sarcopenia: origins and clinical relevance. *J Nutr.* 1997;127:S990–S991.
6. Cruz-Jentoft AJ, Baeyens JP, Bauer JM, et al. Sarcopenia: European consensus on definition and diagnosis. *Age Ageing.* 2010;39:412–423.
7. Cummings SR, Studenski S, Ferrucci L. A diagnosis of dismobility – giving mobility clinical visibility: a mobility working group recommendation. *JAMA.* 2014;311:2061–2062.
8. Studenski S, Perera S, Patel K, et al. Gait speed and survival in older adults. *JAMA.* 2011;305:50–58.
9. Stucki G, Bickenbach J, Gutenbrunner C, Melvin J. Rehabilitation: the health strategy of the 21st century. *J Rehabil Med.* 2017. https://doi.org/10.2340/16501977-2200.
10. Fielding RA, Vellas B, Evans WJ, et al. Sarcopenia: an undiagnosed condition in older adults. Current consensus definition: prevalence, etiology, and consequences. International Working Group on Sarcopenia. *J Am Med Dir Assoc.* 2011;12:249–256.
11. Studenski SA, Peters KW, Alley DE, et al. The FNIH sarcopenia project: rationale, study description, conference recommendations, and final estimates. *J Gerontol A Biol Sci Med Sci.* 2014;69:547–558.
12. Chen LK, Liu LK, Woo J, et al. Sarcopenia in Asia: consensus report of the Asian Working Group for Sarcopenia. *J Am Med Dir Assoc.* 2014;15:95–101.
13. Chen LK, Lee W-J, Peng L-N, et al. Recent advances in sarcopenia research in Asia: 2016 update from the Asian Working Group for Sarcopenia. *J Am Med Dir Assoc.* 2016;17:767.e1–767.e7.
14. Laurentani F, Ruso C, Bandinelli S, et al. Age-associated changes in skeletal muscles and their effects on mobility: an operational diagmnosis of sarcopenia. *J Appl Physiol.* 2003;95:1851–1860.
15. Malmstrom TK, Morley JE. SARC-F: a simple questionnaire to rapidly diagnose sarcopenia. *J Am Med Dir Assoc.* 2013;14:531–532.
16. Yoshida D, Suzuki T, Shimada H, et al. Using two different algorithms to determine the prevalence of sarcopenia. *Geriatr Gerontol Int.* 2014;14(suppl 1):46–51.
17. Landi F, Cruz-Jentoft AJ, Liperoti R, et al. Sarcopenia and mortality risk in frail older persons aged 80 years and older: results from ilSIRENTE study. *Age Ageing.* 2013;42:203–209.
18. Ryu M, Jo J, Lee Y, Chung Y-S, Kim K-M, Baek W-C. Association of physical activity with sarcopenia and sarcopenic obesity in community-dwelling older adults: the Fourth Korea National Health and Nutrition Examination Survey. *Age Ageing.* 2013;42:734–740.
19. Cruz-Jentoft AJ, Landi F, Schneider SM, et al. Prevalence of and interventions for sarcopenia in ageing adults: a systematic review. Report of the International Sarcopenia Initiative (EWGSOP and IWGS). *Age Ageing.* 2014;43:748–759.
20. Joseph A-M, Adhihetty PJ, Leeuwenburgh C. Beneficial effects of exercise on age-related mitochondrial dysfunction and oxidative stress in skeletal muscle. *J Physiol.* 2016:5105–5123.
21. Demontis F, Piccirillo R, Goldberg AL, Perrimon N. The influence of skeletal muscle on systemic aging and lifespan. *Aging Cell.* 2013;12:943–949.
22. Frontera WR, Hughes VA, Fielding RA, et al. Aging of skeletal muscle: a 12-yr longitudinal study. *J Appl Physiol.* 2000;88:1321–1326.
23. Reid KF, Pasha E, Doros G, et al. Longitudinal decline of lower extremity muscle power in healthy and mobility-limited older adults: influence of muscle mass, strength, composition, neuromuscular activation and single fiber contractile properties. *Eur J Appl Physiol.* 2014;114:29–39.
24. Hughes VA, Frontera WR, Wood M, et al. Longitudinal muscle strength changes in older adults: influence of muscle mass, physical activity and health. *J Gerontol Biol Sci.* 2001;56A:B209–B217.
25. Reid KF, Doros G, Clark DJ, et al. Muscle power failure in mobility-limited older adults: preserved single fiber function despite lower whole muscle size, quality and neuromuscular activation. *Eur J Appl Physiol.* 2012;112:2289–2301.
26. Dahlqvist JR, Vissing CR, Hedermann G, Thomsen C, Vissing J. Fat replacement of paraspinal muscles with aging in healthy adults. *Med Sci Sports Exerc.* 2017;49:595–601.
27. Rantakokko M, Mänty M, Rantanen T. Mobility decline in old age. *Exerc Sport Sci Rev.* 2013;41:19–25.
28. Bean JF, Kiely DK, Herman S, et al. The relationship between leg power and physical performance in mobility-limited older people. *J Am Geriatr Soc.* 2002;50:461–467.
29. Frontera WR, Krivickas L, Suh D, et al. Skeletal muscle fiber quality in older men and women. *Am J Physiol.* 2000;279:C611–C618.
30. Frontera WR, Reid KF, Phillips EM, et al. Muscle fiber size and function in elderly humans: a longitudinal study. *J Appl Physiol.* 2008;105:637–642.
31. Krivickas LS, Dorer DJ, Ochala J, Frontera WR. Relationship between force and size in human single muscle fibers. *Exp Physiol.* 2011;96(5):539–547.
32. López-Otín C, Blasaco MA, Partridge L, Serrano M, Kroemer G. The hallmarks of aging. *Cell.* 2013;153:1194–1217.

33. Verdijk LB, Koopman R, Schaart G, Meijer K, Savelberg HH, van Loon LJ. Satellite cell content is specifically reduced in type II skeletal muscle fibers in the elderly. *Am J Physiol Endocrinol Metab.* 2007;292:E151–E157.

34. McKay BR, Ogborn DI, Baker JM, Toth KG, Tarnopolsky MA, Parise G. Elevated SOCS3 and altered IL-6 signaling is associated with age-related human muscle stem cell dysfunction. *Am J Physiol Cell Physiol.* 2013;304:C717–C728.

35. Venturelli M, Morgan GR, Donato AJ, et al. Cellular aging of skeletal muscle: telomeric and free radical evidence that physical inactivity is responsible and not age. *Clin Sci.* 2014;127:415–421.

36. Weisleder N, Brotto M, Komazaki S, et al. Muscle aging is associated with compromised Ca^{2+} spark signalling and segregated intracellular Ca^{2+} release. *J Cell Biol.* 2006;174:639–645.

37. de Magalhães JP, Curado J, Chruch GM. Meta-analysis of age-related gene expression profiles identifies common signatures of aging. *Bioinformatics.* 2009;25:875–881.

38. Tan L-J, Liu S-L, Lei S-F, Papasian CJ, Deng H-W. Molecular genetic studies of gene identification for sarcopenia. *Hum Genet.* 2012;131:1–31.

39. Zykovich A, Hubbard A, Flynn JM, et al. Genome-wide DNA methylation changes with age in disease-free human skeletal muscle. *Aging Cell.* 2014;13:360–366.

40. Tiainen K, Sipilä S, Alen M, et al. Shared genetic and environmental effects on strength and power in older female twins. *Med Sci Sports Exerc.* 2005;37:72–78.

41. Miller MS, Bedrin NG, Callahan DM, et al. Age-related slowing of myosin-actin cross-bridge kinetics is sex-specific and predicts decrements in whole skeletal muscle performance in humans. *J Appl Physiol.* 2013;115:1004–1014.

42. Li M, Ogilvie H, Ochala J, et al. Aberrant post-translational modifications compromise human myosin motor function in old age. *Aging Cell.* 2015;14:228–235.

43. Brocca L, McPhee JS, Longa W, et al. Structure and function of human muscle fibers and muscle proteome in physically active older men. *J Physiol.* 2017. https://doi.org/10.1113/JP274148.

44. Booth FW, Laye MJ, Roberts MD. Lifetime sedentary living accelerates some aspects of secondary aging. *J Appl Physiol.* 2011;111:1497–1504.

45. Peterson MD, Rhea MR, Sem A, Gordon PM. Resistance exercise for muscular strength in older adults: a meta analysis. *Ageing Res Ver.* 2010;9:226–237.

46. Bean JF, Kiely DK, LaRose S, O'Neill E, Goldstein R, Frontera WR. Increased velocity exercise specific to task (InVEST) training vs. the National Institute on Aging's (NIA) strength training program: changes in limb power and mobility. *J Gerontol A Med Sci.* 2009;64A:983–991.

47. Reid KF, Martin KI, Doros G, et al. Comparative effects of low and high intensity power training for improving lower extremity power and physical performance in mobility-limited older adults. *J Gerontol.* 2015;70:374–380.

48. Dickinson JM, Volpi E, Rasmussen BB. Exercise and nutrition to target protein synthesis impairments in aging skeletal muscle. *Exerc Sport Sci Rev.* 2013;41:216–223.

49. Kim H, Suzuki T, Saito K, Kojima N, Hosoi E, Yoshida H. Long-term effects of exercise and amino acid supplementation on muscle mass, physical function, and falls in community-dwelling elderly Japanese sarcopenic women; a 4-year follow-up study. *Geriatr Gerontol Int.* 2016;16:175–181.

CHAPTER 3

Osteoporosis and Fragility Fracture

JAE-YOUNG LIM, MD, PHD • JAEWON BEOM, MD, PHD •
SANG Y. LEE, MD, PHD

INTRODUCTION

As elderly subjects increase in number, the physical impairments and disability associated with falls and fragility fractures constitute major threats to health in older age and increase healthcare and socioeconomic burdens.[1] Osteoporotic fractures or fragility fractures have been recognized as geriatric conditions associated with various and complex problems that significantly compromise whole-body conditions and functions in addition to the musculoskeletal problems due to fracture per se.[2] If a fracture is not treated early, the fracture may trigger serious conditions leading to death.

The most common cause of osteoporotic fracture is a fall-related injury. Epidemiologic data and the healthcare systems regarding the occurrence of falls, risk factors for falls, and postfall outcomes in older adults show that such problems are already of major international concern. Comprehensive and systematic rehabilitation can minimize complications and increase the success of medical and surgical treatments, thereby lowering the extent of impairment.

This chapter focuses on the rehabilitative management of hip and vertebral fractures, which are the most common fragility fractures causing severe dysfunction in the very elderly (who are at greatest risk).

OSTEOPOROSIS

Definition and Diagnosis of Osteoporosis in the Geriatric Population

Osteoporosis is defined as "a disease characterized by low bone mass and structural deterioration of bone tissue that increase the risk of fracture due to weakened bone strength" by the National Institutes of Health Consensus Development Panel.[3] Bone strength is determined by bone density and quality. Bone quality is determined by the bone turnover rate, bone microarchitecture and mineralization, etc., but these are rarely used to diagnose osteoporosis because it is difficult to measure bone quality in a clinical setting. However, as up to 80% of bone strength is attributable to bone density, measurement of bone density is useful for diagnosing osteoporosis. Therefore, diagnosis of osteoporosis is currently achieved by assessment of bone density (in g/cm^2) as measured by dual-energy X-ray absorptiometry. The standard criterion defining and diagnosing osteoporosis is a T-score of ≤ -2.5 at the lumbar spine, femoral neck, or total hip as revealed by bone mineral density (BMD) measurements[3] (Table 3.1).

The T-score as a reference standard of the World Health Organization (WHO) criteria was calculated using the young normal mean (white females aged 20–29 years). The WHO definition may be applied properly to postmenopausal females but was not developed for males or premenopausal females.[4] In terms of a reference standard for males, controversy exists as to whether it is appropriate to use BMD data from young healthy males (a sex-specific T-score) or young healthy females. However, the accumulated evidence suggests that both bone strength and the relative risks of fracture at the same femoral neck BMD are similar between males and females.[5,6] The 2013 update from the International Society for Clinical Densitometry

TABLE 3.1 World Health Organization Criteria for Clinical Diagnosis of Osteoporosis	
BMD T-Score	**Diagnosis**
T-score ≥ −1	Normal
−1 > T-score > −2.5	Low bone mass
T-score ≤ −2.5	Osteoporosis
T-score ≤ −2.5 with existing fracture	Severe osteoporosis

BMD, bone mineral density.
From NIH Consensus Development Panel on Osteoporosis Prevention, Diagnosis, and Therapy. Osteoporosis prevention, diagnosis, and therapy. *JAMA*. 2001;285(6):785–795; with permission.

recommends the use of a uniform Caucasian (non–race adjusted) female reference for males of all ethnic groups. In addition, if local reference data are available, they should be used to calculate only Z-scores but not T-scores.[7]

Epidemiology and Risk Factors

With advancing age, BMD decreases and the prevalence of osteoporosis increases. It is estimated that over 200 million subjects worldwide suffer from the disease.[8] It is estimated that the annual number of osteoporotic hip fractures worldwide will rise from 1.66 million to 6.26 million by the year 2050. Approximately 30% of all postmenopausal females in the United States and Europe have osteoporosis.[9] In Sweden 6.3% of males and 21.2% of females aged 50–80 years have been classified as osteoporotic.[10] Currently, in Asian countries, the incidence of osteoporosis is relatively low compared with that in Western countries. However, according to projections by the WHO, the Asian population will consist of 900 million males and females aged ≥65 years by the year 2050. As a result, although only 30% of all hip fractures worldwide occurred in Asia in 1990, this figure will be more than 50% by 2050.[11]

Osteoporosis in aging societies experiencing prolonged life spans has already attracted a great deal of interest in terms of risks and management; many research and clinical reports have appeared. In particular, the consequences of osteoporosis are worse for older adults; the number of osteoporotic fractures increases with age, as do the risks of fracture-related morbidity and mortality.[12] The rate of bone loss is approximately 1% per year after 30s and higher during the perimenopausal period (bone loss commences before menopause). In approximately, 50% of subjects aged 65–69 years, the bone mineral content falls below the fracture threshold, which is the 90th percentile for proximal femoral BMD for hip fractures and that of the spine for vertebral fractures, respectively. Almost all individuals aged ≥85 years exhibit bone mineral contents that have reached the fracture thresholds, and most elderly females are at risk of fracture. Osteoporosis causes approximately 9 million fractures annually worldwide, of which more than 4.5 million occur in the Americas and Europe. The estimated lifetime risk for a wrist, hip, or vertebral fracture is approximately 30%–40% in developed countries.

Primary osteoporosis has been known to be associated with major risk factors including advanced age, female sex, low body weight/body mass index, early menopause, low calcium and/or vitamin D intake,

TABLE 3.2
Commonly Prescribed Medications Lowering Bone Mineral Density and Possible Mechanisms

Drug Class	Mechanism of Action
Glucocorticoids	Decreased bone formation and increased bone resorption
Proton pump inhibitors	Unknown but may be due to decreased intestinal absorption of calcium
Anticonvulsants (phenytoin, carbamazepine, phenobarbital, valproic acid)	Uncertain but may include inactivation of vitamin D
Levothyroxine (oversupplementation)	Increase in both the number and turnover rate of bone turnover units
Aromatase inhibitors	Reduced estrogen production leading to increased bone resorption
GnRH agonists	Prevent the production of LH and FSH, thereby decreasing testosterone and estradiol and leading to increased bone resorption
Serotonin selective reuptake inhibitors	Uncertain
Thiazolidinediones	Decreased bone formation
Heparin	Osteoblast inhibition with decreased bone formation; increased bone resorption

FSH, follicle-stimulating hormone; *GnRH*, gonadotropin-releasing hormone agonist; *LH*, luteinizing hormone.

and a sedentary lifestyle. Secondary osteoporosis may be the consequence of endocrine and metabolism disorders (e.g., hypogonadism, hypercortisolism, hyperparathyroidism, hyperthyroidism, and/or anorexia), lymphoproliferative disorders, intestinal malabsorption, rheumatoid arthritis, renal failure, and/or certain drugs (e.g., corticosteroids, selective serotonin reuptake inhibitors, anticoagulants, antidiabetic medications, anticonvulsants, and proton pump inhibitors). For example, the main culprits in male drug-induced osteoporosis are glucocorticoids and androgen deprivation therapy (ADT).[13]

Commonly prescribed medications that decrease BMD and the potential associated mechanisms of action are summarized in Table 3.2.

TABLE 3.3
Common Laboratory Findings in Primary and Secondary Osteoporosis

	Calcium	Phosphate	PTH	ALP
Primary osteoporosis	NC	NC	NC	NC
Primary hyperparathyroidism	Inc	Dec	Inc	Inc
Malignant hypercalcemia	Inc	NC	Dec	Inc
Vitamin D insufficiency	Dec or NC	Dec or NC	Inc or NC	Inc or NC
Osteomalacia	Dec	Dec	Inc	Inc

ALP, alkaline phosphatase; *Dec*, decreased; *Inc*, increased; *NC*, not changed; *PTH*, parathyroid hormone.

Recently, fracture risk prediction algorithms, such as the fracture risk assessment tool (FRAX), have been widely used to predict osteoporotic fractures. FRAX is used diagnostically to evaluate the 10-year probability of bone fracture (www.sheffield.ac.uk/FRAX).[14] The FRAX tool was developed in 2008 by the WHO to calculate the overall risk of fracture (in both females and males) by reference to several clinical risk factors, with or without the measurement of BMD. The clinical risk factors included in the FRAX algorithm are age, sex, weight, height, a previous fracture, a parental hip fracture, current smoking status, glucocorticoid use, rheumatoid arthritis, secondary osteoporosis, and alcohol intake (≥ 3 units/day).

Workup and Management of Osteoporosis
Approaches
Clinical history taking of patient's complaints, any medical history relevant to bone metabolism, accompanying diseases, medication use, and family history (osteoporosis, breast cancer) are obtained from the patient. Physical examination should begin with an inspection of the patient. Thoracic kyphosis, a dowager hump, and a history of height loss increase the suspicion of vertebral fracture. In addition, examination of active and passive range of motion (ROM) is necessary to determine whether bone and/or joint pathology may also be present.[3,15]

Laboratory studies
Laboratory studies are performed to establish baseline conditions or to exclude secondary causes of osteoporosis. A complete blood count and serum levels of calcium, phosphate, alkaline phosphatase, 25(OH)-vitamin D, and creatine are measured at baseline. The serum levels of calcium, phosphate, and alkaline phosphatase are usually normal in patients with primary osteoporosis. Severe hypercalcemia may

TABLE 3.4
Bone Turnover Markers in Osteoporosis

Bone Resorption Markers	Bone Formation Markers
Hydroxyproline	Bone-specific alkaline phosphatase
Pyridinolines	Osteocalcin
N-terminal cross-linking telopeptide	C-terminal propeptide of type I collagen
C-terminal cross-linking telopeptide	Procollagen type I N-terminal propeptide

reflect an underlying malignancy or hyperparathyroidism; hypocalcemia can contribute to osteoporosis. Inadequate vitamin D levels can predispose to osteoporosis. Liver function tests and measurements of the levels of thyroid-stimulating hormone, parathyroid hormone, luteinizing hormone, and follicle-stimulating hormone are also need to be checked. Elevated parathyroid hormone levels and sex hormone deficiencies are secondary causes of osteoporosis (Table 3.3).

Bone-specific alkaline phosphatase, osteocalcin, urine hydroxyproline have all been evaluated as possible markers of bone turnover[16,17] (Table 3.4). Such markers may be useful to monitor patients and aid in decision-making as to when therapy should be recommenced, but they still have limited clinical utility.[18] The International Osteoporosis Foundation and the International Federation of Clinical Chemistry and Laboratory Medicine Working Group recommend the use of one bone formation marker (serum procollagen type I N propeptide, s-PINP) and one bone resorption marker (serum C-terminal cross-linking telopeptide of type I collagen, s-CTX) as reference markers.[19]

Treatment of osteoporosis

Various pharmacologic and nonpharmacologic therapies have been developed to prevent and delay osteoporosis. Here, we will review the latest trends in pharmacotherapy; rehabilitation and exercise management will be discussed in later parts of this chapter. The generic drug names, dosages, instructions for administration, precautions, and side effects are summarized in Table 3.5.

Bisphosphonates. Bisphosphonates are the most common drugs to treat osteoporosis. All second- and third-generation bisphosphonates (alendronate, risedronate, ibandronate, and zoledronate) with nitrogen-containing side chains are powerful antiresorptive agents that effectively limit osteoclast-mediated bone resorption, increasing BMD and reducing fracture rates.[20] Oral bisphosphonates are minimally absorbed by the intestine (1% bioavailability) and should thus be taken on an empty stomach and accompanied by sufficient calcium intake. Therefore,

intravenous preparations affording high bioavailability are advantageous in terms of therapeutic effects in some geriatric patients with especially poor drug bioavailability and poor compliance. Both oral and intravenous formulations of ibandronate are available.[20] Zoledronate is frequently used as an intravenous bisphosphonate administered once a year for the treatment of osteoporosis.[21] Although this treatment is well established, routine use of zoledronate is limited because of the cost and concerns regarding adverse effects such as nephrotoxicity and cardiotoxicity. In particular, zoledronate is contraindicated in patients with creatinine clearance < 35 mL/min. Oral ibandronate is relatively safe in geriatric patients with chronic kidney disease.

Parathyroid hormone therapy. Anabolic agents stimulating bone formation are ideal therapies for patients with osteoporosis. The only anabolic agent currently approved by the Food and Drug Administration (FDA) is teriparatide or PTH 1-34, which effectively treats

TABLE 3.5
Pharmacologic Treatment for Osteoporosis

Medication	Treatment Dosage	Instructions for Administration and Precautions	Side Effects
BISPHOSPHONATES			
Alendronate	10 mg once daily, 70 mg once weekly	Take first thing in the morning Take with full glass of plain water Wait for >30 min to eat; take other medications Sit upright/stand for over 30 min Caution with renal dysfunction	Esophagitis, heartburn, difficulty swallowing, headache, fever, etc.
Risedronate	5 mg once daily, 35 mg once weekly	See above	See above
Ibandronate	Oral: 2.5 mg once daily, 150 mg once monthly, 3 mg once every 3 months	See above	See above renal toxicity, injection site reaction, ocular inflammation; rarely, osteonecrosis of jaw
Zoledronate	5 mg infused over 15 min, yearly	Take Ca and Vitamin D if insufficient in diet Caution with renal dysfunction	See above (alendronate) Acute-phase reaction (headache, myalgias, fever)
HORMONE THERAPY			
Teriparatide	20 mcg SQ everyday	Contraindicated in hyperparathyroidism and open epiphyses	Muscle cramps, spasm, dizziness, sore throat
MONOCLONAL ANTIBODY			
Denosumab	60 mg SQ everyday	Caution with patients with impaired immune system	Eczema, flatulence; rarely, cellulitis

osteoporosis, significantly reducing the fracture risk, and has excellent safety profiles. However, it can be inconvenient to administer, as daily subcutaneous injections are required.[16]

Denosumab. Denosumab is an antiresorptive agent limiting osteoclast-mediated bone resorption. The FDA has approved the drug for the treatment of osteoporosis and to prevent bone loss in males on ADT who are at high risk of fracture.[22] Denosumab is a fully human monoclonal antibody that specifically binds to receptor activator of nuclear factor κ-B ligand (RANKL), the master regulatory molecule required for osteoclast formation and activity, thereby preventing RANKL from binding to the osteoclast receptor, RANK. Thus, osteoclastogenesis and bone-resorbing activity are inhibited and bone resorption is markedly suppressed. Freemantle et al. showed that denosumab was more effective at reducing the occurrence of vertebral fractures than were raloxifene, risedronate, and alendronate. The long-term efficacy and toxicity of denosumab need to be explored in studies that include longer follow-up periods than those of previous works.[23]

FALLS AND FRAGILITY FRACTURES

Injuries caused by falls, the leading cause of nonfatal injuries and the third leading cause of fatal injuries in the United States, have increased in recent years. The WHO defines fragility fracture as a fracture occurring during an activity that would not normally injure a young healthy bone (i.e., a fall from standing height or less). Of all fragility fractures, the care and rehabilitation of patients with hip fractures pose critical challenges in terms of functional outcomes and medical costs in a superaged society. More attention must be paid to mortality and morbidity profiles, loss of independence, and their resulting clinical and socioeconomic impacts.

Epidemiology

Several epidemiologic studies have explored the incidence of falls and fall-related injuries; the findings are diverse. One study reported that one-third of subjects aged >65 years fall at least once each year, as do half of those aged >80 years.[24] A special supplement of the NHIS (National Health Interview Survey), one of the largest health surveys in the United States, noted that 12% of community-dwelling adults reported falling in the previous year, yielding a total estimate of 80 million falls per year and a rate of 37.2 falls per 100

person-years. The incidence of falls in a cross-sectional public survey was 13% among the community-dwelling elderly. Furthermore, approximately 20% of falls required medical attention, and approximately 10% caused fractures.[25] Among fragility fractures, hip fracture is the most catastrophic for patients and their families and the most expensive to treat. It is estimated that the incidence of hip fracture will rise from 1.66 million worldwide in 1990 to 6.26 million by 2050.[26] Vertebral fracture is the most common fragility fracture, reducing health-related quality of life by causing back pain as well as decreasing physical capabilities and perceived general health and emotional status. The epidemiologic data on vertebral fractures differ from report to report largely because only one-quarter to one-third of vertebral fractures are clinically recognized at the time of occurrence and lateral spine imaging is required.[27] Wrist fracture is more prevalent in younger old women. Such fractures are not just fractures; they are warnings of further fragility fractures in the future. Both vertebral fractures and nonhip nonvertebral fractures should also be considered clinically important and financially significant.

Outcomes of Fragility Fractures

After hip fracture in-hospital mortality was 1.6%, 1-month mortality 9.6%, and 6-month mortality 13.5%, another 12.8% patients required constant assistance to ambulate.[28] The 1-year mortality rates were variable, ranging from 11.5% to 33% depending on the study design (prospective or retrospective) and institutions and countries where the studies were conducted.[29–33] The most common postoperative complications were chest infection (9%) and heart failure (5%).[33] The risk factors for death after hip fracture were increased age, male sex, multiple comorbidities, and cognitive disorders.[29,34–36] Functional outcomes such as mobility and living independence are critical when evaluating the success of geriatric rehabilitation in patients experiencing fall-related fragility fractures (Fig. 3.1). Individuals with hip fractures suffer increased long-term disability and functional dependence; most older adults do not reattain their preinjury functional levels. One Japanese study found that the proportion of patients who could walk outdoors alone with or without an assistive device was 68% before the fracture and was reduced to 51% by 120 days postfracture.[37] Of patients hospitalized for hip fractures, only 60% had recovered their prefracture walking ability 6 months later.[38]

Recurrent or repeated fractures, a second or subsequent fracture at any site after the initial fracture, are

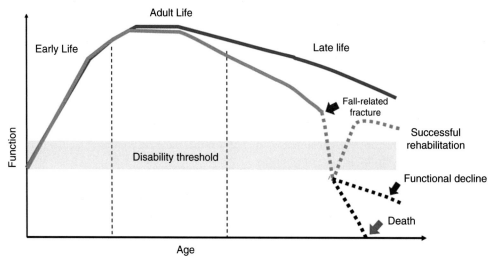

FIG. 3.1 Consequences of fall-related fracture.

associated with higher mortality and a greater risk of admission to a nursing care facility, compared with the primary fracture events.[39] The refracture rate of vertebral fractures was 16.6%, and the rate of refracture 1 year after surgery in patients with hip fractures was 3.19%–5.16%.[40]

ORTHOPEDIC TREATMENT

Of the various fragility fractures, the management of hip fractures, which constitute major burdens on public health systems, and vertebral fractures causing back pain and dysfunction is the principal topic of this section.

Preoperative Care

Most patients with hip fractures are delivered to emergency rooms. The fracture should be diagnosed by taking history and performing the necessary physical examination. With the patient supine, and the leg held in external rotation and abduction, the leg appears to be shortened. Pain is elicited on gentle internal and external rotation of the lower leg and thigh. A fracture may be suspected if groin pain is elicited on axial loading and the patient is unable to perform an active straight leg raise. Ecchymosis is rarely present initially. Plain X-rays are the most widely used imaging technique for the diagnosis of hip fractures. To diagnose occult fractures, magnetic resonance imaging is the gold standard but is neither as readily available, nor as inexpensive

as computed tomography (CT). Therefore, emergency CT scan should be used instead. Because they are older patients, the presence of medical and neurologic disorders should be checked before surgery and appropriate measures be taken. To minimize complications, such as muscle weakness and pressure ulcers, accurate assessment is essential. Although the use of pretreatment traction has been reported to reduce preoperative pain and to reduce further fracture displacement, its effectiveness thereof remains unclear; traction has been reported to increase the requirement for analgesic anti-inflammatory agents.[41] Care should also be taken to prevent the development of pressure ulcers, deep vein thrombosis (DVT), and pneumonia. The optimal time to surgery remains unclear, but surgical fixation should not be delayed very long to reduce complications associated with the fracture.

Perioperative Care Before and After Surgery

Perioperative time (preoperative and postoperative time) is defined as the time from immediately before surgery to the end of postoperative medical stabilization. During this period, various surgical treatments, prevention of early complications that may develop after surgery, and medical treatment are important components of management.

Orthopedic management

Hip fractures are classified as femur neck fractures, intertrochanteric fractures, or subtrochanteric

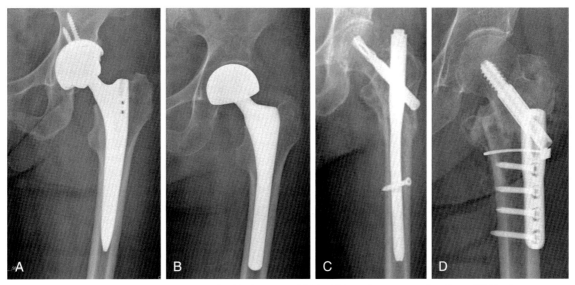

FIG. 3.2 Various surgical treatments for hip fractures. **(A)** Total hip replacement arthroplasty, **(B)** bipolar hemiarthroplasty, **(C)** proximal femoral nail antirotation, and **(D)** compression screw fixation.

fractures according to the fracture site. Femoral neck fractures are classified according to the anatomical location of the fracture and the extent of displacement. Structurally, such fractures may be classified as impacted, nondisplaced, or displaced fractures. The Garden's classification system is most commonly used in clinical practice to assess the fracture type and severity. Fractures are divided into four types depending on the presence or absence of displacement and the extent of displacement. Type 1 and 2 fractures are associated with good prognoses. Type 3 and 4 fractures (displaced fractures) potentially cause complications such as avascular necrosis. Nonsurgical treatment should be applied cautiously, because the patient cannot perform joint movement or tolerate weight-loading for a considerable period of time. In terms of surgical treatment, various methods are used depending on the patient's condition, level of activity, combined disease status, age, and the preference of the surgeon. Of the surgical methods used for hip fracture treatment, internal fixation using metal plates or pins is widely used to treat nondisplaced fractures. Replacement arthroplasty is usually performed to treat femoral neck fractures. Intertrochanteric or extracapsular fractures associated with displacement may undergo replacement arthroplasty or internal fixation, but the optimum treatment remains controversial (Fig. 3.2). Postoperative rehabilitation differs by surgical procedure. When compression screw fixation is used to treat comminuted fractures, weight-bearing is often not permitted for several days to weeks, to allow adequate bone union. On the other hand, replacement arthroplasty enables earlier mobilization and provides superior functional outcomes, compared with those of internal fixation in elderly patients with unstable fractures.

Osteoporotic vertebral compression fractures in the thoracic or lumbar spine cause serious acute back pain, especially during postural changes. Bed rest for longer than a few days is not recommended for those with stable fractures, because immobilization can trigger muscular weakness in the spine and lower extremities. Appropriate spinal orthoses and analgesics aid in reducing the pain induced by spinal motion. The efficacies of the various vertebral augmentation techniques, including percutaneous vertebroplasty and balloon kyphoplasty, remain controversial, although they may relieve acute or chronic back pain in some patients.[42–44] If no neurologic deficit is apparent, early initiation of rehabilitation program including balance training and strengthening exercises can help accelerate functional recovery after compression fractures.

Other fragility fractures of the wrist (mainly the distal radius) and proximal humerus often require reduction and internal fixation.

Postoperative complications

Thromboembolic disease. The incidence of DVT after hip fracture surgery is increasing. Proximal thrombosis has been reported in up to 27% of patients, and the incidence of fatal pulmonary embolism during the first 3 months has increased from 1.4% to 7.5%.[45] The lack of sufficient sensitivity associated with physical examination renders a diagnosis of DVT difficult. If persistent edema is apparent, but there is no evidence of inflammation or pain in the thigh or lower leg, combined with elevated D-dimer level, a diagnosis of DVT may be made by ultrasound Doppler imaging or CT angiography.[46] If DVT is evident, low doses of heparin are more appropriate for minimizing bleeding side effects. The National Institute for Health and Care Excellence guideline suggests that venous thromboembolism (VTE) prophylaxis should be combined with mechanical and pharmacologic treatments when caring for patients undergoing hip fracture surgery. Mechanical VTE prophylaxes include antiembolism stockings, foot impulse devices, and intermittent pneumatic compression devices. Mechanical VTE prophylaxis should be continued until the patient's mobility is no longer significantly reduced since admission. The guideline recommends the addition of pharmacologic VTE prophylaxis for patients with a low risk of bleeding, using either low molecular weight heparin or unfractionated heparin (for patients with severe renal impairment or established renal failure). Pharmacologic VTE prophylaxis is continued until the patient no longer exhibits significantly reduced mobility (generally 5–7 days).[47] In some Asian countries including Korea, VTEs are relatively uncommon, arising in only 5.1% of all cases in one study.[48] Patients at an increased risk of bleeding are often treated via nonpharmacologic methods, such as early mobilization, antithrombotic stockings, or pump therapy, without the prescription of prophylactic thrombolytic agents.

Infection. Infection is one of the most serious complications after fracture treatment. If a deep infection develops, bone union may be impossible, and the internal fixator or artificial joint should be removed and the necrotic tissues be resected. Apart from infectious symptoms such as fever and chills, persistent pain around the hip joint, pain associated with joint motion, and an increased erythrocyte sedimentation rate should raise a suspicion of infection, which must then be investigated meticulously and treated with antibiotics. Prescription of prophylactic antibiotics for patients with hip fractures was found to reduce the incidence of deep infections and urinary tract infections.[49]

Delirium. Delirium is a relatively common problem during hospitalization for hip fracture treatment and is one of the major factors prolonging hospitalization and increasing the medical costs. Delirium is characterized by the sudden appearance of disturbance(s) in consciousness and changes in cognitive function, with the symptoms rising and falling over a single day. It is essential to identify and eliminate the cause of delirium. Maintenance of O_2 saturation (>95%), blood pressure (systolic blood pressure > 90 mmHg), electrolyte balance, postoperative pain control, and bladder and bowel functions; good nutrition; and early rehabilitation are important to prevent delirium. Nonpharmacologic intervention is the mainstay of delirium treatment. Haloperidol is a recognized first-generation drug, and olanzapine, risperidone, and quetiapine fumarate are second-generation drugs.[50] However, such medications should be final options, prescribed only when patients may harm themselves or others. Further details of delirium appear in Chapter 13, Geriatric Psychiatric and Cognitive Disorders: Depression, Dementia, and Delirium.

REHABILITATION IN ACUTE CARE
Establishment of a Postoperative Rehabilitation Program

A specific and stepwise postoperative rehabilitation program should be established by every institution engaged in geriatric interventions. An integrated rehabilitation program applied after hip fracture surgery is essential for elderly patients, and such programs have recently become established in several countries.

In the United Kingdom, models of orthogeriatric care have become well established. Perioperative orthopedic management is followed by early postoperative transfer to a geriatric orthopedic rehabilitation unit. The identification of appropriate patients may be left to orthopedic staff, specialist orthogeriatric liaison nurses, or geriatricians on their rounds. The extent of orthopedic input to the rehabilitation ward depends on how soon patients are moved from acute wards; ready access to orthopedic advice is vital if the momentum of rehabilitation is to be maintained. A weekly visit by a surgeon at a predictable time allows multidisciplinary team members to describe their concerns and problems and discuss X-rays with the specialist. Alternatively, an orthopedic liaison nurse may visit the rehabilitation ward to give advice, adjust plaster casts, and liaise with orthopedic surgeons.[51]

In Korea, a multidisciplinary fragility fracture care program (particularly for those with hip fractures) staffed by physiatrists, geriatricians, and orthopedic surgeons has been established since the mid-2000s. Recently, a nationwide, multicenter fracture liaison service launched a standardized, fracture-integrated rehabilitation management of the hip joint (FIRM-HIP) program to aid the elderly. This is based on the critical features of fragility fracture rehabilitation in both hospital and community settings. Patients receive FIRM-HIP care, which consisted of physical therapy (lower limb strengthening and gait training using assistive device, twice daily), occupational therapy (several sessions during admission), training in fall prevention, and discharge planning advice for 2–3 weeks after hip surgery (Table 3.6). No serious event has been reported among patients who received FIRM-HIP care. At an average of 6–7 days postoperatively, patients are transferred to the department of rehabilitation medicine. After FIRM-HIP care, we found that mobility scores, competence when engaged in the activities of daily living (ADL), quality-of-life scores, and frailty scores all improved significantly.[52]

Rehabilitation in the acute phase and subacute phase

The goal of rehabilitation of patients in the acute and subacute phases is to get them out of bed as soon as possible and to make them stand and walk using walking aids. At this stage, recovery of joint ROM and strength, pain control, and training in ADLs are all required. In addition, planning for functional recovery and discharge should commence.

The modified Barthel index can be used to assess competence in terms of ADLs. Screening tests detecting cognitive dysfunction and dementia should be applied. Elderly patients exhibit limitations in the performance of daily activities because of comorbidities and cognitive decline. As comprehensive management is thus required, interest is growing in the formation of standardized protocols using team and multidisciplinary approaches.

Early mobilization (within 24 h after surgery) is required. Exercise is essential to prevent DVT, pressure

---

TABLE 3.6
An Example of Integrated Rehabilitation Management for Hip Fracture

Goal	Items of Rehabilitation Management
Prevention of complications	Delirium: pain management, cessation of medications aggravating delirium, and environmental modification Pressure ulcer: education for position change and prevention of shear stress (to caregiver) Pneumonia: sputum expectoration and education of respiratory training Cystitis: early removal of an indwelling catheter, evaluation of bladder function, and urinalysis Evaluation of nutritional status and nutritional support
Mobility training and exercise	Wheelchair ambulation: 1–2 days after operation Tilt table training, standing frame, and parallel bar standing (if patients cannot walk premorbidly) Gradual increase in weight-bearing and early initiation of walker gait (if patients can walk premorbidly) Cane gait if mobility function improves Hip range of motion exercise: careful for patients who underwent total hip arthroplasty or hemiarthroplasty Isotonic strengthening exercise using machine and rubber band—Stationary bicycle is not applied for patients who underwent replacement arthroplasty Balance training: using instrument and machine
Occupational therapy	Training for activities of daily living: bedside activity, transfer, sit-up and sit-to-stand, dressing, wearing shoes, toileting, etc.
Early supported discharge	Determination of transfer to other hospital or discharge to home Home exercise education Architectural barrier removal when visiting home Community liaison: providing information for community liaison, sharing patients' information with local hospitals, and regular functional evaluation after discharge

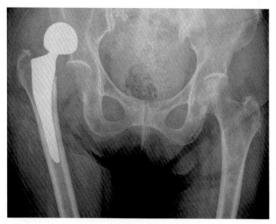

FIG. 3.3 An example of right hip dislocation developed 3 weeks after bipolar hemiarthroplasty.

ulcers, and atelectasis. Patients may commence with ankle pumping and then restore ROM via passive and active assistive exercise. After the patient attains a standing posture and balance using a parallel bar, rehabilitation training features walking with a walker or cane. In patients who underwent replacement arthroplasty via a posterolateral approach, internal rotation, adduction, and hyperflexion (>90 degrees) of the hip joint should be avoided for 2–3 months after surgery to prevent dislocation of the metallic femoral head (Fig. 3.3). Furthermore, ADL training must continue in the home or rehabilitation facility, and cognitive rehabilitation may be required depending on the extent of cognitive decline.

It is essential that ADL training is subdivided into small manageable activities; application of the whole activities should be performed only after training for each part is complete. The use of walking aids is important for elderly patients because of poor balance, loss of muscle strength and endurance, and visual and sensory dysfunctions. For example, a walker, cane, long-handled reacher to cope with reduced ROM caused by surgery, handle in the bath, bath chair, and auxiliary chair to raise the toilet seat height may all be helpful. It is necessary to evaluate and remove architectural barriers at home before discharge. Thresholds and stairs that compromise walking, lack of space between furniture, and inappropriate lighting all need consideration and modification.

Early active, active assistive, and isometric exercises are required for the hip extensors, flexors, and abductors. Isometric contraction of the quadriceps

muscles is also beneficial, for example, by placing objects under the knee. Such strengthening exercises aid walking via muscular retraining. Vigorous resistive exercise is not recommended at this phase. During the early postoperative period, straight leg raising exercises need to be avoided, because this may increase the rotational torque on the internal fixator of the replaced joint.

COMMUNITY CARE AND LONG-TERM CARE

Loss of functional independence is a well-known long-term sequela after a fragility fracture.[53] Functional outcomes are particularly poor for those who already live in nursing homes.[54] However, deterioration in the health-related quality of life is common in patients who have suffered fragility fractures.[55] Longitudinal studies have found that the functional status of such patients declined following the tapering of rehabilitation services.[56] Relative immobility following discharge contributes to balance deterioration and muscle weakness, increasing the likelihood of subsequent fractures. Recent clinical trials showed that the long-term functional outcomes afforded by geriatric rehabilitation services delivered after surgery to treat fragility fractures included significantly better mobility and ADL scores.[57-59] However, the evidence supporting long-term functional improvement after the regular rehabilitation period remains weak. A metaanalysis of 11 studies failed to demonstrate any improvement in long-term functional outcomes after the implementation of rehabilitation or orthogeriatric models of care.[60] Therefore, a few months of geriatric rehabilitation after fragility fracture surgery may not be enough to achieve the previous levels of function; continuous community-based rehabilitation services are required.

Exercise
Home-Based Exercise
Notably, a prospective cohort study found that most (75%) patients receiving standard care for fractured hips did not even meet a very low target of return to the prior level of function at 12 months postoperatively.[61] Therefore, home-based exercise is an essential component of long-term care after fragility fractures. To this end, the ProMo Trial[59] randomized 81 hip fracture patients to standard care or a year-long home-based program including evaluation/modification of environmental hazards, guidance in terms of safe walking,

pain management, progressive implementation of a multicomponent home exercise program, and physical activity counseling. The program reduced the overall disability of the elderly after hip fracture. Orwig et al. developed an exercise program featuring 12 months of home-based aerobic and strength training after hip fracture surgery.[62] The program increased activity levels and modestly improved bone density, compared with usual care. However, in contrast to their hypotheses, no significant changes in muscle mass, strength, ADL independence, or physical function were observed. Thus, there is as yet no evidence that such all-inclusive programs are effective compared with shorter-term, robust strength training (as described earlier).[54] Notably, the lack of supervision, the fact that multiple exercise modalities are required, and the fact that the patients are at home likely reduce training intensity, even if adherence is good, explaining the observed lack of efficacy.

Community-based exercise
Interest is increasing in booster exercise program that continue beyond the regular rehabilitation period for patients with hip fractures who are returning to the community. These programs can be divided into two groups: exercise training conducted at home and that conducted in the community. A systematic review comparing home- and community-based programs[63] found that the effect sizes for community-based interventions were larger and were more likely to be statistically significant, explained by higher exercise intensity and the availability of more sophisticated equipment in community-based, extended exercise facilities. However, the subgroup comparisons should be interpreted with caution, as the differences between the two groups might be due to confounding factors rather than the interventional setting. It is true, however, that group settings enhance social interaction among patients sharing the same condition, which may enhance participation in more intensive community-based programs, reduce costs, and improve motor learning skills.[64,65]

Nutrition
General malnutrition is both very prevalent (40%–80% of hospitalized patients with hip fractures) and one of the strongest predictors of poor outcomes after fracture.[66] Oral nutritional supplements can help elderly patients recover after hip fracture surgery and reduce perioperative complications. An interdisciplinary treatment program evaluating 162 hip fracture patients found that mobility and functional outcomes improved in ≥60% of patients who were malnourished on admission and then randomized to the experimental intervention.[67] It is not surprising that such a modest intervention, without attention paid to the cause of malnutrition, changes to the residential environment, or ongoing nutritional support, improved clinically relevant long-term outcomes and even resulted in weight gain. Finally, a controlled trial in the Netherlands evaluated the cost-effectiveness of a multicenter, randomized controlled trial of regular dietary counseling and oral nutritional supplementation for 3 months, postoperatively delivered to 152 patients with hip fracture.[68] Cost-effectiveness was considered significant for weight gain but not quality-adjusted life years.

In addition, a high-protein diet may impact bone health positively via several mechanisms including increased intestinal calcium absorption, stimulation of insulin-like growth factor-1, and enhanced lean body mass.[69] Despite previous concerns that an increase in dietary protein triggers calcinuria to an extent impairing calcium balance or induces a shift in systemic pH (thus increasing osteoclastic bone resorption), the studies have consistently shown that higher protein intake was associated with a higher bone density and lower fracture risk. Protein supplementation after hip fracture increased the BMD and muscle strength and decreased complications and the length of hospital stay. Increased protein intake (via diet or supplements) may also be beneficial for the treatment of sarcopenia (which is common in elderly cohort)[70] and, if given near the time of resistance training sessions, may enhance anabolic adaptation to such training. This was vital in a frail hip fracture cohort in whom standard application of resistance training, even at high intensity, may not result in muscle hypertrophy.[71]

Vitamin D
All patients with fragility fractures should have their 25-hydroxy-vitamin D levels assessed and corrected to a steady state of >32 ng/mL.[72] Many oral supplements are available. There is no universal agreement on either the ideal supplement or the dosing schedule. Vitamin D supplements come in two forms: ergocalciferol (vitamin D2) (from plants and yeasts) and cholecalciferol (vitamin D3) (from animal sources and production in the skin).[73] After repletion of vitamin D levels, patients are advised to take 2000 IU cholecalciferol (vitamin D3) daily for long term in addition

to any vitamin D contained in their multivitamin or calcium supplements. A metaanalysis of vitamin D3 regimens showed that 25-hydroxy-vitamin D levels of 32–44 ng/mL afforded optimal health benefits and were achieved only when 1800–4000 IU vitamin D3 were taken daily.[74] Mean serum calcium levels were not adversely affected by dosing regimens of up to 10,000 IU vitamin D3 daily.[75]

Mobile Outreach Program

At the University of Minnesota and Regions Hospital, Geriatric Fracture Program was established in 2004 and featured an in-hospital fracture liaison service, a bone health and secondary fracture prevention service, and an on-site orthopedic clinical service: "Mobile Outreach." This model shares decision-making via high-quality communication with patients and their families, which is a cornerstone of the program. Orthopedic care is provided for the frailest patients, including those whose orthopedic needs are often nonsurgical and for whom public transport access is difficult. In the present era of bundled payments and the growth of advanced practice providers, Mobile Outreach afforded a new opportunity to improve the care and outcomes of a growing population of patients with fragility fractures.[76] Further investigations to reveal the cost-effectiveness of the program should be needed.

FALL PREVENTION

The occurrence of falls is multifactorial in nature. It results from a combination of extrinsic factors related to the environment and intrinsic factors related to individual physical and cognitive conditions.[77] Such intrinsic factors include muscle strength, flexibility, balance, gait, and mobility, all of which are potentially modifiable by adequate and effective interventions. Geriatric physiatrists should review their prescription of medications that may increase the risk of falls (antihistamines or sleeping pills). Vitamin D is recommended for patients at risk of vitamin D deficiency. Physiatrists should also conduct a comprehensive geriatric assessment to identify impaired mobility and dementia, both of which contribute to the risk of falling. Further details of fall are described in Chapter 4, Fall Prevention and Intervention.

Fall Risk Measurements

Many possible predictors of fall-associated fractures are known; the timing of the associations between these risk factors and the actual fracture remains unclear.[78] It is evident that a previous fracture (at a different site)

is a risk factor for a future fracture; this risk is highest immediately after the initial event and subsequently decreases over time.[2,79–81] This was well demonstrated recently.[79] The authors suggested that the risk of a major osteoporotic fracture after the first major osteoporotic fracture was 2.7-fold greater than the risk in the general population at 1 year and decreased to 1.4-fold after 10 years. The risk of a second major osteoporotic fracture increased by 4% with each year of age. Furthermore, prior fractures continue to be an important predictor of fracture risk for up to 10 years, even in models adjusted for age, BMD, and other clinical risk factors.[82] Further studies are needed to define the determinants of imminent risk (e.g., whether the type of fracture affects the future risk, and whether the risks identified are responsive to medical intervention). To date, a previous fracture is the strongest predictor of a future fracture.

Clinicians can also perform more targeted assessments of balance and gait features that directly impact the fall risk. The Timed Up and Go (TUG) test is an extension of the comfortable gait speed test that incorporates the additional components of rise from a chair and a turn. Prospective data gathered over 1 year showed that the TUG was particularly sensitive when used to predict future falls in older women with a history of vertebral fractures.[83] The Berg Balance Scale (BBS) is a performance-based measure of the ability to complete 14 mobility tasks that are thought to be representative of typical daily tasks. Each task is scored on a scale of 0 (unable to complete the task) to 4 (able to do the task independently), with a maximum score of 56. The BBS has been useful for predicting falls in the frail elderly.[84] Measurement of the comfortable gait speed is a simple method to assess dynamic balance that can be performed in any clinic, hallway, or room, and it has shown strong prediction of future disability, institutionalization, and even mortality.[85] Gait speed is also a significant predictor of falls; 0.8 m/s was an optimal cutoff for identifying at-risk individuals.[86] Gait speed measures typical aspects of postural maintenance, required for basic upright balance and simple ambulation. However, as is true of single measure, critical information may be lost or overlooked if an inappropriate incorrect assessment tool is chosen and a functionally impaired area is thus not assessed.[87]

Interventions to Prevent Falls

Physical exercise significantly prevents falls and fractures in the ambulatory elderly.[88] Several systematic reviews and metaanalyses have emphasized and demonstrated the beneficial effects of physical exercise programs on falls and fracture prevention in community-dwelling older adults.[89-91] Exercise improves strength, endurance, muscle flexibility, and postural balance. Therefore, exercise not only reduces physical disability and functional limitations in older adults but also aids in the maintenance of mechanisms that prevent imminent falls.[92] In contrast, the effect of exercise on fall and fracture prevention in long-term care residents remains controversial. A recent Cochrane review suggested that exercise was not effective in preventing falls in long-term care residents.[93] However, the review was limited in terms of the studies selected for the evaluation; these studies included not only specific exercise interventions but also general fall prevention programs in which exercise was just one component of the entire program. This may affect the validity of conclusions drawn in terms of a specific role for exercise in fall prevention (the primary outcome).[92] A more recent systematic review suggested that combined, frequent, and long-term exercise programs are effective to prevent falls in long-term care facilities, but no effect of exercise on fracture prevention was noted.[92] It was also reported that exercise was more effective when programs lasted for >6 months with two to three exercise sessions weekly.

One clinical trial evaluated the effect of an exercise program on falls by nursing home residents.[94] The program featured a combination of balance exercises and progressive resistance training using ankle weights and dumbbells. Each session commenced with 20 min of balance exercises in a standing position, and walking if possible. Progressive resistance training was of nine different standardized types using the "10 repetitions maximum (10 RM)" as a marker for approximately 75% maximum voluntary contraction and included all major muscle groups of the upper and lower extremities. The exercises were done in two sets, each comprising 10 repetitions. Participants can progress to a maximum of 10 kg ankle weights and 5 kg upper extremity weights. Instructors increased the load as tolerated based on the 10-RM data. This program reduced the fall rate of the intervention group (relative risk = 0.55) compared with the control group. Schnelle et al. described an easier and thus more feasible fall prevention exercise program for clinical settings, termed Functional Incidental Training. The program targeted continence, physical activity, and mobility endurance.[95] Participants were encouraged to walk or, if not ambulatory, to wheel their chairs, and to repeat sit-to-stands up to eight times with minimal human

assistance. When in bed, upper body resistance training (arm curls or arm raises) was performed. Target goals were individually set and adjusted on a weekly basis. Although this intervention may seem too simple, the intervention group exhibited significantly better functional outcomes than those of the control group (in terms of strength and mobility endurance) and a 10% reduction in the incidence of acute conditions. Therefore, no matter how simple the exercises are, it can positively work on fall prevention.

CONCLUSION

Those involved in rehabilitation for falls and osteoporotic fracture must have a good understanding of osteoporosis, falls, fragility fracture, and pre-, peri-, and postoperative care. Multidisciplinary integrated rehabilitation programs are paving the way by which practitioners to provide appropriate postoperative care and improve the quality of life after hip fracture surgery. There is no easy path to fall prevention. However, the first step is clinical awareness and evaluation of the risk of falls. In addition, the risk can be minimized by the exercise programs included in community-based fall prevention programs.

REFERENCES

1. Verma SK, Willetts JL, Corns HL, et al. Among community-dwelling adults in the United States. *PLoS One.* 2016;11(3):e0150939.
2. Johnell O, Kanis JA, Oden A, et al. Fracture risk following an osteoporotic fracture. *Osteoporos Int.* 2004;15(3):175–179.
3. Nih Consensus Development Panel on Osteoporosis Prevention, Diagnosis, Therapy. Osteoporosis prevention, diagnosis, and therapy. *JAMA.* 2001;285(6):785–795.
4. Bernabei R, Martone AM, Ortolani E, Landi F, Marzetti E. Screening, diagnosis and treatment of osteoporosis: a brief review. *Clin Cases Miner Bone Metab.* 2014;11(3):201–207.
5. Srinivasan B, Kopperdahl DL, Amin S, et al. Relationship of femoral neck areal bone mineral density to volumetric bone mineral density, bone size, and femoral strength in men and women. *Osteoporos Int.* 2012;23(1):155–162.
6. Johnell O, Kanis JA, Oden A, et al. Predictive value of BMD for hip and other fractures. *J Bone Miner Res.* 2005;20(7):1185–1194.
7. TISFC Densitometry. *2013 ISCD Official Positions – Adult;* 2013. https://www.iscd.org/official-positions/2013-iscd-official-positions-adult/.
8. Cooper C, Campion G, Melton 3rd LJ. Hip fractures in the elderly: a world-wide projection. *Osteoporos Int.* 1992;2(6):285–289.

9. Randell A, Sambrook PN, Nguyen TV, et al. Direct clinical and welfare costs of osteoporotic fractures in elderly men and women. *Osteoporos Int.* 1995;5(6):427–432.

10. Kanis JA, Johnell O, Oden A, Jonsson B, Dawson A, Dere W. Risk of hip fracture derived from relative risks: an analysis applied to the population of Sweden. *Osteoporos Int.* 2000;11(2):120–127.

11. Lau EM. Osteoporosis–a worldwide problem and the implications in Asia. *Ann Acad Med Singap.* 2002;31(1):67–68.

12. Kanis JA, Johnell O. The burden of osteoporosis. *J Endocrinol Invest.* 1999;22(8):583–588.

13. Laurent M, Gielen E, Claessens F, Boonen S, Vanderschueren D. Osteoporosis in older men: recent advances in pathophysiology and treatment. *Best Pract Res Clin Endocrinol Metab.* 2013;27(4):527–539.

14. McCloskey EV, Harvey NC, Johansson H, Kanis JA. FRAX updates 2016. *Curr Opin Rheumatol.* 2016;28(4):433–441.

15. Lim SY, Lim JH, Nguyen D, et al. Screening for osteoporosis in men aged 70 years and older in a primary care setting in the United States. *Am J Mens Health.* 2013;7(4):350–354.

16. Watts NB, Adler RA, Bilezikian JP, et al. Osteoporosis in men: an Endocrine Society clinical practice guideline. *J Clin Endocrinol Metab.* 2012;97(6):1802–1822.

17. Kuo TR, Chen CH. Bone biomarker for the clinical assessment of osteoporosis: recent developments and future perspectives. *Biomark Res.* 2017;5:18.

18. Wheater G, Elshahaly M, Tuck SP, Datta HK, van Laar JM. The clinical utility of bone marker measurements in osteoporosis. *J Transl Med.* 2013;11:201.

19. Vasikaran S, Cooper C, Eastell R, et al. International Osteoporosis Foundation and International Federation of Clinical Chemistry and Laboratory Medicine position on bone marker standards in osteoporosis. *Clin Chem Lab Med.* 2011;49(8):1271–1274.

20. Drake MT, Clarke BL, Lewiecki EM. The pathophysiology and treatment of osteoporosis. *Clin Ther.* 2015;37(8):1837–1850.

21. Black DM, Delmas PD, Eastell R, et al. Once-yearly zoledronic acid for treatment of postmenopausal osteoporosis. *N Engl J Med.* 2007;356(18):1809–1822.

22. Cummings SR, San Martin J, McClung MR, et al. Denosumab for prevention of fractures in postmenopausal women with osteoporosis. *N Engl J Med.* 2009;361(8):756–765.

23. Freemantle N, Cooper C, Diez-Perez A, et al. Results of indirect and mixed treatment comparison of fracture efficacy for osteoporosis treatments: a meta-analysis. *Osteoporos Int.* 2013;24(1):209–217.

24. Sleet DA, Moffett DB, Stevens J. CDC's research portfolio in older adult fall prevention: a review of progress, 1985-2005, and future research directions. *J Saf Res.* 2008;39(3):259–267.

25. Stevens JA, Mack KA, Paulozzi LJ, Ballesteros MF. Self-reported falls and fall-related injuries among persons aged>or=65 years–United States, 2006. *J Saf Res.* 2008;39(3):345–349.

26. Dhanwal DK, Dennison EM, Harvey NC, Cooper C. Epidemiology of hip fracture: worldwide geographic variation. *Indian J Orthop.* 2011;45(1):15–22.

27. Schousboe JT. Epidemiology of vertebral fractures. *J Clin Densitom.* 2016;19(1):8–22.

28. Hannan EL, Magaziner J, Wang JJ, et al. Mortality and locomotion 6 months after hospitalization for hip fracture: risk factors and risk-adjusted hospital outcomes. *JAMA.* 2001;285(21):2736–2742.

29. Mitchell R, Harvey L, Brodaty H, Draper B, Close J. One-year mortality after hip fracture in older individuals: the effects of delirium and dementia. *Arch Gerontol Geriatr.* 2017;72:135–141.

30. Guerra MT, Viana RD, Feil L, Feron ET, Maboni J, Vargas AS. One-year mortality of elderly patients with hip fracture surgically treated at a hospital in Southern Brazil. *Rev Bras Ortop.* 2017;52(1):17–23.

31. Yoon HK, Park C, Jang S, Jang S, Lee YK, Ha YC. Incidence and mortality following hip fracture in Korea. *J Korean Med Sci.* 2011;26(8):1087–1092.

32. Muraki S, Yamamoto S, Ishibashi H, Nakamura K. Factors associated with mortality following hip fracture in Japan. *J Bone Miner Metab.* 2006;24(2):100–104.

33. Roche JJ, Wenn RT, Sahota O, Moran CG. Effect of comorbidities and postoperative complications on mortality after hip fracture in elderly people: prospective observational cohort study. *BMJ.* 2005;331(7529):1374.

34. Ishidou Y, Koriyama C, Kakoi H, et al. Predictive factors of mortality and deterioration in performance of activities of daily living after hip fracture surgery in Kagoshima, Japan. *Geriatr Gerontol Int.* 2017;17(3):391–401.

35. Cenzer IS, Tang V, Boscardin WJ, et al. One-year mortality after hip fracture: development and validation of a prognostic index. *J Am Geriatr Soc.* 2016;64(9):1863–1868.

36. Li SG, Sun TS, Liu Z, Ren JX, Liu B, Gao Y. Factors influencing postoperative mortality one year after surgery for hip fracture in Chinese elderly population. *Chin Med J (Engl).* 2013;126(14):2715–2719.

37. Tsuboi M, Hasegawa Y, Suzuki S, Wingstrand H, Thorngren KG. Mortality and mobility after hip fracture in Japan: a ten-year follow-up. *J Bone Joint Surg Br.* 2007;89(4):461–466.

38. Magaziner J, Hawkes W, Hebel JR, et al. Recovery from hip fracture in eight areas of function. *J Gerontol A Biol Sci Med Sci.* 2000;55(9):M498–M507.

39. Tinetti ME, Williams CS. Falls, injuries due to falls, and the risk of admission to a nursing home. *N Engl J Med.* 1997;337(18):1279–1284.

40. Beraldi R, Masi L, Parri S, Partescano R, Brandi ML. The role of the orthopaedic surgeon in the prevention of refracture in patients treated surgically for fragility hip and vertebral fracture. *Clin Cases Miner Bone Metab.* 2014;11(1):31–35.

41. Rosen JE, Chen FS, Hiebert R, Koval KJ. Efficacy of preoperative skin traction in hip fracture patients: a prospective, randomized study. *J Orthop Trauma.* 2001;15(2):81–85.

42. Buchbinder R, Osborne RH, Ebeling PR, et al. A randomized trial of vertebroplasty for painful osteoporotic vertebral fractures. *N Engl J Med.* 2009;361(6):557–568.

43. Sun H, Li C. Comparison of unilateral and bilateral percutaneous vertebroplasty for osteoporotic vertebral compression fractures: a systematic review and meta-analysis. *J Orthop Surg Res.* 2016;11(1):156.

44. Tan HY, Wang LM, Zhao L, Liu YL, Song RP. A prospective study of percutaneous vertebroplasty for chronic painful osteoporotic vertebral compression fracture. *Pain Res Manag.* 2015;20(1):e8–e11.

45. Fisher WD, Agnelli G, George DJ, et al. Extended venous thromboembolism prophylaxis in patients undergoing hip fracture surgery – the SAVE-HIP3 study. *Bone Joint J.* 2013;95-B(4):459–466.

46. Girasole GJ, Cuomo F, Denton JR, O'Connor D, Ernst A. Diagnosis of deep vein thrombosis in elderly hip-fracture patients by using the duplex scanning technique. *Orthop Rev.* 1994;23(5):411–416.

47. *Venous Thromboembolism: Reducing the Risk for Patients in Hospital.* 2015. https://www.nice.org.uk/guidance/cg92/chapter/1-recommendations.

48. Lee YK, Choi YH, Ha YC, Lim JY, Koo KH. Does venous thromboembolism affect rehabilitation after hip fracture surgery? *Yonsei Med J.* 2013;54(4):1015–1019.

49. LeBlanc KE, Muncie Jr HL, LeBlanc LL. Hip fracture: diagnosis, treatment, and secondary prevention. *Am Fam Physician.* 2014;89(12):945–951.

50. Lee HB, Oldham MA, Sieber FE, Oh ES. Impact of delirium after hip fracture surgery on one-year mortality in patients with or without dementia: a case of effect modification. *Am J Geriatr Psychiatry.* 2017;25(3):308–315.

51. *British Orthopaedic Association and British Geriatrics Society. The care of patients with fragility fracture.* British Orthopaedic Association. 2007.

52. Lee SY, Beom J. Letter to the editor: specific and stepwise postoperative rehabilitation program is needed in the elderly after hip fracture surgery. *Ann Geriatr Med Res.* 2016;20(4):233.

53. Magaziner J, Simonsick EM, Kashner TM, Hebel JR, Kenzora JE. Predictors of functional recovery one year following hospital discharge for hip fracture: a prospective study. *J Gerontol.* 1990;45(3):M101–M107.

54. Neuman MD, Silber JH, Magaziner JS, Passarella MA, Mehta S, Werner RM. Survival and functional outcomes after hip fracture among nursing home residents. *JAMA Intern Med.* 2014;174(8):1273–1280.

55. Randell AG, Nguyen TV, Bhalerao N, Silverman SL, Sambrook PN, Eisman JA. Deterioration in quality of life following hip fracture: a prospective study. *Osteoporos Int.* 2000;11(5):460–466.

56. Young Y, Xiong K, Pruzek RM. Longitudinal functional recovery after postacute rehabilitation in older hip fracture patients: the role of cognitive impairment and implications for long-term care. *J Am Med Dir Assoc.* 2011;12(6):431–438.

57. Prestmo A, Hagen G, Sletvold O, et al. Comprehensive geriatric care for patients with hip fractures: a prospective, randomised, controlled trial. *Lancet (Lond, Engl).* 2015;385(9978):1623–1633.

58. Lahtinen A, Leppilahti J, Harmainen S, et al. Geriatric and physically oriented rehabilitation improves the ability of independent living and physical rehabilitation reduces mortality: a randomised comparison of 538 patients. *Clin Rehabil.* 2015;29(9):892–906.

59. Edgren J, Salpakoski A, Sihvonen SE, et al. Effects of a home-based physical rehabilitation program on physical disability after hip fracture: a randomized controlled trial. *J Am Med Dir Assoc.* 2015;16(4):350.e351–350.e357.

60. Deschodt M, Flamaing J, Haentjens P, Boonen S, Milisen K. Impact of geriatric consultation teams on clinical outcome in acute hospitals: a systematic review and meta-analysis. *BMC Med.* 2013;11:48.

61. Lloyd BD, Williamson DA, Singh NA, et al. Recurrent and injurious falls in the year following hip fracture: a prospective study of incidence and risk factors from the Sarcopenia and Hip Fracture study. *J Gerontol Ser A, Biol Sci Med Sci.* 2009;64(5):599–609.

62. Orwig DL, Hochberg M, Yu-Yahiro J, et al. Delivery and outcomes of a yearlong home exercise program after hip fracture: a randomized controlled trial. *Arch Intern Med.* 2011;171(4):323–331.

63. Auais MA, Eilayyan O, Mayo NE. Extended exercise rehabilitation after hip fracture improves patients' physical function: a systematic review and meta-analysis. *Phys Ther.* 2012;92(11):1437–1451.

64. McNevin NH, Wulf G, Carlson C. Effects of attentional focus, self-control, and dyad training on motor learning: implications for physical rehabilitation. *Phys Ther.* 2000;80(4):373–385.

65. Shea CH, Wulf G, Whitacre C. Enhancing training efficiency and effectiveness through the use of dyad training. *J Mot Behav.* 1999;31(2):119–125.

66. Resnick B, Beaupre L, McGilton KS, et al. Rehabilitation interventions for older individuals with cognitive impairment post-hip fracture: a systematic review. *J Am Med Dir Assoc.* 2016;17(3):200–205.

67. Li HJ, Cheng HS, Liang J, Wu CC, Shyu YI. Functional recovery of older people with hip fracture: does malnutrition make a difference? *J Adv Nurs.* 2013;69(8):1691–1703.

68. Wyers CE, Reijven PL, Evers SM, et al. Cost-effectiveness of nutritional intervention in elderly subjects after hip fracture. A randomized controlled trial. *Osteoporos Int.* 2013;24(1):151–162.

69. Fiatarone Singh MA. Exercise, nutrition and managing hip fracture in older persons. *Curr Opin Clin Nutr Metab Care.* 2014;17(1):12–24.

70. Hida T, Ishiguro N, Shimokata H, et al. High prevalence of sarcopenia and reduced leg muscle mass in Japanese patients immediately after a hip fracture. *Geriatr Gerontol Int.* 2013;13(2):413–420.

71. Singh NA, Quine S, Clemson LM, et al. Effects of high-intensity progressive resistance training and targeted multidisciplinary treatment of frailty on mortality and nursing home admissions after hip fracture: a randomized controlled trial. *J Am Med Dir Assoc.* 2012;13(1):24–30.

72. Bischoff-Ferrari HA. Vitamin D and fracture prevention. *Endocrinol Metab Clin North Am.* 2010;39(2):347–353. Table of contents.

73. Bukata SV, Kates SL, O'Keefe RJ. Short-term and long-term orthopaedic issues in patients with fragility fractures. *Clin Orthop Relat Res.* 2011;469(8):2225–2236.

74. Bischoff-Ferrari HA, Shao A, Dawson-Hughes B, Hathcock J, Giovannucci E, Willett WC. Benefit-risk assessment of vitamin D supplementation. *Osteoporos Int.* 2010;21(7):1121–1132.

75. Bischoff-Ferrari HA, Dawson-Hughes B, Staehelin HB, et al. Fall prevention with supplemental and active forms of vitamin D: a meta-analysis of randomised controlled trials. *BMJ.* 2009;339:b3692.

76. Switzer JA, Bozic KJ, Kates SL. Geriatric fracture care: future trajectories: a 2015 AOA critical issues symposium. *J Bone Joint Surgery Am.* 2017;99(8):e40.

77. Halil M, Ulger Z, Cankurtaran M, et al. Falls and the elderly: is there any difference in the developing world? A cross-sectional study from Turkey. *Arch Gerontol Geriatr.* 2006;43(3):351–359.

78. Kanis JA, Cooper C, Rizzoli R, et al. Identification and management of patients at increased risk of osteoporotic fracture: outcomes of an ESCEO expert consensus meeting. *Osteoporos Int.* 2017;28.

79. Johansson H, Siggeirsdottir K, Harvey NC, et al. Imminent risk of fracture after fracture. *Osteoporos Int.* 2017;28(3):775–780.

80. Johnell O, Oden A, Caulin F, Kanis JA. Acute and long-term increase in fracture risk after hospitalization for vertebral fracture. *Osteoporos Int.* 2001;12(3):207–214.

81. Ryg J, Rejnmark L, Overgaard S, Brixen K, Vestergaard P. Hip fracture patients at risk of second hip fracture: a nationwide population-based cohort study of 169,145 cases during 1977-2001. *J Bone Miner Res.* 2009;24(7):1299–1307.

82. Giangregorio LM, Leslie WD, Manitoba Bone Density P. Time since prior fracture is a risk modifier for 10-year osteoporotic fractures. *J Bone Miner Res.* 2010;25(6):1400–1405.

83. Morris R, Harwood RH, Baker R, Sahota O, Armstrong S, Masud T. A comparison of different balance tests in the prediction of falls in older women with vertebral fractures: a cohort study. *Age Ageing.* 2007;36(1):78–83.

84. Kim SG, Kim MK. The intra- and inter-rater reliabilities of the short form Berg balance scale in institutionalized elderly people. *J Phys Ther Sci.* 2015;27(9):2733–2734.

85. Studenski S, Perera S, Patel K, et al. Gait speed and survival in older adults. *JAMA.* 2011;305(1):50–58.

86. Abellan van Kan G, Rolland Y, Andrieu S, et al. Gait speed at usual pace as a predictor of adverse outcomes in community-dwelling older people an International Academy on Nutrition and Aging (IANA) Task Force. *J Nutr Health Aging.* 2009;13(10):881–889.

87. Persad CC, Cook S, Giordani B. Assessing falls in the elderly: should we use simple screening tests or a comprehensive fall risk evaluation? *Eur J Phys Rehabil Med.* 2010;46(2):249–259.

88. Donald IP, Pitt K, Armstrong E, Shuttleworth H. Preventing falls on an elderly care rehabilitation ward. *Clin Rehabil.* 2000;14(2):178–185.

89. Petridou ET, Manti EG, Ntinapogias AG, Negri E, Szczerbinska K. What works better for community-dwelling older people at risk to fall? a meta-analysis of multifactorial versus physical exercise-alone interventions. *J Aging Health.* 2009;21(5):713–729.

90. Sherrington C, Tiedemann A, Fairhall N, Close JC, Lord SR. Exercise to prevent falls in older adults: an updated meta-analysis and best practice recommendations. *N S W Public Health Bull.* 2011;22(3–4):78–83.

91. Sherrington C, Whitney JC, Lord SR, Herbert RD, Cumming RG, Close JC. Effective exercise for the prevention of falls: a systematic review and meta-analysis. *J Am Geriatr Soc.* 2008;56(12):2234–2243.

92. Silva RB, Eslick GD, Duque G. Exercise for falls and fracture prevention in long term care facilities: a systematic review and meta-analysis. *J Am Med Dir Assoc.* 2013;14(9):685–689. e682.

93. Cameron ID, Murray GR, Gillespie LD, et al. Interventions for preventing falls in older people in nursing care facilities and hospitals. *Cochrane Database Syst Rev.* 2010;(1):CD005465.

94. Becker C, Kron M, Lindemann U, et al. Effectiveness of a multifaceted intervention on falls in nursing home residents. *J Am Geriatr Soc.* 2003;51(3):306–313.

95. Schnelle JF, Kapur K, Alessi C, et al. Does an exercise and incontinence intervention save healthcare costs in a nursing home population? *J Am Geriatr Soc.* 2003;51(2):161–168.

CHAPTER 4

Fall Prevention and Intervention

MOOYEON OH-PARK, MD • MICHELLE DIDESCH, MD

INTRODUCTION

Falls are highly prevalent[1] and a significant concern among older adults worldwide. Falls, however, are not part of the normal aging process. Rather, they reflect the combined effect of illness, medications, and environmental hazards.[2] Falls in older adults can lead to devastating consequences of additional morbidity, loss of independence, institutionalization, and even death. Falls also affect self-esteem and confidence in older adults, compromising their quality of life. The direct cost for fall injuries in the United States was estimated at around $31 billion in 2015.[3,4] Literature has shown that systematic fall risk assessment, targeted intervention, exercise programs, and environmental modifications can significantly reduce falls among older adults. This chapter will provide an overview of the epidemiology and risk factors of falls as well as a practical guide for fall prevention and intervention among older adults in community and institutional settings.

DEFINITION OF FALLS

Although falls can be easily recognized when they occur, the term "fall" can hold different meanings for older adults and healthcare providers. For example, most older adults often associate falls with a physical loss of balance but rarely as a side effect of medications. In addition, both older adults and healthcare providers tend to focus on the consequences of falls, which can result in dismissing noninjurious falls, thereby missing an opportunity for early intervention.[5]

The World Health Organization defines a fall as *an event that results in a person coming to rest inadvertently on the ground or floor or other lower level.*[6] The Kellogg International Working Group on the Prevention of Falls by the Elderly includes this additional phrase to the definition: *other than as a consequence of the following: sustaining a violent blow, loss of consciousness, sudden onset of paralysis, as in a stroke, an epileptic seizure.*[2]

Slips and trips are terms often used by older adults as synonyms for falls. A slip is "sliding of the support leg" and a trip is an "impact of the swinging leg with an external object or a body part."[5] These events may result in falls but are not synonymous with falls.

A clear definition of falls must be used to improve the effectiveness of screening high-risk individuals and to improve the validity of fall research. A list of International Statistical Classification of Diseases and Related Health Problems (ICD)-10 codes is included in Table 4.1; consistency in diagnostic coding will also help improve clinical research.

EPIDEMIOLOGY OF FALLS
Fall Rates and Risks

A variety of methods are used to determine and report falls, which makes it challenging for healthcare providers to compare fall rates or risks among different care settings. Rate of falls is defined as "the total number of falls per unit of person time that falls were monitored (e.g., falls per person year)." Risk of falling is calculated as the number of fallers during a given time.[7] It is important to recognize how the fall rate and risk are calculated to understand the epidemiology of falls and the effectiveness of interventions.

Falling is a common problem for older adults. Approximately 30% of persons aged ≥65 years suffer a fall each year.[8,9] After 75 years of age, fall rates increase up to 50% per year with an increase in concomitant injury and mortality.[1,10,11] Unfortunately, after an initial fall, the risk of a repeat fall within a year is 66%.[9]

Despite this high prevalence, older adults are often reluctant to discuss falls with their healthcare providers because of the fear of losing their independence. In the community, women fall more frequently than men. Although this may be related to physical factors such as bone mineral density and lower-extremity strength, this statistic is skewed because women are

TABLE 4.1
ICD-10 Codes for Falls

History of falling[a]	Z91.81
Repeated falls[b]	R29.6
Falls divided by etiology	W00–W19[c]
Ice and snow	W00
Slipping, tripping, and stumbling	W01
Collision with another person	W03
While being carried or supported by others	W04
From nonmoving wheelchair, nonmotorized scooter, and motorized mobility scooter[d]	W05
From bed	W06
From chair	W07
From other furniture	W08
On/from playground equipment	W09
On/from stairs, steps, curb, incline, escalator	W10
On/from ladder	W11
On/from scaffolding	W12
From/out/through building, balcony, bridge, roof, floor, window	W13
From tree	W14
From cliff	W15
Into water	W16
Other specific etiologies including falling into hole, into well, in shower	W17–W18
Unspecified	W19

[a]Indicates fall risk.
[b]Can be used for acute fall when etiology is still being explored.
[c]Further specifications needed for initial encounter, subsequent encounter, sequela, fall level, and secondary injury.
[d]Fall from powered moving wheelchair: V00.811; fall from moving motorized mobility scooter: V00.831; fall from nonmotorized scooter: V00.141.
From the Centers for Medicare & Medicaid Services. *2018 ICD-10 CM and GEMs*. Available at: https://www.cms.gov/Medicare/Coding/ICD10/2018-ICD-10-CM-and-GEMs.html; with permission.

BOX 4.1
2014 Centers for Disease Control and Prevention Statistics on Falling in the United States Among Noninstitutionalized Adults Aged 65 Years and Older

- Falls are the leading cause of fatal and nonfatal injuries
- Approximately 30% older adults reported falls in the past year
- 29 million total falls reported
- 7 million associated injuries and 27,000 fatalities due to falls
- 2.8 million patients treated in emergency departments
- 800,000 hospitalized
- Women reported more falls than men (30.3% vs. 26.5%, respectively)
- Women reported more fall-related injuries than men (12.6% vs. 8.3%, respectively)

Data from Bergen G, Stevens MR, Burns ER. Falls and fall injuries among adults aged ≥65 years – United States, 2014. *Morb Mortal Wkly Rep*. 2016;65(37):993–998.

Fall risk and rates vary considerably among settings, with a higher incidence of falls in long-term care facilities. The fall rate for elderly individuals living in the community is estimated at 20%–40% per year (Box 4.1). This rate is at least twice as high in older adults living in long-term care, with a higher incidence of serious complications. Interestingly, in these facilities, male residents are reported to fall more frequently and sustain more injuries than female residents.[7] This finding is in contrast to the sex differences seen among community-dwelling adults. Most falls in long-term care facilities occur in the resident's room or bathroom, with 41% during transfers and 36% while walking.[7] These are theoretically preventable events.

The higher rate of falls in institutionalized settings is multifactorial. Those living in a long-term care facility may have more risk factors for falling than healthy older adults living in the community, such as more medical comorbidities, difficulty sleeping, and higher rates of delirium. Given the potential serious complications of a fall, additional efforts should be made to prevent falls in long-term care facilities.

Outcomes of Falls

Fortunately, most falls do not result in serious physical injury. However, approximately 10%–25% result in serious injury.[10,13] The risk of injury and mortality

more likely than men to report falls and seek medical attention. Despite the higher reporting rates among females, most falls are not reported in both men and women, and fall prevention is discussed even less.[12] Research on the incidence of falling is also affected by recall bias, which likely underestimates the true scope of this issue.

from falls increases with age. Falls remain the leading cause of fatal injuries among older adults[1]; however, the majority of deaths secondary to falls are considered preventable.[10] Falls are also the most common cause of trauma-related hospital admissions among older adults. The main reasons for hospitalization after falls include traumatic brain injury (TBI) and orthopedic injuries such as hip, forearm, and humerus fractures.[8,11] Although a minority of falls result in serious physical injuries, even those that appear to have no physical effects often have serious social and psychologic consequences.

Orthopedic Injuries

Although the proportion of falls that result in fracture is low, the absolute number of older people who suffer fractures is high and places heavy burdens on the patient and the healthcare system. The acute management of fractures is complicated by severe pain, impaired mobility, and impaired function. Even after acute treatment of a fracture, persistent pain, decreased function, avascular necrosis, delayed bone healing, and osteoarthritis are a few of the possible sequelae.[14]

Fracture patterns depend on fall mechanism and intensity. Wrist fractures tend to be more prevalent in individuals aged 65–75 years, whereas hip fractures are more prevalent after 75 years of age. This statistic may be due to the differing mechanisms of injury depending on the age-group. When quick protective reflexes are intact, individuals tend to brace themselves from the impact of the fall using their upper extremities. This predisposes them to upper-extremity fractures. However, delayed protective reflexes result in falls to the side, predisposing individuals to hip fractures. These delayed protective reflexes may be secondary to a combination of decreased strength, impaired balance and coordination, and cognitive changes.[10,14]

Low femoral bone mineral density and increased fall energy are also associated with a higher risk of hip fracture. One hypothesis is that elderly individuals with an increased fear of falling tend to stiffen their muscles while falling, which can increase the fall impact. A decrease in muscle mass and strength is associated with impaired balance, decreased soft tissue, and increased bone mineral density loss. Fragility fractures are further described in Chapter 3, Osteoporosis and Fragility Fracture. Although factors such as osteoporosis are considered risk factors for postfall fracture, falling itself is considered a stronger risk factor.[14,15] Therefore, fall prevention is a key first step to decreasing fracture rates.

Unfortunately, these orthopedic injuries result in significant morbidity and mortality. One-third of patients with wrist fractures have persistently decreased function for 6 months.[16] The consequences of hip fractures can be even more detrimental than those of other fractures. The mortality rate in the first 6 months after a hip fracture is reportedly up to 20%. In particular, the risk of mortality is associated with infections such as pneumonia or sepsis. Therefore, extra care should be taken to avoid these secondary complications, including simple measures such as early mobilization and incentive spirometry.[14,15] One in four individuals end up in long-term care after a hip fracture, and the majority are unable to return to their prior functional level.[15] It is notable that the prognosis of older adults who suffer a hip fracture in the hospital is worse than that in the community.[7] Returning to baseline function after a fall requires a multifactorial approach that includes improving psychosocial well-being, effectively utilizing support systems, and maintaining medical stability and adequate pain control.

Traumatic Brain Injury

Falls are now the leading cause of TBI for all age-groups based on the recent Morbidity and Mortality Weekly Report on 2013 surveillance data from the Centers for Disease Control and Prevention (CDC). The highest rate of combined TBI-related emergency department visits, hospitalizations, and deaths was observed among persons aged ≥75 years (2232.2 per 100,000) followed by those 0–4 years (1591.5) and those 15–24 years (1080.7).[17] The number and rate of TBI-related hospitalizations among individuals aged ≥75 years showed an increase of 27% from 2007 to 2013, primarily due to increasing falls. In the aging population, these findings support a significant increase in fall-related TBI that results in hospitalizations and deaths. Increasing public health attention to this issue is needed.[17]

Common pathologies include traumatic subdural hemorrhage, subarachnoid hemorrhage, and concussion. The use of antiplatelet and anticoagulant medications, cerebral atrophy, and chronic cerebrovascular disease associated with aging all contribute to this medically complex picture. Older age increases mortality and morbidity after TBI. In an Australian study, 13% of all hospitalizations in the elderly due to TBI resulted in death; this was most commonly associated with subdural hemorrhage.[18] A cohort study using the National Study on the Costs and Outcomes of Trauma database showed that older adults (aged 75–84 years) had a 32% increased risk of in-hospital death and more than 2.3 times increased risk of withdrawal of therapy compared with younger patients of the same injury severity, comorbidities, and sex.[19] Elderly patients, even those with less severe injuries, have lengthier hospitalizations than younger patients. In addition, there is a heightened concern about neurologic deterioration, which is more often delayed in its clinical presentation, and evidence of slower functional gains and increased dependence compared with younger patients.[20] One study showed that 1 year post-TBI, 70%–75% of those aged <50 years had good recovery, whereas only 20% of those aged ≥60 years had good recovery.[21] Possible modifiable factors to explain these worse outcomes in older adults include a lower intensity of care in older patients with TBI and the lack of an organized multisystemic approach.[19] Given the poorer outcome, elderly patients not surprisingly have higher rates of institutionalization after TBI.[22]

Spinal Cord Injury

While motor vehicle accidents remain the leading cause of spinal cord injury (SCI), falls are the second leading cause and are increasing in prevalence, especially among patients ≥60 years of age. There has been a significant increase in the incidence of SCI among those ≥65 years of age from 3.1% to 13.2% when comparing data from 1970s to data from 2010–2014. In fact, falls are the leading cause of SCI in individuals ≥50 years of age.[23,24] SCI in the older adult from a fall tends to result in incomplete tetraplegia. The most common mechanism of injury is cervical hyperextension on an already spondylotic spine, which can result in clinical central cord syndrome. In central cord syndrome, the upper extremities are more affected than the lower extremities. Falls resulting in SCI are most commonly from the same level.[25-27] As is the case with TBI, older adults who suffer an SCI tend to have longer and more complicated hospital stays than younger patients.[26]

Postfall Syndrome ("Postfall Anxiety Syndrome")

Postfall syndrome is a combination of fear of falling again and fear of losing one's independence. Unfortunately, this combination may result in self-induced restraints in physical activity, which results in an ongoing cycle of increasing frailty and unintentional increases in fall risk. Activity restriction due to fear of falling is an independent predictor for worsening disability.[28]

The presence and severity of fear of falling can be assessed using the Modified Fall Efficacy Scale

(MFES), which asks older adults to rate their confidence (0 being the lowest, 10 being the highest) in performing 14 indoor and outdoor daily activities. The final score is the average confidence score across these different activities (range, 0–10). The mean score (range) of the MFES for healthy older women is 9.8 (9.2–10).[29,30]

RISK FACTORS FOR FALLS

An older person may fall for different reasons depending on his/her age, health status, level of mobility, and residential setting (i.e., living in the community vs. a long-term care facility). Risk factors for falls in the elderly are frequently multifactorial. It is important to use a systematic approach to identifying risk factors when assessing a patient who is at risk for falling (Box 4.2). In a survey, older adults reported balance impairments, weather, inattention, medical conditions, and surface hazards as their main risk factors for falls. Less than 3% of older adults thought that medications could put them at risk of falls and that education about medications would be warranted.[5]

Risk factors for falls among older adults residing in long-term care facilities include older age, higher care demands, incontinence, male sex, prior falls, slow reaction times, and psychoactive medications. Risk factors for older adults in acute care hospitals include gait difficulty, confusion with agitation, urinary incontinence, previous falls, and psychotropic medications.[7] A systematic review of falls among 1924 older adults in rehabilitation facilities identified the following risk factors summarized in Box 4.3.[31]

Intrinsic Risk Factors

First, there are intrinsic factors that place elderly individuals at higher risk for falls including changes in gait, vision, hearing, cognition, and balance that are part of the aging process.[32] As mentioned earlier, females fall more frequently in the community, whereas males have higher fall rates in long-term care facilities. In addition, a history of falls is a strong risk factor for recurrent falls.[13,33]

Many medical conditions increase one's risk for falls. Cardiovascular instabilities, such as orthostasis, arrhythmias, and syncope, can result in sudden-onset falls. Neurologic illnesses, including stroke, peripheral neuropathies, radiculopathies, and movement disorders, affect gait and balance. Endocrinological and renal issues can result in hyponatremia and hypoglycemia, which may acutely increase one's

---

BOX 4.2
Risk Factors for Falls in Older Adults

Female sex (among community-dwelling adults)
Previous fall
Visual changes
Hearing loss
Cognitive deficits
Alcohol/substance use
Cardiovascular
  Orthostasis
  Arrhythmias
  Syncope
  Dizziness
  Low ejection fraction
  Coronary artery insufficiency/myocardial
    infarction
  Carotid stenosis
Neurologic injuries that can affect gait or balance,
  including:
  Stroke
  Parkinson's disease
  Nervous system tumor
  Postpolio syndrome
  Multiple sclerosis
  Spinal cord injury
  Neuropathies
  Radiculopathies
  Vertebrobasilar insufficiency (drop attacks)
  Vestibular disturbance (peripheral or central)
  Seizure
Musculoskeletal
  Sarcopenia
  Osteoarthritis
  Foot deformities

Renal/genitourinary
  Hypovolemia
  Urinary incontinence
Endocrine
  Hypoglycemia
  Hyponatremia
  Hypothyroidism
Pharmacology
  Psychoactive medications
    Antidepressants (e.g., SSRIs, TCAs)
    Antipsychotics
    Sedatives, hypnotics (i.e., benzodiazepines, sleep
      medications)
    Anticonvulsants
  Antihypertensives
  Antiarrhythmics
  Pain medication
  Polypharmacy
Hematologic
  Anemia
Extrinsic factors
  Rugs
  Cords
  Lighting
  Stability of furniture and banisters
  Steps
  Wet surfaces
  Lack of adaptive equipment such as hand rails, raised
    toilet seats
  Footwear
SSRIs, selective serotonin reuptake inhibitors; *TCAs*,
tricyclic antidepressants.

BOX 4.3
Risk Factors for Falling Among Older Adults in Rehabilitation Facilities

- Carpet flooring
- Vertigo
- Being an amputee
- Confusion
- Cognitive impairment
- Stroke
- Sleep disturbance

- Anticonvulsants
- Tranquilizers
- Antihypertensive medications
- Previous falls
- Need for transfer assistance
- Age 71–80 years

From Vieira ER, Freund-Heritage R, da Costa BR. Risk factors for geriatric patient falls in rehabilitation hospital settings: a systematic review. *Clin Rehabil*. 2011;25(9):788–799; with permission.

fall risk. Musculoskeletal disorders including osteo-arthritis and sarcopenia may affect gait and transfers.

Over the past two decades, the role of cognition in locomotion and falls has been increasingly recognized. Poor performance during cognitive and walking dual tasks predicts falls,[34] and poor executive function is predictive of increased fall risk in community-residing older adults.[35] These findings may have ramifications in the development of novel interventions to reduce the risk of falls in older adults.

Extrinsic Risk Factors

Medications affecting the nervous system and muscles also increase fall risk.[10] In particular, poly-pharmacy and use of psychotropic medications are associated with higher fall rates.[36] They can affect balance and reaction time. Even antidepressants previously considered safe in the elderly, such as selective serotonin receptor inhibitors, are associated with an increased risk of fall.[15,37,38] In clinical practice, some of these medications may be necessary; however, careful monitoring with gradual titration would be recommended. Finally, other extrinsic factors include home setup and footwear. Lighting, rugs, cords, and steps should all be considered in the assessment of fall risk. In addition, appropriate footwear can provide increased stability.

SCREENING AND ASSESSMENT FOR FALL RISK

Falls among older adults are largely preventable in 30%–40% of cases, and healthcare providers including physicians, nurses, therapists, and pharmacists can play an important role by discussing falls with older patients and providing appropriate interventions.[39] Effective fall prevention has the potential to reduce serious fall-related injuries, emergency department visits, hospitalizations, nursing home placements, and functional decline. Most effective fall reduction programs start with a systematic fall risk assessment that can lead to targeted interventions. Healthcare providers should be aware of underreporting of falls by older adults, particularly older male patients in the community, and proactively ask about falls.[12] A multifactorial fall risk assessment is primarily recommended for older adults who are at high risk of falling during the initial screening process (Boxes 4.4 and 4.5). Considering the complex nature of falls, interdisciplinary collaboration may be initiated at the assessment and to guide interventions. The recommendations from the American Geriatrics Society,

British Geriatrics Society,[37] and Stopping Elderly Accidents, Deaths, and Injuries (STEADI)[44,45] developed by the CDC are summarized in Fig. 4.1.

INTERVENTIONS
Older Community-Dwelling Adults

It is ideal for health professionals to assess fall risk and directly implement interventions or ensure that these interventions are provided by other qualified professionals (Box 4.6). Once the causes or risk factors of falling are identified, interventions can be instituted.[37] For example, if postural hypotension is noted, the discontinuation of medication that excessively lowers the blood pressure and ensuring proper hydration are important aspects of treatment. For older adults with gait or balance abnormalities, investigation of the underlying neurologic or musculoskeletal etiologies is essential before or in parallel with assessing the need for walking aids, orthoses, and gait and balance training. During the in-office gait and balance evaluation, rehabilitation specialists may identify specific impairments including proximal lower-limb muscle weakness from deconditioning, joint pain or instability, or limb-length discrepancies. Physical therapy, shoe lifts, or bracing can effectively address modifiable factors in many cases. The following are the commonly included components of multifactorial interventions. The subset of these components can be used to target the identified risk factors. For practical purposes, the STEADI initiative stresses the completion of two interventions during a single patient visit: (1) review of medications with modifications to those that increase fall risk (anticonvulsants, antidepressant, antipsychotics, benzodiazepines, opioids, sedatives-hypnotics, anticholinergics, antihistamines, muscle relaxants, blood pressure medications) and (2) the recommendation of a daily vitamin D supplement with/without calcium cosupplementation.[1,45]

Interventions to reduce the fear of falling

A Matter of Balance is an 8-week cognitive-behavioral program that works on strategies to decrease the fear of falling and increase physical activity. Through the program, participants gradually learn to conceptualize falls and fear of falling as controllable entities. They set manageable activity goals and engage in exercise to improve overall balance and strength. In addition, they learn to modify their external environment to decrease fall risk. A Matter of Balance program significantly improves functional performance (i.e., Timed Up and Go, Performance-Oriented Mobility Assessment) and reduces the physical risk of falls.[47,48]

BOX 4.4
Key Recommendations for the Initial Screening for Fall Risk in Community-Dwelling Adults ≥65 Years of Age

- All older individuals should be asked about:
  - whether they have fallen in the past year
  - whether they have difficulty with walking or balance
  - whether they worry about falling
- Multifactorial fall assessment should be performed for individuals with:
  - repeated falls
  - a fall requiring medical attention

- gait or balance impairments
- poor performance on a standardized gait and balance tests
- Gait and balance evaluation should be done for:
  - any older adult who falls

Older individuals with only a single fall and no subjective or objective difficulty on gait and balance evaluation DO NOT require a multifactorial fall risk assessment.

BOX 4.5
Multifactorial Fall Risk Assessment for High-Risk Group

- Focused history
  - Fall frequency
  - Injuries and other consequences of falls
  - Circumstances of fall(s):
    - sudden change in position from lying down or sitting, suggestive of orthostatic hypotension
    - slip or trip from gait instability, balance impairment, vision deficits, or environmental hazards
    - drop attack without loss of consciousness (vertebrobasilar insufficiency, knee instability, leg weakness)
    - after looking sideways or up, suggestive of vascular etiology such as carotid sinus or arterial compression
    - sudden loss of consciousness, such as from seizure or syncope
  - Symptoms associated with falls:
    - dizziness (cardiovascular issue such as orthostatic hypotension or arrhythmia, vestibular etiology, medication side effect)
    - palpitations (cardiac arrhythmia)
  - Medication review:
    - prescribed and over-the-counter medications including supplements
  - Risk factors:
    - Medical history including osteoporosis, known cardiovascular disease, acute or chronic urinary incontinence
- Physical Examination
  - Gait, mobility, and balance assessment (see Table 4.2 for details)
  - Recommendation from the Stopping Elderly Accidents, Deaths, and Injuries Initiative of the Centers for Disease Control (CDC)

- Timed Up and Go (TUG) Test[40,41]
- Chair Stand Test[42] (optional)
- 4-Stage Balance Test[43] (optional)
- Recommendation from American Geriatrics Society/British Geriatrics Society (any of the following):
  - TUG
  - Berg Balance Scale
  - Performance-Oriented Mobility Assessment
- Lower-extremity joint evaluation (range of motion, instability, tenderness, effusions)
- Neurologic assessment (cognitive testing, extrapyramidal and cerebellar function, muscle strength, sensation including proprioception, reflexes, peripheral nerve evaluation)
- Cardiovascular examination: Check for orthostatic hypotension and examine heart rate and rhythm while assessing for murmurs
- Visual acuity
- Inspection and evaluation of feet and footwear
- Functional assessment
  - Evaluation of gait and mobility with the use of assistive devices as needed
  - Assessment of activities of daily living performance with the use of adaptive equipment as needed
  - Individual's own perception of functional ability
  - Fear of falling (FOF): Impact of FOF and assessment if fear is appropriate and beneficial or negative and contributing to lack of physical activity and poor quality of life
- Environmental assessment
  - Home safety (i.e., area rugs or electrical cords on the floor)

Data from Panel on Prevention of Falls in Older Persons, American Geriatrics Society and British Geriatrics Society. Summary of the updated American Geriatrics Society/British Geriatrics Society clinical practice guideline for prevention of falls in older persons. *J Am Geriatr Soc.* 2011;59(1):148–157.

TABLE 4.2
Gait and Balance Evaluation Tools

Tools	Description	Mean Value (Range)	Cutoff for High Risk of Falls		
Timed Up and Go Test	Measures the time (s) that a person takes to stand up from an arm chair, walk a distance of 3 m, turn, walk back, and sit down again in the chair (higher score indicating worse balance) Time to complete: <5 min	7–11: older men 7–12: older women living in the community	≥12 s Check also for • Slow tentative pace • Little or no arm swing • Steadying self on walls • Shuffling • En bloc turning • Not using assistive device properly		
30-Second Chair Stand Test	Tests leg strength and endurance Records the number of times the patient stands in 30 s from a chair without arm support Time to complete: a few minutes	Below the average score on the right indicates a high risk for falls	**Age (years)**	**Men**	**Women**
			60–64	<14	<12
			65–69	<12	<11
			70–74	<12	<10
			75–79	<11	<10
			80–84	<10	<9
			85–89	<8	<8
			90–94	<7	<4
4-Stage Balance Test	Assesses static balance Person is asked to stand in four progressively more challenging positions without using an assistive device • Stand with feet side by side • Place the instep of one foot so it is touching the big toe of the other foot • Place one foot in front of the other, heel touching toe • Stand on one foot Time to complete: a few minutes		An older adult who cannot hold the tandem stance ≥10 s is at risk of falling		
Berg Balance Scale	Tests balance 14 items, each scored from 0 to 4 (total score, 0–56) Higher score indicates better balance Time to complete: 15–20 min	50–55 for community-dwelling older adults	<45–49 indicates high risk for falls		
Performance-Oriented Mobility Assessment (POMA)	Total score range 0–28 with POMA-balance subscale (12) and POMA-gait subscale (16) Higher score indicates better balance Time to complete: 15 min	25–27 for age 65–79 years	19–23 indicates moderate risk for falls <19 indicates high risk for falls		

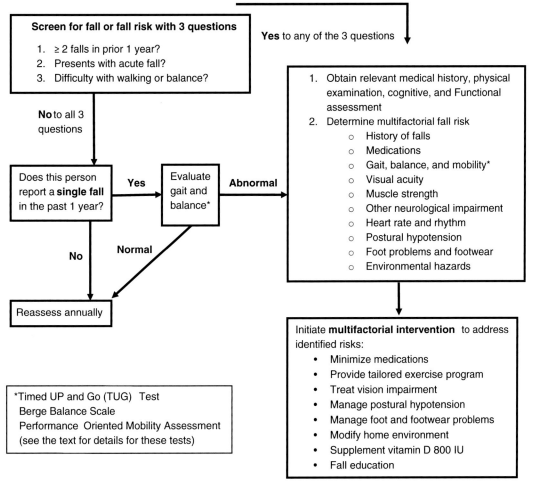

FIG. 4.1 Algorithm for fall screening and intervention in community-dwelling older adults. (Adapted from Panel on Prevention of Falls in Older Persons, American Geriatrics Society and British Geriatrics Society. Summary of the updated American Geriatrics Society/British Geriatrics Society clinical practice guideline for prevention of falls in older persons. *J Am Geriatr Soc.* 2011;59(1):150; with permission.)

Older Adults in Long-Term Care Facilities

Fall incidence in long-term care facilities is three times higher than that in the community, with a rate of 1.5 falls (range: 0.2–3.6) per bed per year.[7]

- The level of evidence for interventions in this population is not as strong as that for older community-dwelling adults. The similar principle of multifactorial intervention is considered to reducefalls.

- An exercise program should be implemented with caution, considering the risk of injury in older adults with frailty.
- Vitamin D supplementation effectively reduces fall rate for residents with low baseline vitamin D levels.[7] Vitamin D supplementation ≥800 IU daily should be provided to individuals with proven or suspected vitamin D deficiency and to those at increased risk of falls.
- Hip protector pads reportedly reduce hip fractures by 60%, although compliance can be an issue.[49]

BOX 4.6
Components of Effective Interventions

- Recommended with good to fair evidence[10]:
  - Adaptation or modification of the home environment[37]
    - Assessment and intervention provided by a healthcare professional
    - Elimination of home hazards (i.e., loose rugs or electrical cords)
    - Sufficient lighting
    - Bathroom modifications (i.e., grab bars, raised toilet seat)
    - Secured banisters
    - Working accessible alarm systems
    - US Consumer Product Safety Commission provides a Safety for Older Consumers–Home Safety Checklist for further details[43]
  - Withdrawal or minimization of psychoactive medications (strongest evidence compared with reduction in other medications)[37]
  - Sedative hypnotics and anxiolytics
  - Antipsychotics and antidepressants
- Selective serotonin reuptake inhibitors affect fall risk as much as tricyclic antidepressants
  - Exercise[37,39,46]
    - Overall, exercise reduces the rate of falls by 21%–40% with greater effects seen from exercise programs that challenge balance and involve >3 h of exercise per week[46]
    - Exercise types: Combination of balance, strength, and gait training
      - Flexibility and endurance training should not be the only component of exercise program
    - Strength training: Chair rise exercise by Stopping Elderly Accidents, Deaths, and Injuries can be done at home and repeated 10–15 times
    - Balance training: Standing on one foot 10–15 times for 10 s for each leg. Safety tip: Have a sturdy chair or a person nearby to hold onto in case the patient feels unsteady. Walking heel to toe for 20 steps; performing back leg raises 10–15 times, side leg raises 10–15 times, and a balance (tandem) walk

- Most effective exercise programs are implemented for >12 weeks
- Both group and individual (home) exercises are effective for fall prevention
- Exercise may be more effective in conjunction with other interventions
- Management of postural hypotension[10,37]:
  - Keeping head of bed raised at night to avoid orthostasis when rising
  - Wearing elastic stockings to reduce lower-extremity venous pooling
  - Getting up slowly or sitting on the side of the bed for a few minutes before standing
  - Avoiding heavy meals or vigorous physical activity in hot weather
  - Increasing blood volume by increasing dietary salt if not medically contraindicated
  - If above measures are not effective and no medical contraindications, fludrocortisone 0.1 mg/day or α-1 agonist (midodrine 2.5 mg three times a day) can be trialed
- If cataract surgery is indicated, it should be expedited to reduce fall risks in older women
- Dual-chamber cardiac pacing in individuals with cardioinhibitory carotid sinus hypersensitivity with repeated unexplained falls
- Vitamin D 800 IU supplementation daily should be provided for those with vitamin D deficiency or those at risk of falls
- Fair evidence but no recommendation for or against the intervention
  - Reduction in total number or doses of medications
  - Vision intervention
    - Multifocal lenses should be avoided during ambulation, especially when attempting stairs
  - Management of foot problems and footwear
    - Trial footwear with a relatively low heel and high surface contact area
  - Education tailored to individual cognitive level and language
    - Education should NOT be provided as a single intervention

Older Adults in Hospitals and Rehabilitation Facilities

A 2012 Cochrane review showed that multifactorial interventions in hospitals reduced the fall rate (number of falls over a given time) by 31%.[7] Risk of falling (number of fallers during a given time) also showed a decreasing trend but no statistically significant difference. Further studies are needed to confirm the effectiveness of multifactorial interventions in acute care hospitals or rehabilitation facilities.

Older Individuals With Cognitive Impairment[37]

There is insufficient evidence to provide recommendations regarding fall prevention techniques in older adults with dementia.

Implementing Fall Prevention Programs as a Public Health Intervention

Although interventions targeting multiple fall risk factors could reduce fall rates by up to 40%, only 8% of physicians implemented fall prevention screenings according to clinical practice guidelines.[50] The frequently reported barriers to implementing fall screening included time constraints during visits, higher priority of other medical issues, lack of educational materials, cost, and lack of referral sources.[50] In 2011, health department and health system partnerships in Oregon and New York used CDC funding to implement STEADI in their primary care practices. Before implementing STEADI, healthcare providers rarely discussed falls with older patients. After the implementation, approximately 65% and 50% of all adult patients were screened and assessed for fall risk in New York and Oregon, respectively.[1]

To overcome the barriers to fall prevention program implementation, the Centers for Medicare & Medicaid Services offers incentives for healthcare providers to provide fall prevention activities and links fall prevention quality measures through the Physician Quality Reporting System in the Merit-Based Incentive Program (see Box 4.7).[1,51]

Cost-Effectiveness of Fall Prevention

Withdrawal of psychotropic medications and group tai chi classes are the least costly and most effective single interventions for the prevention of hip fractures. Home modifications also provide good value in fall prevention for their cost.[52] The use of a primary fall prevention program has been advocated at the state level using the existing aging service infrastructure.

> ### BOX 4.7
> ### Centers for Medicare & Medicaid Services Provides Incentives to Physicians to Implement Fall Prevention Programs
>
> - Welcome to Medicare preventive visit: One-time initial examination within the first year after Medicare enrollment. Coverage for fall screening, safety, and functional evaluation
> - Annual wellness visit: Preventive care service including fall prevention
> - Two quality measures for falls in the Physician Quality Reporting System
>   - Fall risk assessment
>   - Fall plan of care

Data from Bergen G, Stevens MR, Burns ER. Falls and fall injuries among adults aged >65 years – United States, 2014. *Morb Mortal Wkly Rep.* 2016;65(37):993–998.

Pennsylvania's Department of Aging has offered a fall prevention program, entitled "Healthy Steps for Older Adults," since 2005; to date, 40,000 older adults have been screened for fall risk.[53] This program was associated with a 17% reduction in fall rate after adjusting for risk factors[54] and a savings of $840 for the estimated hospitalization and emergency department care costs per program participant[53] relative to the comparison group.

Technological Applications and Novel Interventions for Fall Prevention

Compliant flooring is a promising strategy for preventing fall-related injuries. A recent review showed that compliant flooring can reduce fall-related impact forces but minimally affects standing and walking balance. The findings from the pilot studies reported that compliant flooring may be a cost-effective strategy; however, it may result in increased physical demands for healthcare workers (i.e., increased force required for nurses to push a medication cart).[55]

In hospitals and long-term care facilities, bed rails or restraints have been used to prevent falls, particularly among older patients with cognitive impairment. However, bed rails or restraints have shown to be ineffective in preventing falls and even harmful to older patients. Fall prevention sensor systems (i.e., bed-exit alarms) have also been developed to alert patients, caregivers, and healthcare professionals that a patient is leaving a bed unassisted. However, a high false alarm rate can be a burden. Details of fall prevention technology can be found in Chapter 16, Assistive Technology for Geriatric Population.

Exercise interventions using video games are also used for fall prevention. Exercise-based video games aim to improve the compliance of exercise interventions by using recreation, social interactions, and performance feedback. Older fallers are more likely to take incorrect steps such as in the wrong direction, be slower to initiate stepping responses, and be distracted when stepping while doing other tasks.[56] Dance Dance Revolution is an exercise game with repetitive stepping in all directions at varying speeds that requires balance, coordination, and attention.[56] Two to three exercise game sessions of 15–20 min duration for 8 weeks showed improvements in reaction time and physical function in community-dwelling older adults.

Interventions to improve mobility and reduce falls among older adults have traditionally focused on the physical domain. Researchers are currently investigating whether cognitive training as a complementary intervention can improve mobility in older adults with promising preliminary findings.[57,58] Considering the low adherence to physical exercise programs, cognitive remediation may serve as an attractive alternative or complementary intervention to the traditional approach.

CONCLUSION

Falls are highly prevalent, and fall rates are expected to increase as the global population ages. The consequences of falls include devastating injuries or death, but in addition, falls can also trigger loss of confidence, decreased independence, and reduced quality of life among older adults. The systematic screening of fall risks using public guidelines should be routinely implemented in all primary and rehabilitation settings as the first step toward effective fall prevention. Multifactorial fall interventions should be implemented for individuals at high risk of falling with an emphasis on medication reconciliation, resistance and balance exercises, vitamin D intake, and environmental modifications. Communication among multiple disciplines, the patient, and the family about their roles is critical to a successful fall prevention and intervention program.

REFERENCES

1. Bergen G, Stevens MR, Burns ER. Falls, fall injuries among adults aged >/=65 years – United States, 2014. *Morb Mortal Wkly Rep.* 2016;65(37):993–998.

2. Gibson MJ, Andres RO, Isaacs B, Radebaugh T. The prevention of falls in later life. A report of the Kellogg International Work Group on the prevention of falls by the elderly. *Dan Med Bull.* 1987;34(suppl 4):1–24.

3. https://www.cdc.gov/homeandrecreationalsafety/falls/adultfalls.html.

4. Burns ER, Stevens JA, Lee R. The direct costs of fatal and non-fatal falls among older adults – United States. *J Saf Res.* 2016;58:99–103.

5. Zecevic AA, Salmoni AW, Speechley M, Vandervoort AA. Defining a fall and reasons for falling: comparisons among the views of seniors, health care providers, and the research literature. *Gerontologist.* 2006;46(3):367–376.

6. *World Health Organization Fact Sheet.* http://www.who.int/mediacentre/factsheets/fs344/en/.

7. Cameron ID, Gillespie LD, Robertson MC, et al. Interventions for preventing falls in older people in care facilities and hospitals. *Cochrane Database Syst Rev.* 2012;12:CD005465.

8. Organization WH. *WHO Global Report on Falls Prevention in Older Age.* Geneva: World Health Organization; 2008.

9. Vieira ER, Palmer RC, Chaves PH. Prevention of falls in older people living in the community. *BMJ (Clin Res Ed).* 2016;353:i1419.

10. Rubenstein LZ. Falls in older people: epidemiology, risk factors and strategies for prevention. *Age Ageing.* 2006;35(suppl 2):ii37–ii41.

11. Finlayson ML, Peterson EW. Falls, aging, and disability. *Phys Med Rehabil Clin North Am.* 2010;21(2):357–373.

12. Stevens JA, Ballesteros MF, Mack KA, Rudd RA, DeCaro E, Adler G. Gender differences in seeking care for falls in the aged Medicare population. *Am J Prev Med.* 2012;43(1):59–62.

13. Peel NM. Epidemiology of falls in older age. *Can J Aging.* 2011;30(1):7–19.

14. Marks R, Allegrante JP, Ronald MacKenzie C, Lane JM. Hip fractures among the elderly: causes, consequences and control. *Ageing Res Rev.* 2003;2(1):57–93.

15. Cummings-Vaughn LA, Gammack JK. Falls, osteoporosis, and hip fractures. *Med Clin North Am.* 2011;95(3):495–506.

16. Vergara I, Vrotsou K, Orive M, et al. Wrist fractures and their impact in daily living functionality on elderly people: a prospective cohort study. *BMC Geriatr.* 2016;16:11.

17. Taylor CA, Bell JM, Breiding J. Traumatic brain injury-related emergency department visits, hospitalizations, and deaths – United States, 2007 and 2013. *Morb Mortal Wkly Rep Surveill Summ.* 2017;66(9):1–16. Centers for Disease Control and Prevention https://www.cdc.gov/mmwr/volumes/66/ss/ss6609a1.htm?s_cid=ss6609a1_w.

18. Harvey LA, Close JC. Traumatic brain injury in older adults: characteristics, causes and consequences. *Injury.* 2012;43(11):1821–1826.

19. Thompson HJ, Rivara FP, Jurkovich GJ, Wang J, Nathens AB, MacKenzie EJ. Evaluation of the effect of intensity of care on mortality after traumatic brain injury. *Crit Care Med.* 2008;36(1):282–290.

20. Thompson HJ, McCormick WC, Kagan SH. Traumatic brain injury in older adults: epidemiology, outcomes, and future implications. *J Am Geriatr Soc.* 2006;54(10): 1590–1595.

21. Rothweiler B, Temkin NR, Dikmen SS. Aging effect on psychosocial outcome in traumatic brain injury. *Arch Phys Med Rehabil.* 1998;79(8):881–887.

22. Testa JA, Malec JF, Moessner AM, Brown AW. Outcome after traumatic brain injury: effects of aging on recovery. *Arch Phys Med Rehabil.* 2005;86(9):1815–1823.

23. Chen Y, He Y, DeVivo MJ. Changing demographics and injury profile of new traumatic spinal cord injuries in the United States, 1972-2014. *Arch Phys Med Rehabil.* 2016;97(10):1610–1619.

24. DeVivo MJ, Chen Y. Trends in new injuries, prevalent cases, and aging with spinal cord injury. *Arch Phys Med Rehabil.* 2011;92(3):332–338.

25. Weingarden SI, Graham PM. Falls resulting in spinal cord injury: patterns and outcomes in an older population. *Paraplegia.* 1989;27(6):423–427.

26. Chen Y, Tang Y, Allen V, DeVivo MJ. Fall-induced spinal cord injury: external causes and implications for prevention. *J Spinal Cord Med.* 2016;39(1):24–31.

27. Stevenson CM, Dargan DP, Warnock J, et al. Traumatic central cord syndrome: neurological and functional outcome at 3 years. *Spinal Cord.* 2016;54(11):1010–1015.

28. Deshpande N, Metter EJ, Lauretani F, Bandinelli S, Guralnik J, Ferrucci L. Activity restriction induced by fear of falling and objective and subjective measures of physical function: a prospective cohort study. *J Am Geriatr Soc.* 2008;56(4):615–620.

29. Hill KD, Schwarz JA, Kalogeropoulos AJ, Gibson SJ. Fear of falling revisited. *Arch Phys Med Rehabil.* 1996;77(10): 1025–1029.

30. Hill K, Schwarz J, Flicker L, Carroll S. Falls among healthy, community-dwelling, older women: a prospective study of frequency, circumstances, consequences and prediction accuracy. *Aust N Z J Public Health.* 1999;23(1):41–48.

31. Vieira ER, Freund-Heritage R, da Costa BR. Risk factors for geriatric patient falls in rehabilitation hospital settings: a systematic review. *Clin Rehabil.* 2011;25(9):788–799.

32. Kwan E, Straus SE. Assessment and management of falls in older people. *Can Med Assoc J.* 2014;186(16): E610–E621.

33. Beegan L, Messinger-Rapport BJ. Stand by me! Reducing the risk of injurious falls in older adults. *Clevel Clin J Med.* 2015;82(5):301–307.

34. Verghese J, Buschke H, Viola L, et al. Validity of divided attention tasks in predicting falls in older individuals: a preliminary study. *J Am Geriatr Soc.* 2002;50(9):1572–1576.

35. Holtzer R, Friedman R, Lipton RB, Katz M, Xue X, Verghese J. The relationship between specific cognitive functions and falls in aging. *Neuropsychology.* 2007;21(5):540–548.

36. Park H, Satoh H, Miki A, Urushihara H, Sawada Y. Medications associated with falls in older people: systematic review of publications from a recent 5-year period. *Eur J Clin Pharmacol.* 2015;71(12):1429–1440.

37. Panel on Prevention of Falls in Older Persons AGS, British Geriatrics S. Summary of the updated American Geriatrics Society/British Geriatrics Society clinical practice guideline for prevention of falls in older persons. *J Am Geriatr Soc.* 2011;59(1):148–157.

38. Allain H, Bentue-Ferrer D, Polard E, Akwa Y, Patat A. Postural instability and consequent falls and hip fractures associated with use of hypnotics in the elderly: a comparative review. *Drugs Aging.* 2005;22(9):749–765.

39. Gillespie LD, Robertson MC, Gillespie WJ, et al. Interventions for preventing falls in older people living in the community. *Cochrane Database Syst Rev.* 2012;(9): CD007146.

40. https://www.cdc.gov/steadi/pdf/TUG_Test-a.pdf.

41. Barry E, Galvin R, Keogh C, Horgan F, Fahey T. Is the timed up and go test a useful predictor of risk of falls in community dwelling older adults: a systematic review and meta-analysis. *BMC Geriatr.* 2014;14:14.

42. https://www.cdc.gov/steadi/pdf/30_Second_Chair_Stand _Test-a.pdf.

43. *Consumer Product Safety Commission Safety for Older Consumers – Home Safety Checklist.* https://www.cpsc.gov/s3fs-public/701.pdf.

44. Stevens JA, Phelan EA. Development of STEADI: a fall prevention resource for health care providers. *Health Promot Pract.* 2013;14(5):706–714.

45. *STEADI – Older Adult Fall Prevention.* https://www.cdc.gov/ steadi/.

46. Sherrington C, Michaleff ZA, Fairhall N, et al. Exercise to prevent falls in older adults: an updated systematic review and meta-analysis. *Br J Sports Med.* 2017;51(24):1750–1758.

47. National Council on Aging. *Program Summary: A Matter of Balance.* https://www.ncoa.org/resources/program-summary-a-matter-of-balance/.

48. Chen TY, Edwards JD, Janke MC. The effects of the A matter of balance program on falls and physical risk of falls, Tampa, Florida, 2013. *Prev Chronic Dis.* 2015;12:E157.

49. Kannus P, Parkkari J, Niemi S, et al. Prevention of hip fracture in elderly people with use of a hip protector. *N Engl J Med.* 2000;343(21):1506–1513.

50. Jones TS, Ghosh TS, Horn K, Smith J, Vogt RL. Primary care physicians perceptions and practices regarding fall prevention in adult's 65 years and over. *Accid Anal Prev.* 2011;43(5):1605–1609.

51. *Welcome to Medicare Preventive Visit.* https://www.medicareinteractive.org/get-answers/medicare-covered-services/preventive-care-services/welcome-to-medicare-preventive-visit.

52. Frick KD, Kung JY, Parrish JM, Narrett MJ. Evaluating the cost-effectiveness of fall prevention programs that reduce fall-related hip fractures in older adults. *J Am Geriatr Soc.* 2010;58(1):136–141.

53. Albert SM, Raviotta J, Lin CJ, Edelstein O, Smith KJ. Cost-effectiveness of a statewide falls prevention program in Pennsylvania: healthy steps for older adults. *Am J Manag Care.* 2016;22(10):638–644.

54. Albert SM, King J, Boudreau R, Prasad T, Lin CJ, Newman AB. Primary prevention of falls: effectiveness of a statewide program. *Am J Public Health*. 2014;104(5):e77–e84.

55. Lachance CC, Jurkowski MP, Dymarz AC, et al. Compliant flooring to prevent fall-related injuries in older adults: a scoping review of biomechanical efficacy, clinical effectiveness, cost-effectiveness, and workplace safety. *PLoS One*. 2017;12(2):e0171652.

56. Schoene D, Lord SR, Delbaere K, Severino C, Davies TA, Smith ST. A randomized controlled pilot study of home-based step training in older people using videogame technology. *PLoS One*. 2013;8(3):e57734.

57. Verghese J, Mahoney J, Ambrose AF, Wang C, Holtzer R. Effect of cognitive remediation on gait in sedentary seniors. *J Gerontol A Biol Sci Med Sci*. 2010;65(12): 1338–1343.

58. Verghese J, Ayers E, Mahoney JR, Ambrose A, Wang C, Holtzer R. Cognitive remediation to enhance mobility in older adults: the CREM study. *Neurodegener Dis Manag*. 2016;6(6):457–466.

CHAPTER 5

Central Nervous System Disorders Affecting Mobility in Older Adults

CAROL LI, MD • BLESSEN C. EAPEN, MD • CARLOS A. JARAMILLO, MD, PHD • DAVID X. CIFU, MD

AGING AND CENTRAL NERVOUS SYSTEM

A discussion of normal age-related changes in the central nervous system (CNS) system may be approached from an anatomic, physiologic, or functional perspective. Anatomically, there is reduction of brain mass, dilation of ventricles, widening of sulci, and shrinkage of gyri, as well as decline and changes in cell number, size, structure, and degree of myelination of white matter over time that affects neurotransmission and efficiency that affect the CNS in a nonuniform pattern, including selectively affecting certain brain regions.[1,2] More specifically, brainstem nuclei have been shown to retain the full complement of neurons, whereas neuronal loss in the substantia nigra and locus ceruleus has been identified to correlate with age. An estimated decrease in conduction velocities of 1–2 m per second per decade after the fifth decade of sensory and motor nerves, as well as loss of myelin sheaths within the central and peripheral nervous systems, has also been reported.[3,4] Functionally, a combination of decreased core strength and tight hip flexors can affect overall posture and the ability to ambulate efficiently. Age-related changes in auditory and visual systems may lead to distortion in interpreting signals accurately, thus leading to inaccurate input to the CNS and impairment in balance and higher risk for falls.

Current research suggests that the levels of physiologic and structural abnormalities in the CNS are not usually directly proportional to the amount of functional impairment observed in aging.[1] In fact, despite the known CNS changes with aging, some individuals may survive well into old age without much functional loss, whereas others may not. It has been suggested that neuroplasticity of CNS is one of the major driving forces that produce this variability in functional performance, thus supporting the concept that aging is not a homogenous process.[1] The appropriate reaction and function of a healthy aging adult requires a balancing act of sensory and motor input, processing this input intellectually or automatically at a motor level, and being able to select the correct motor reaction in the setting of the surrounding environment. When these processes are altered at any level because of secondary factors that may be seen in older adults such as chronic exposure to toxins, inadequate nutritional status, or the burden of neurologic disease, there may be a production of cumulative changes that result in far greater functional deficits than those associated with known normal age-related changes in CNS. Thus, as with all aspects of geriatric medicine and rehabilitation, it is important to realize that the translation of anatomy and physiology to function and disability is not direct and a comprehensive approach is required to understand and address functional problems related to the complex nature of aging and the CNS.

Visual and Auditory Changes

The most rapid decline in visual acuity and incidence of ocular disease occurs after age 60 years.[1] Both pathologic and normal aging of the eye arise from tissue changes within the eye. Loss of accommodation ability and flexibility, also known as presbyopia, owing to changes in connection between the lens and ciliary body, is often the first sign of an aging visual system. One may also see loss of central vision from retinal aging and macular degeneration, visual field loss and glaucoma that may result from optic nerve damage, cataracts forming from lens degeneration, and poor night vision from overall decrease in visual clarity.[5] Other comorbidities that commonly occur in the aging population, such as diabetes and hypertension, can also affect ocular health and further compound visual deficits.

Hearing loss is also common in the aging population, and the rate of disabling hearing loss, either of peripheral or central etiologies, can quadruple for adults aged 55–64 years when compared with adults aged 45–54 years.[3] The inner ear is composed of three major structures, semicircular canals, vestibule, and cochlea, which all play an important role in maintaining balance and equilibrium. In general, all structures can be affected adversely with age. Dizziness is a commonly experienced condition and affects about a quarter of the US geriatric population.[6] Peripheral vestibular dysfunction is one of the most frequent causes of dizziness and imbalance in older individuals, which leads to an increase in the risk of falls and subsequent injuries. Similar to ocular health, abnormalities in metabolic, vascular, and renal systems, nutritional deficiencies, inflammations, infections, medications, and head trauma, can secondarily affect the auditory system.

The identification of changes in the visual and auditory systems that accompany aging can help modify and assist in the selection of the most appropriate therapeutic interventions, as well as provide an understanding regarding psychosocial implications of such deficits. For example, even though hearing loss does not directly cause motor deficits, if the eighth cranial nerve is involved, the vestibular system will be affected and contribute to vertigo that can cause gait imbalance and increase the risk of falling. Furthermore, when the processing of visual and auditory senses is altered, in combination with cognitive deficits, it may impair the utility of these systems as modalities for motor and procedural learning. From a psychosocial standpoint, hearing loss affects not only the function of the individual but also communication with family members, thereby potentially isolating them from social and occupational opportunities and relationships, which can further diminish the quality of life.

Sensory and Motor Changes

Age-associated degeneration of dorsal column nuclei has been demonstrated in some rodent studies,[7] which may explain the propensity of impairment in light touch sensation, vibration, and proprioception seen in older individuals. Demyelination of nerve fibers or axonal loss can lead to generalized peripheral neuropathy (PN), which has an overall prevalence of 1% in the general population, but the prevalence increases to 7% in the elderly.[8] Older patients with PN are at a greater risk of falls, and more so in unfamiliar environments. Individuals with other comorbidities in conjunction with PN have worse baseline functioning than those with similar comorbidities without PN. The details of peripheral nervous system disorders are described in Chapter 6.

It is well known that there is a loss of motor units and muscle fibers during aging,[9] resulting in a decrease in overall muscle mass and loss of force per unit area, which causes a significant but not completely irreversible decrease in muscle strength, as resistance training

has been shown to improve strength and function even in the very old.[10] The process and details of sarcopenia are further discussed in Chapter 3. In addition to causing neuromuscular changes that contribute to activity limitations, the decline in central processing of external stimuli may also affect motor planning and performance. Motor system function involves complex interactions between the premotor and motor areas of the frontal lobes, basal ganglia, cerebellum, brainstem, and spinal cord. Loss of neuroplasticity may also be a limiting factor in the ability of an aging CNS to adapt, learn, coordinate, and refine motor control. Studies have shown that there is a decrease in the recruitment of frontal brain regions and impaired modulation of corticospinal excitability that can lead to prolonged reaction times and a delay in generation, anticipation, and preparation of motor responses.[11]

Cognitive, Memory, and Behavioral Changes

Cognitive abilities are highly variable among individuals, and this variability increases among older adults.[1,2,8,12] Although there are significant individual differences, generally speaking, what is known as "fluid intelligence" that involves problem solving, executive functioning, multitasking, abstract reasoning, and episodic memory declines with age, whereas "crystallized intelligence" that includes procedural and semantic memory remains stable. It is also documented that a reduction in adrenergic function and deterioration of excitatory neurotransmitters can lead to age-related decline in working memory,[13] whereas slower cognitive capabilities and impaired attentiveness have been associated with poorer oxygen supply.[14] Although there is an age-related decline in memory performance, disabling intellectual decline is not an inevitable or expected consequence of aging, and it should be considered significant pathology. Dementia and depression are also common in the elderly population; however, they are not part of the normal aging process. Although the topic of neuropsychological and objective metrics for formal cognitive evaluation is complex in general, the main challenge is the variable nature of cognitive deficits seen in aging, in the setting of multiple medical comorbidities or variable neurologic recovery after a CNS insult.

Medication Metabolism Changes

Age-related changes in pharmacokinetics and pharmacodynamics can lead to more frequent and severe side effects in the elderly population.[5] Further details on this topic are described in Chapter 9 of this book. The key changes include (1) an increase in adipose tissue,

(2) a decrease in total body water, and (3) a decrease in hepatic and renal clearance, all of which can prolong a medication's biologic half-life and increase serum concentrations. In addition, there is an increase in sensitivity to several classes of medications, including psychotropics, anticoagulants, and cardiovascular drugs.[15] This increase in sensitivity to medications, such as neuroleptics and other CNS altering medications, can further increase the risk of falls and/or delirium among vulnerable older adults.

EPIDEMIOLOGY OF NEUROLOGIC DISORDERS IN GERIATRIC POPULATION

According to the most recent data from the Population Reference Bureau, the elderly population comprises 46.2 million in 2014 or 14.5% of the US population and is anticipated to more than double by 2060. Neurologic disorders, including neuropsychiatric, cerebrovascular disease, and infectious etiologies, contribute to 6.3% of global burden of disease and are projected to double by year 2030,[16] which reflects an increasing demand and the importance of addressing CNS disorders in the geriatric population.

CENTRAL NERVOUS SYSTEM DISORDERS THAT AFFECT GERIATRIC POPULATIONS

Cerebrovascular Disease (Stroke)

According to the Centers for Disease Control and Prevention, an individual has a stroke every 40 s and a death from stroke occurs every 4 min in the United States.[17] Along with musculoskeletal disorders, stroke is a major cause of serious long-term disability and reduces mobility in more than half of the stroke survivors over age 65 years.[17] Risk factors are similar for both old and young populations, including hypertension, hyperlipidemia, diabetes, heart disease, family history of stroke, and previous stroke or transient ischemic attack (TIA). Functional outcomes and prognosis are worse among older adults, because of the combination of comorbidities and frailty. The 2-year survival rate is also lower in the very old (85 years and above) with a history of recurrent stroke as compared with women and younger males aged 65–69 years with a history of one stroke[18]; however, access to advanced medical care and inpatient rehabilitation have been shown to be associated with significant functional gains and higher return to the community for patients with stroke over 85 years.[19]

Most strokes are ischemic, and anticoagulant therapy may be indicated in cases of cardiac emboli, TIA, atrial fibrillation, or prothrombotic states. Although the fear of increased bleeding risk in elderly patients who are at a high fall risk requires the clinician to weigh the risk and benefits of antithrombotic therapy, American College of Chest Physicians guideline recommendations of initiating oral anticoagulation remains strong, especially given the increased thromboembolic and stroke risk with age.[20,21] Stroke risk stratification can be assessed with scoring systems such as the $CHADS_2$ (congestive heart failure, hypertension, age $\geq$75 years, diabetes, stroke [double weight]) for patients with atrial fibrillation. It is also important to consider other risk factors for bleeding and intracranial hemorrhage (ICH), such as hypertension, anticoagulation intensity, previous cerebral ischemia, and advanced age,[21] when weighing the risks of anticoagulation therapy. The standard 3 months of anticoagulation treatment for acute venous thromboembolism (VTE) is associated with a 2%–3% increase in major bleeding (defined by episode of bleeding that requires transfusion or hospitalization, stroke, myocardial infarction, or death) events per year, and the rate nearly doubles for populations over 65 years.[22] However, in other studies, elderly patients who were determined to be high fall risk who were being treated for VTE with anticoagulation were not at an increased risk of bleeding when compared with low fall risk groups[23] but had an increased risk for nonmajor bleeding and not major bleeding.[24] Studies comparing the use of aspirin and warfarin showed comparable risk for ICH in elderly patients, and vigilant modification of other ICH risk factors can enhance the safety of anticoagulants, such as warfarin, in the elderly population.[21] In addition to being aware of these risks, physical activity should not be discouraged for elderly patients on anticoagulants, as it has been shown that moderate and even high vigorous level of physical activity in this population is associated with a decreased risk of major bleeding when compared with those who had low physical activity.[25]

Clinical presentation of a stroke varies depending on the location of lesion. The various stages of motor recovery post stroke have been well described by Brunnstrom, Sawner, and Lavigne and can facilitate appropriate therapeutic intervention. Clinical practice guidelines for stroke rehabilitation approaches have been described[26]; however, when considering stroke rehabilitation for the elderly population, the severity of neurologic deficits, other medical comorbidities that may affect overall endurance and participation with therapies, and learning potential in the setting of superimposed cognitive deficits must be considered to determine the intensity of rehabilitation and develop a comprehensive and customized treatment program.

TABLE 5.1

Assessment Tools of Dementia and Mild Cognitive Impairment (MCI)

Assessment Tool	Description	Sensitivity, Specificity
Mini-mental status examination (MMSE)	Measures cognitive function in areas of memory, attention and calculation, language, and visual construction. Score of 23–24 or less is abnormal	55%–78% sensitivity,[85–87] 100% specificity[77] for the detection of mild dementia (MMSE > 26) 18% sensitivity for the detection of MCI[87]
General practitioner assessment of cognition	9-item cognitive questions and 6 informant questions to assess change over time	Strong sensitivity and specificity over MMSE for dementia screening in the primary care setting 81%–98% sensitivity and 72%–95% specificity[88]
Montreal cognitive assessment	Assesses attention/concentration, executive functions, conceptual thinking, memory, language, calculation, and orientation on a 30-point scale. Score less than 25 is abnormal	Sensitive and specific for MCI in the setting of normal MMSE scores 90% sensitivity for MCI[87] 100% sensitivity for mild Alzheimer dementia (AD)[87] 87% specificity for both MCI and mild AD[87]
Memory impairment screen	4-item scale, does not include visuospatial and executive function evaluation	High construct validity for memory impairment, good sensitivity and specificity and positive predictive value for AD and other dementias 42.9% sensitivity and 98% specificity for AD[89]

Data from Sheehan B. Assessment scales in dementia. *Ther Adv Neurol Disord*. 2012;5(6):349–358 and Ismail Z, Rajji TK, Shulman KI. Brief cognitive screening instruments: an update. *Int J Geriatr Psychiatry*. 2010;25(2):111–120.

Neurodegenerative Disorders

Dementia

Dementia, also known as major neurocognitive disorder, is defined as an irreversible global decline of a nonorganic etiology that interferes with functional independence involving at least one or more cognitive domains: (1) learning and memory, (2) language, (3) executive function, (4) complex attention, (5) perceptual motor, and (6) social cognition.[27] A report by the World Health Organization in 2012 documented 35.6 million people living with dementia worldwide, a number expected to double by 2030. Alzheimer dementia is the most common type of dementia in older adults, representing 65% of dementia cases.[28] Mild cognitive impairment (MCI), associated with cognitive decline abnormal for normal aging that does not interfere with daily functioning, has been described, although not in all cases, as a risk factor for progression to dementia.[28–30] Several assessment tools are available for evaluating dementia and MCI (Table 5.1). The value of these assessment tools may differ depending on the population age and living setting (community, nursing home) and may require different cutoff scores for accurate diagnosis of cognitive impairment.[31] Further details of dementia are described in Chapter 13 of this book.

Parkinson disease

Parkinson disease (PD) is a progressive neurodegenerative disorder affecting the dopaminergic neurons of substantia nigra and locus coerulus. PD affects 1% of the population older than 60 years.[4] Diagnosis is based on clinical criteria, and the etiology is currently unknown. Parkinsonian features are commonly associated with medications[32] (Table 5.2), but they are also associated with trauma-related degenerative issues (i.e., chronic traumatic encephalopathy), environmental toxins (manganese, carbon monoxide), structural lesions in the basal ganglia, neurodegenerative disorders such as dementia with Lewy bodies, progressive supranuclear palsy, multiple system atrophy, cortical-basal ganglionic degeneration, or brain iron accumulation.[33]

Classic motor symptoms include tremor at rest, rigidity, and bradykinesia, which often present unilaterally before progressing to the other side of the body.[33] The combination of rigidity and bradykinesia may give patients with PD a sense of weakness even if no weakness can be detected on physical examination. Other parkinsonian signs include reduced arm swing, impaired rapid limb movement, micrographia, reduced voice, masked facies, and reduced spontaneous gesturing. As the condition progresses, severe akinesia, pain, freezing, falls, and signs of postural instability become more prominent, making it more difficult to distinguish from other causes of parkinsonism. Although there are several different diagnostic criteria described in the literature for PD, expert opinion is still considered the gold standard and guidelines have been proposed by the Movement Disorder Society to assist with

TABLE 5.2
Medications Associated With Parkinsonism

Medication		Notes
Typical antipsychotics	Phenothiazine Chlorpromazine Prochlorperazine Perphenazine Fluphenazine Promethazine Haloperidol Pimozide Sulpiride	• The most common cause of extrapyramidal symptoms (EPS) • Frequently causes symptoms days to weeks after medication initiation
Atypical antipsychotics	Risperidone Olanzapine Ziprasidone Aripiprazole	• The risk of EPS and aggravation of parkinsonism are lower than with typical antipsychotics • Selective serotonin-2A (S2A) activity more than on dopamine (D2) receptors • Risperidone has high binding to S2A but fast dissociation with D2 receptors in a dose-dependent manner • Of all atypical antipsychotics, clozapine and quetiapine have the lowest risk of drug-induced parkinsonism
Dopamine antagonists	Reserpine Tetrabenazine	
Antiemetics	Metoclopramide Levosulpiride Clebopride	• Blocks peripheral D2 receptors in the gut, area postrema, and central D2 receptors • Levosulpiride causes more parkinsonian features than other EPS • Metoclopramide is frequently associated with tardive dyskinesia
Calcium channel blocker	Flunarizine Cinnarizine	• The exact mechanism of inducing parkinsonism is unclear • May reduce dopamine neurotransmission directly by acting on central D2 receptors
Antiepileptics	Valproic acid	• Parkinsonian features found in 5% of patients with long-term use • Possible role in oxidative stress and mitochondrial dysfunction
Others: mood stabilizers, antidepressants	Lithium Citalopram Sertraline Paroxetine	• Infrequent cause of parkinsonism • Lithium can decrease dopamine in the striatum and increase cholinergic activity by inhibiting acetylcholinesterase

Adapted from Shin HW, Chung SJ. Drug-induced Parkinsonism. *J Clin Neurol*. 2012;8(1):16; with permission.

diagnosis for both clinical and research settings.[34] Generally speaking, there is a consensus that presence of rest tremor, improvement of symptoms with levodopa lasting 5 years, levodopa-induced dyskinesia, progressive disorder lasting 10 years, and absence of features suggestive of other forms of parkinsonism is suggestive of PD. The neurodegenerative process of PD often is asymptomatic until dopamine depletion greater than 50%, and as a result, many studies have described "preclinical" or "prodromal" symptoms that are vague and nonspecific that can occur before the more classic motor symptoms manifest.[33] These nonspecific symptoms may include widespread pain involving muscles and joints, hypertension, mood disorders, unilateral action dystonia, constipation, rapid eye movement sleep behavior disorder, hyposmia, anosmia, and nonspecific limb weakness that can lead to extensive workup for neuropathy or radiculopathy.[35-39] Dementia related to Lewy body deposition may be seen in up to one-third of patients with PD. Pathophysiology of dementia in PD is not clearly understood, although studies have identified potential cerebrospinal fluid (CSF) biomarkers for cognitive impairment in PD.[40,41]

The shuffling and festinating gait (FSG) patterns are classic and pathognomonic presentations of gait disturbances in patients with PD. The mechanism to sustain normal posture and locomotion involves activation of frontal and parahippocampal gyri providing input to brainstem via the basal ganglia to initiate gait. It is a complex interaction and delicate balance between central processing and sensory input modulation to produce appropriate involuntary and voluntary muscle movements. Functional magnetic resonance imaging (MRI) findings show altered activities of these normal pathways and activation of less efficient pathways in PD. Balash et al.[42] organized PD gait disturbance variety by stages (see Table 5.3).

Episodic gait patterns such as FSG and freezing of gait (FOG) are brief, involuntary movements that are present in later stages and frequently interfere with gait synchronicity. FSG is defined as uncontrolled forward propulsion with rapid small steps, with a sensation of "being pushed."[43] FOG is characterized by brief (lasting less than 30 s)[42] periods of inability to initiate or maintain locomotion with tremor in legs. FOG also contributes to the overall postural instability, which in combination with greater hesitancy for turning when changing direction of ambulation, can increase the risk

for falls, which may be a sign of disease progression. In later stages of PD, FOG becomes the most disabling motor symptom; however, visual/sensory and mental tricks have shown promising results in reducing these episodes.[44,45] The decrease in proprioception and sensory feedback that results in FOG may lead to an increase in visual kinesthesia as a maladaptive compensation for the loss of function and create a more exaggerated dependence on visual feedback and control to help with initiating movement. In other words, external cues may act as a way to replace and compensate for the lack of internal cues from the basal ganglia via the thalamus to the primary and supplementary motor cortex.[46] This can possibly explain the mechanism of why visual cues may be beneficial. In advanced stages of PD, falls become the chief complaint of most patients and caregivers[42] as a result of increasing postural instability paired with decreased gait continuity. Other exacerbating factors include the presence of urge urinary incontinence increasing the risk for falls by six times than in those with PD without urge incontinence.[47]

Medications that promote dopamine action and decrease cholinergic effect are typically first line, although surgical options, such as deep brain stimulation (DBS), are also available. It is important to note that patients with PD with dementia or psychiatric/behavioral symptoms are less likely candidates for DBS.[4] Rehabilitation is primarily supportive in addressing deficits related to mobility, fall risk, fine motor control, cognition, speech, swallowing, and mood, particularly as the disease progresses. Physical exercise, including resistance training, has been shown to slow but not stop the disease progression[5,48] and exercise-induced motor recovery due to an increase in dopamine transporters[49] but not restoration of dopamine in the nigrostriatal pathway itself in animal models.[50] Core strengthening exercises should be prioritized given that abdominal muscle weakness has been shown to be more significant than other muscles in the body.[51] Music-based movement therapy and dance, such as tango,[52] have also shown positive effects.[53]

Multiple sclerosis

Multiple sclerosis (MS) is a chronic demyelinating, inflammatory, and immune-mediated CNS disorder that results in neurologic and neuropsychological dysfunction. MS can also mimic other neurologic, rheumatologic, and vascular diseases, which makes MS primarily a diagnosis of exclusion. The average age of onset is 30 years, and it is considered one of the most common disabling neurologic conditions of young and middle-aged adults, but the variable nature of clinical

TABLE 5.3 Clinical Staging of Parkinson Disease Gait Patterns	
	Clinical Gait Features
Stage 1	• Short step length • ↓Gait speed, arm swing • ↑Stride-to-stride variability • Hesitancy with turning and initiation of movement • Bradykinesia
Stage 2	• Shuffling with ↑bradykinesia • Weakness to hip flexion and ankle plantarflexion affecting presswing and "toe off" in stance phase • Dual tasking derangement (i.e., unable to talk while walking) • ↑↑Stride-to-stride variability
Stage 3	• Freezing of gait • Festinating gait • ↑↑Hesitancy with turning and initiation of movement, higher risk for falling
Stage 4	• ↑↑Falls • ↓↓Stride length due to poor toe clearance • Knee and ankle contractures causing excessive knee flexion in stance and "walking on toes"

From Balash Y, Hausdorff JM, Gurevich T, et al. Gait disorders in Parkinson's disease. In: Pfeiffer RF, Wszolek ZK, Ebadi M, eds. *Parkinson's Disease*. 2nd ed. Boca Raton: CRC Press; 2013; with permission.

presentation and disease course makes it challenging to predict prognosis for the disease's effect on the aging population. Although onset is rare for adults over 50 years, about 10%–15% of people with MS who have the primary progressive type are typically over the age of 40 years,[1] and a wide range of 5%–64% are categorized as having a "benign" course,[54] which has been defined and described in different ways.[55] Initial symptoms may include motor, sensory or autonomic dysfunction, ataxia, vision changes, optic neuritis, fatigue, bladder incontinence, or mood disturbances. Because fatigue is one of the most common presenting symptoms and may often precede a relapse, it can be challenging to determine if fatigue is "normal" for aging or pathologic in an older patient with MS. Fatigue can be due to sleep disturbances, depression, and heat intolerance. Depression is simultaneously the most common mental health issue in the aging population and the most common mood disturbance associated with MS. Patients with MS-related depression have a higher suicide risk because of psychosocial issues rather than the severity or duration of MS.[56] In addition, although patients with MS have a normal lifespan, medical comorbidities affect persons with MS earlier than their peers,[57] which significantly decreases their overall quality of life. Aging patients with MS are forced to consider nursing home placement with fear of caregiver strain burden and loss of autonomous control at an earlier age compared with other patients with long-term disability.

Early in the disease course, MS is characterized by inflammation and relapses of episodic neurologic dysfunction with partial to total recovery, but the neurodegenerative process is what leads to progression of disability over time. Diagnosis is based on objective neurologic findings and at least one relapse, as described by the McDonald Criteria.[58] MRI findings and CSF studies (i.e., presence of oligoclonal bands) can be supportive, but they have limited specificity and no gold standard to validate these tests and there may be a tendency to overtreat and overdiagnose.[54] In addition, although the physiologic process of aging may also produce hyperintense signals in the subcortical region on MRI, knowing that MS lesions typically involve the ventricles, brainstem, corpus callosum, cerebellum, and spinal cord can be helpful in differentiating pathology in the older adult with MS.[1] Disease-modifying agents, such as interferons, can be used as long-term management, but weighing the risk versus benefit is important before prescribing these agents because of adverse side effects, such as flulike symptoms, blood and bone marrow abnormalities, and thyroid dysfunction, that may further increase the risk of falls in older adults.

Cognitive deficits occur in about 50%–60% of patients with MS; however, there is no direct correlation between cognitive deficits and physical disability, disease duration, or course of the disease,[59,60] although a high baseline cognitive capacity may be protective.[61] Pharmacologic options, such as donepezil, ginkgo biloba, memantine, and rivastigmine, have been studied; however, they have limited efficacy in improving memory performance.[62-66] MS-related cognitive dysfunction is also highly individualized and variable, with memory and learning dysfunction and slowed processing speed as the most common cognitive-related deficits, which can affect multiple aspects of a patient's activities of daily living. Thus an individualized, comprehensive, and interdisciplinary approach must be used when developing a rehabilitation regimen for elderly patients with MS.

Traumatic Brain Injury in the Elderly

Traumatic brain injury (TBI) in the elderly accounts for 80,000 emergency department visits annually, and over 50% of cases are due to falls. The highest rates of TBI-related hospitalizations, morbidity, and mortality occur in adults older than 75 years, making geriatric TBI an important public health concern. Age-related biochemical and physiologic changes may predispose this demographic to a higher stress response and inflammation after TBI.[67,68] Medical comorbidities, such as cardiac disease, requiring anticoagulation and coagulopathies can further increase bleeding risk and the development of ICHs after a fall, which can be related to syncope, gait imbalance, orthostatic hypotension, PN, malnutrition, electrolyte disturbances, or side effects from polypharmacy. Subdural hematomas resulting from trauma to bridging veins are most frequent. The cost of immediate medical care and length of rehabilitation required to achieve the same level of outcomes rises above that of the general population, despite less favorable outcomes.[67,69,70] Although older age, medical comorbidities, gender, and preadmission functional ability have been identified as factors that negatively affect recovery and prognosis after TBI, these variables are not as well studied in the geriatric population.[71] An integrated program to address both cognitive and neuromuscular impairments within the context of premorbid functional status is the recommended rehabilitation approach for this population.

Normal Pressure Hydrocephalus

Normal pressure hydrocephalus (NPH) is a disease of the elderly, most commonly affecting adults 65 years and older, and the prevalence increases after age 80 years.[72]

It is defined as a type of communicating hydrocephalus with normal intracranial pressure. The etiology and pathogenesis for NPH can be idiopathic, but cerebrovascular disease, such as stroke, TBI, and cardiovascular disease causing inflammatory changes in the CNS, have also been proposed to alter the flow and absorption of CSF.[73,74] The clinical triad of gait imbalance, altered mental status, and urinary incontinence is well described; however, these symptoms can also be nonspecific and presentation may be more subtle, thus a high clinical suspicion and ruling out other causes of dementia is necessary.

Gait apraxia, most commonly seen as short stride, low speed, and wide based, is the earliest and most predominant symptom of NPH and has the greatest chance of improvement after shunting.[75] Gait improves by 64% 3 months after shunting and by 26% at 3 years[76]; more specifically, the gait velocity increases by 20% after CSF tapping.[77] Thus gait improvement after temporary removal of CSF is an important aspect of criteria to meet for shunt surgery. It is interesting to note that there are some similarities between gait disturbances noted in PD and NPH. For example, both conditions may have decreased steps, rigidity of lower extremities, flexed posture, and impaired postural reflexes. However, comparative analysis between PD and NPH have shown NPH to have significantly slower velocity and stride length and increased step width and outward rotation of foot to contribute to a broad-based gait that is not seen in PD,[77] although both conditions shared loss of balance, short stride, and slowness, with parkinsonian features being the main distinguishing features between NPH and PD groups.[78] In addition, although the NPH group did worse on the walk test, the symptom duration was shorter than in patients with PD,[77,78] which is consistent with the progressive nature of PD as described in the previous section. In addition, external sensory cues that help improve gait imbalances in patients with PD have minimal to no effect on patients with NPH.[77] These overlaps in gait impairment and differences in response to therapeutic interventions in both the NPH and PD patient populations may challenge the idea that gait alterations are isolated to basal ganglia pathology. Radiographic findings of ventriculomegaly disproportionate to the amount of cerebral atrophy can be seen, without elevation in the CSF pressure.

Treatment involving surgical shunting in patients over the eighth decade is described as a safe procedure[79]; however, results may vary. As discussed earlier, surgical shunting may be a treatment of choice when gait imbalance improves after CSF tapping,[5] whereas coexisting depression may not be as responsive to shunting.[80]

There is strong evidence that shunting improves all aspects of NPH, although not all with equal efficacy, including cognition.[81–84] Common complications after shunting include shunt malfunction causing obstruction or overdrainage, infection, wound dehiscence near the abdomen, and subdural hematoma. Symptoms of overdrainage include "muffled" hearing and, on dedicated imaging, evidence of thin subdural effusions.[84] Headaches that worsen with sitting and standing, but that improves with lying down, are the most common symptom of overdrainage and can be corrected by raising the shunt setting.[84] For this reason, periodic brain imaging is recommended in the first 6–12 months after surgery to monitor for changes.[84] Shunt malfunction resulting in obstruction can occur in up to 30% of patients,[84] and rarely an emergency if detected and treated early on. Nearly half who have a shunt will require revision within 3 years secondary to infection and shunt malfunction.[76] In the elderly population, transient worsening weeks to months after the initial shunt surgery may not always indicate shunt malfunction and may require additional workup for other etiologies and comorbidities.

CONCLUSION/SUMMARY

CNS disorders that affect the elderly population are complex clinical conditions and present with a wide variety of symptoms. To design an effective strategy to treat these conditions, the rehabilitation expert must have a comprehensive understanding of the nervous system as well as the normal and abnormal aging process. With increasing global burden of CNS disorders in the aging population, there is a growing need for the development of treatment and rehabilitation programs that optimize function and assist with caregiver support.

REFERENCES

1. Umphred DA, Lazaro RT. Aging and the central nervous system. In: Kauffman TL, Barr JO, Moran M, eds. *Geriatric Rehabilitation Manual*. Edinburgh: Churchill Livingstone Elsevier; 2008:21–30.
2. Jiang X, et al. Individual differences in cognitive function in older adults predicted by neuronal selectivity at corresponding brain regions. *Front Aging Neurosci*. 2017;9:103.
3. *Quick Statistics About Hearing*. National Institute of Deafness and Other Communication Disorders; 2017. https://www.nidcd.nih.gov/health/statistics/quick-statistics-hearing.
4. Cuccurullo S, Lee J. *Physical Medicine and Rehabilitation Board Review*. 3rd ed. New York: Demos Medical; 2015:877–891.

5. Jaramillo C. The geriatric patient. In: Braddom RL, ed. *Physical Medicine and Rehabilitation*. St. Louis: Elsevier Health Sciences; 2016:653–664.

6. Iwasaki S, Yamasoba T. Dizziness and imbalance in the elderly: age-related decline in the vestibular system. *Aging Dis*. 2015;6(1):38–47.

7. Johnson JE, et al. A fine structural study of degenerative changes in dorsal column nuclei of aging mice, lack of protection by vitamin E. *J Gerontol*. 1975;20(4):395–411.

8. Morse CK. Does variability increase with age? An archival study of cognitive measures. *Psychol Aging*. 1993;8:156–164. https://doi.org/10.1037/0882-7974.8.2.156.

9. Faulkner JA, Larkin LM, Claflin DR, Brooks SV. Age-related changes in the structure and function of skeletal muscles. *Clin Exp Pharmacol Physiol*. 2007;34:1091–1096.

10. Doherty T. Invited review: aging and sarcopenia. *J Appl Physiol*. 2003;95(4).

11. Cuypers K, et al. Age-related differences in corticospinal excitability during a choice reaction time task. *Age*. 2013;35(5):1705–1719. *PMC*. Web. 23 Aug. 2017.

12. Spreng RN, Wojtowicz M, Grady CL. Reliable differences in brain activity between young and old adults: a quantitative meta-analysis across multiple cognitive domains. *Neurosci Biobehav Rev*. 2010;34:1178–1194.

13. Strong R, Wood GW, Burke WJ. *Central Nervous System Disorders of Aging: Clinical Intervention and Research*. vol. 33. Raven Press; 1988.

14. Hanninen T, Soininen H. Age associated memory impairment. Normal aging or warning of dementia? *Drugs Aging*. 1997;11(6):480–489.

15. Mangoni A, Jackson S. Age related changes in pharmacokinetics and pharmacodynamics: basic principles and practical applications. *Br J Clin Pharmacol*. 2003;57(1):6–14.

16. Aarli JA, Dua T, Janca A, Muscetta A. *WHO Definition of Neurologic Disorders: Public Health Challenges*. 2006. Available at: http://www.who.int/mental_health/neurology/neurological_disorders_report_web.pdf.

17. Center for Disease Control, Prevention, National Center for Chronic Disease Prevention and Health Promotion, Division for Heart Disease and Stroke Prevention. *Stroke Fact Sheet*. 2017. Available at: https://www.cdc.gov/stroke/facts.htm.

18. Samsa GP, et al. Epidemiology of recurrent cerebral infarction: a medicare claims-based comparison of first and recurrent strokes on 2-year survival and cost. *Stroke*. 1999;30(2):338–349.

19. O'Brien SR, Xue Y. Inpatient rehabilitation outcomes in patients with stroke aged 85 years or older. *Phys Ther*. 2016;96(9):1381–1388.

20. Robert-Ebadi H, Le Gal G, Righini M. Use of anticoagulants in elderly patients: practical recommendations. *Clin Interv Aging*. 2009;4:165–177.

21. Garwood C, Corbett T. Use of anticoagulation in elderly patients with atrial fibrillation who are at risk for falls. *Ann Pharmacother*. 2008;42:523–532.

22. Spencer FA, Gore JM, Lessard D, et al. Venous thromboembolism in the elderly: a community-based perspective. *Thromb Haemost*. 2008;100(5):780–788.

23. Jacques D, et al. Risk of falls and major bleeds in patients on oral anticoagulation therapy. *Am J Med*. 2012;125(8):773–778.

24. Kampfen P, et al. Risk of falls and bleeding in elderly patients with acute venous thromboembolism. *J Intern Med*. 2014;276:378–386.

25. Frey PM, et al. Physical activity and risk of bleeding in elderly patients taking anticoagulants. *Thromb Haemost*. 2014;13:197–205.

26. Winstein CJ, Stein J, Arena R, et al. Guidelines for adult stroke rehabilitation and recovery: a guideline for healthcare professionals from the American Heart Association/American Stroke Association. *Stroke*. 2016;47(6):e98–e169.

27. American Psychiatric Association. *Diagnostic and Statistical Manual of Mental Disorders: DSM-5*. Washington, DC: American Psychiatric Association; 2013.

28. Francis N. Assessment tools for geriatric patients with delirium, mild cognitive impairment, dementia, and depression. *Top Geriatr Rehabil*. 2012;28(3):137–147.

29. Petersen RC, Smith GE, Waring SC, Ivnik RJ, Tangalos EG, Kokmen E. Mild cognitive impairment: clinical characterization and outcome. *Arch Neurol*. 1999;56(3):303–308.

30. Petersen RC. Mild cognitive impairment as a diagnostic entity. *J Int Med*. 2004;256:183–194.

31. Kahle-Wrobleski K, et al. Sensitivity and specificity of the mini-mental state examination for identifying dementia in the oldest-old: the 90+ study. *J Am Geriatr Soc*. 2012;55:284–289.

32. Shin HW, Chung SJ. Drug induced parkinsonism. *J Clin Neurol*. 2012;8(1):15–21.

33. Chou KL, Hurtig HI. Chapter 16: Tremor, rigidity, and bradykinesia. In: *Parkinson's Disease*. 2nd ed. CRC Press; 2012:191–202.

34. Postuma RB, et al. MDS clinical diagnostic criteria for Parkinson's disease. *Mov Disord*. 2015;30(12):1591–1601.

35. Gonera EG, van't Hof M, Berger HJ, van Weel C, Horstink MW. Symptoms and duration of the prodromal phase in Parkinson's disease. *Mov Disord*. 1997;12(6):871–876.

36. Abbott RD, Petrovitch H, White LR, et al. Frequency of bowel movements and the future risk of Parkinson's disease. *Neurology*. 2001;57(3):456–462.

37. Poewe WH, Lees AJ, Stern GM. Dystonia in Parkinson's disease: clinical and pharmacological features. *Ann Neurol*. 1988;23(1):73–78.

38. Schenck CH, Bundlie SR, Mahowald MW. Delayed emergence of a parkinsonian disorder in 38% of 29 older men initially diagnosed with idiopathic rapid eye movement sleep behaviour disorder. *Neurology*. 1996;46(2):388–393.

39. Stern MB, Doty RL, Dotti M, et al. Olfactory function in Parkinson's disease subtypes. *Neurology*. 1994;44(2):266–268.

40. Compta Y, et al. Cerebrospinal tau, phospho-tau, and beta amyloid and neuropsychological functions in Parkinson's disease. *Mov Disord*. 2009;24:2203–2210.

41. Modreneau R, et al. Cross-sectional and longitudinal associations of motor fluctuations and non-motor predominance with cerebrospinal tau and alpha-beta as well as dementia-risk in Parkinson's disease. *J Neurol Sci.* 2017;373:223–229.

42. Balash Y, Hausdorff JM, Gurevich T, Giladi N. Chapter 17: Gait disorders in Parkinson's disease. In: *Parkinson's Disease.* 2nd ed. CRC Press; 2012:203–218.

43. Giladi N, Shabtai H, Simon ES, Biran S, Tal J, Korczyn AD. Construction of freezing of gait questionnaire for patients with Parkinsonism. *Parkinsonism Relat Disord.* 2000;6:165–170.

44. Rubinstein T, Giladi N, Hausdorff JM. The power of cueing, circumvent dopamine deficits: a brief review of physical therapy treatment of gait disturbances in Parkinson's disease. *Mov Disord.* 2002;17:1148–1160.

45. Stern GM, Lander CM, Lees AJ. Akinetic freezing and trick movements in Parkinson's disease. *J Neural Transm.* 1980:137–141.

46. Morris ME, Iansek R, Matyas TA, et al. The pathogenesis of gait hypokinesia in Parkinson's disease. *Brain.* 1994;117:1169–1181.

47. Balash Y, Peretz C, Leibovich G, Herman T, Hausdorff JM, Giladi N. Falls in outpatients with Parkinson's disease: frequency, impact and identifying factors. *J Neurol.* 2005;252(11):1310–1315.

48. Tarsy D, Gordon L. Chapter 51: Clinical diagnostic criteria for Parkinson's disease. In: *Parkinson's Disease.* 2nd ed. CRC Press; 2012:703–712.

49. Smith BA, Goldberg NRS, Meshul CK. Effects of treadmill exercise on behavioral recovery and neural changes in the substantia nigra and striatum of the 1-methyl-4-phenyl-1,2,3,6-tetrahydropyridine-lesioned mouse. *Brain Res.* 2011;1386:70–80.

50. Churchill MJ, Pflibsen L, Sconce MD, Moore C, Kim K, Meshul CK. Exercise in an animal model of Parkinson's disease: motor recovery but not restoration of the nigrostriatal pathway. In: *Neuroscience.* 2017;359:224–247.

51. Scandalis TA, Bosak A, Berliner JC, Helman LL, Wells MR. Resistance training and gait function in patients with Parkinson's disease. *Am J Phys Med Rehabil.* 2001;80(1):38–43.

52. Hackney ME, Earhart GM. Short duration, intensive tango dancing for Parkinson disease: an uncontrolled pilot study. *Complement Ther Med.* 2009;17(4):203–207.

53. De Dreu M, et al. *Partnered Dancing to Improve Mobility for People with Parkinson's Disease.* 2015.

54. Degenhardt A, Ramagopalan SV, Scalfari A, Ebers GC. Clinical prognostic factors in multiple sclerosis: a natural history review. *Nat Rev Neurol.* 2009;5:672–682.

55. Correale J, Ysrraelit MC, Fiol MP. *Curr Neurol Neurosci Rep.* 2012;12:601.

56. Stern M. Aging with multiple sclerosis. *Phys Med Rehabil Clin North Am.* 2005;16:219–234.

57. Buhse M. The elderly person with multiple sclerosis: clinical implications for the increasing life-span. *J Neurosci Nurs.* 2015;47(6):333–337.

58. Shah A, Flores A, Nourbakhsh B, Stüve O. Multiple sclerosis. In: Braddom RL, ed. *Physical Medicine and Rehabilitation.* St. Louis: Elsevier Health Sciences; 2016:1029–1052.

59. Amato MP, Zipoli V, Portaccio E. Cognitive changes in multiple sclerosis. *Expert Rev Neurother.* 2008;8(10):1585–1596.

60. Amato MP, Zipoli V, Portaccio E. Multiple sclerosis-related cognitive changes: a review of cross-sectional and longitudinal studies. *J Neurol Sci.* 2006;245(1-2):41–46.

61. Sumowski JF, Chiaravalloti N, Deluca J. Cognitive reserve protects against cognitive dysfunction in multiple sclerosis. *J Clin Exp Neuropsychol.* 2009;31(8):913–926.

62. Krupp LB, Christodoulou C, Melville P, Scherl WF, MacAllister WS, Elkins LE. Donepezil improved memory in multiple sclerosis in a randomized clinical trial. *Neurology.* 2004;63(9):1579–1585.

63. Krupp LB, Christodoulou C, Melville P, et al. Multicenter randomized clinical trial of donepezil for memory impairment in multiple sclerosis. *Neurology.* 2011;76(17):1500–1507.

64. Lovera J, Bagert B, Smoot K, et al. Ginkgo biloba for the improvement of cognitive performance in multiple sclerosis: a randomized, placebo-controlled trial. *Mult Scler.* 2007;13(3):376–385.

65. Lovera JF, Frohman E, Brown TR, et al. Memantine for cognitive impairment in multiple sclerosis: a randomized placebo-controlled trial. *Mult Scler.* 2010;16(6):715–723.

66. Mäurer M, Ortler S, Baier M, et al. Randomised multicentre trial on safety and efficacy of rivastigmine in cognitively impaired multiple sclerosis patients. *Mult Scler.* 2013;19(5):631–638.

67. Wagner AK, Arenth PM, Kwasnica C, McCullough EH. Traumatic brain injury. In: Braddom RL, ed. *Physical Medicine and Rehabilitation.* St. Louis: Elsevier Health Sciences; 2016:961–998.

68. Wagner AK, McCullough EH, Niyonkuru C, et al. Acute s erum hormone levels: characterization and prognosis after severe traumatic brain injury. *J Neurotrauma.* 2011;28: 871–888.

69. Cifu DX, Kreutzer JS, Marwitz JH, et al. Functional outcomes of older adults with traumatic brain injury: a prospective, multicenter analysis. *Arch Phys Med Rehabil.* 1996;77:883–888.

70. Pennings JL, Bachulis BL, Simons CT, et al. Survival after severe brain injury in the aged. *Arch Surg.* 1993;128:787–793.

71. Thompson HJ, McCormic WC, Kagan SH. Traumatic brain injury in older adults: epidemiology, outcomes, and future implications. *J Am Geriatr Soc.* 2006;54(10):1590–1595.

72. Jaraj D, et al. Prevalence of idiopathic normal-pressure hydrocephalus. *Neurology.* 2014;82(6):1449–1454.

73. Casati M, Arosio B, Gussago C, et al. Down-regulation of adenosine A1 and A2A receptors in peripheral cells from idiopathic normal-pressure hydrocephalus patients. *J Neurol Sci.* 2016;361:196–199.

74. Israelsson H, Carlberg B, Wikkelsö C, et al. Vascular risk factors in INPH: a prospective case-control study (the INPH-CRasH study). *Neurology.* 2017;88(6):577–585.

75. Williams MA, et al. Objective assessment of gait in normal pressure hydrocephalus. *Am J Phys Med Rehabil.* 2008; 87(1):39–45.

76. Hier DB, Michals EA. Chapter 17: Disorders of circulation of cerebrospinal fluid. In: *Hankey's Clinical Neurology.* 2nd ed. CRC Press; 2014:667–678.

77. Stolze H, et al. Comparative analysis of the gait disorder of normal pressure hydrocephalus and Parkinson's disease. *J Neurol Neurosurg Psychiatry.* 2001;70:289–297.

78. Bugalho P, Alves L, Miguel R. Gait dysfunction in Parkinson's disease and normal pressure hydrocephalus: a comparative study. *J Neural Transm.* 2013;120(8):1201–1207.

79. Thompson SD, Shand Smith JD, Khan AA, Luoma AMV, Toma AK, Watkins LD. Shunting of the over 80s in normal pressure hydrocephalus. *Acta Neurochir (Wien).* 2017;159(6):987–994.

80. Israelsson H, Allard P, Eklund A, Malm J. Symptos of depression are common in patients with idiopathic normal pressure hydrcephalus: the INPH-CRasH study. *Neurosurgery.* 2016;78(2):161–168.

81. Thomas G, McGirt MJ, Woodworth G, et al. Baseline neuropsychological profile and cognitive response to cerebrospinal fluid shunting for idiopathic normal pressure hydrocephalus. *Dement Geriatr Cogn Disord.* 2005;20(2-3): 163–168.

82. Katzen H, Ravdin LD, Assuras S, et al. Postshunt cognitive and functional improvement in idiopathic normal pressure hydrocephalus. *Neurosurgery.* 2011;68(2):416–419. https:// doi.org/10.1227/NEU.0b013e3181ff9d01.

83. Hellström P, Klinge P, Tans J, Wikkelsø C. The neuropsychology of iNPH: findings and evaluation of tests in the European multicentre study. *Clin Neurol Neurosurg.* 2012;114(2):130–134. https://doi.org/10.1016/j.clineuro. 2011.09.014.

84. Williams MA, Malm J. Diagnosis and treatment of idiopathic normal pressure hydrocephalus. *CONTINUUM Lifelong Learn Neurol.* 2016;22(2):579–599.

85. Celeste A, Anne-Claire MC. Detection of MCI in the clinic evaluation of the sensitivity and specificity of a computerized test and the MMSE. *Age Aging.* 2009;38(4):455–460.

86. Sabe L, et al. Sensitivity and specificity of the mini-mental state exam in the diagnosis of dementia. *Behav Neurol.* 1993;6(4):207–219.

87. Nasreddine ZS, et al. The montreal cognitive assessment, MoCA: a brief screening tool for mild cognitive impairment. *J Am Geriatr Soc.* 2005;53(4):695–699.

88. Seeher KM, Brodaty H. The general practitioner assessment of cognition (GPCOG). *Cogn Screen Instrum.* 2016:231–239.

89. Modrego P, Gazulla J. The predictive value of the memory impairment screen in patients with subjective memory complaints: a prospective study. *Prim Care Companion CNS Disord.* 2013;15(1). https://doi.org/10.4088/ PCC.12m01435. Published online 2013 Jan 31.

CHAPTER 6

Peripheral Nervous System and Vascular Disorders Affecting Mobility in Older Adults

SEWON LEE, MD • DENNIS D.J. KIM, MD • MOOYEON OH-PARK, MD

Mobility is defined as the ability to move independently and safely from one location to another in a manner that requires intact physical and cognitive function.[1] It is fundamental to healthy aging and quality of life.[2] Impaired mobility in older adults has been associated with cognitive decline, loss of independence, higher rates of depression, fear and anxiety,[3] increased institutionalization, and death.[4,5] Etiologies for impaired mobility in older adults can be roughly categorized into neurologic disorders (central nervous system disorders and peripheral nervous system disorders [PNSD])[6] and nonneurologic disorders such as musculoskeletal disorders and vascular disorders.[7] PNSDs and peripheral vascular disorders (PVDs) are underrecognized by healthcare providers as causes of mobility impairment, although both conditions are increasingly common in an aging population.[8] The presenting symptoms of these conditions are often interpreted as merely aspects of the aging process by patients as well as by healthcare providers, thereby disabling the opportunity to be treated. It is important to recognize and manage these conditions properly to maximize independent mobility in older adults. A diagnosis of PNSD or PVD is largely based on good history taking and physical examination. Electrodiagnosis (Edx), imaging studies, and laboratory testing may confirm the clinical suspicion. Although definitive treatment may be available for some of these conditions, the majority of patients with PNSD or PVD need to manage these conditions via exercise programs, orthosis, and assistive devices. This chapter reviews the practical approaches and physiatric management of older patients with impaired mobility due to PNSD and PVD, focusing on the discussion of the following questions:

- How common are PNSDs and/or PVDs among older adults?
- How do PNSDs and/or PVDs affect mobility in older adults?
- What are the appropriate history components and physical examinations in patients with PNSD and/or PVD?
- How do we select an approach for patients with PNSD and/or PVD based on the clinical information gathered from history and physical examination?
- What diagnostic tests can enhance the evaluation process of older adults with PNSD and/or PVD?
- What are the components of the multidisciplinary management of PNSDs and/or PVDs?
- What conservative treatment options are available for patients with PNSD and/or PVD?

HISTORY TAKING FOR OLDER ADULTS WITH MOBILITY IMPAIRMENT AND SUSPECTED PNSD OR PVD

Questionnaires to screen impaired mobility in the National Health Interview Survey include the categories of difficulty with walking three city blocks, walking a quarter of a mile, walking 10 steps without resting, and/or standing for approximately 20 min.[9] The responses should be interpreted with caution considering the wide range of norms according to age and gender. Other questionnaires for impaired mobility (or dysmobility) include the speed of gait (e.g., being able to safely cross the street[10]), weight change (loss of weight), muscle strength, history of falling, loss of balance, etc. As impaired mobility is often underrecognized by patients and clinicians alike, it is important to consistently review the functional/mobility status of older adult patients during clinic visits. Once the problem of impaired mobility is recognized, collecting information regarding the mode of onset, pattern of progression, and precipitating, aggravating, and relieving factors is useful with regard to addressing other complaints. However, it can be challenging to obtain information pertaining to exacerbating or relieving factors from the older adult population, and healthcare providers must cultivate the skill of effective communication with patience.

PERIPHERAL NERVOUS SYSTEM DISORDERS

Peripheral neuropathy is increasingly common among older adults. According to the National Health and Nutrition Survey, 34.7% of that population complains of sensory impairment after the age of 80 years, as compared with 8.1% at the age of 40–49 years.[11] The prevalence of chronic symmetrical peripheral neuropathy was reported to be approximately 3% among the elderly.[12] Diabetic peripheral neuropathy is the most common form of peripheral neuropathy, and its prevalence is increasing in the aging population. Approximately 50% of diabetic patients older than 60 years of age show evidence of diabetic neuropathy.[13] Overall, myopathies and neuromuscular junction disorders are less common than peripheral neuropathy among older adults. However, some myopathies including statin-associated myopathy,[14] inclusion body myositis (IBM),[15] paraneoplastic myopathy, and neuromuscular transmission disorders (especially presynaptic types) should be recognized as contributors to mobility impairment among older adults. IBM is the most common form of inflammatory myopathy in patients older than 50 years, and it leads to a faster rate of mobility deterioration among older adult patients compared with younger patients. Older patients (60–79 years of age) require a walker for locomotion 5.7 years after the onset of the disease compared with younger patients who tend to need a walker more than 10 years after the onset.[16] Risk of statin-induced myopathy is higher in patients older than 80 years, especially in those with multiple comorbidities, polypharmacy (especially with fibrates and cyclosporine), sarcopenia, and impaired renal and liver function.[17]

Mobility Disability Related to Peripheral Nervous Disorders

Peripheral neuropathy is a well-known risk factor for mobility impairment that is associated with impaired gait, falls, fear of falls, and fall-related injuries.[6] In addition, poor peripheral nerve function has been associated with impaired activities of daily life and late-life disability.[18] The mechanism of mobility impairment in older adults with peripheral neuropathy is multifactorial, including unsteadiness (ataxia), focal muscle weakness (foot dragging, slapping, or knee buckling), fatigue, painful limitations, and/or fear of falls. Unsteady (ataxic) gait is secondary to a loss of proprioception in patients with peripheral polyneuropathy involving large sensory nerve fibers or dorsal root ganglia.[19] Impaired postural stability with increased body sway during the stance phase and displacement of the center of mass during walking was noted in patients with diabetic neuropathy.[20] Foot slapping, dragging, and steppage gait can occur secondary to distal muscle weakness (ankle dorsiflexor). Proximal muscle weakness can manifest as a Trendelenburg gait (secondary to hip abductor weakness), hip lurching (secondary to hip extensor weakness), and knee buckling (knee extensor and hip extensor weakness), depending on the location of the involvement. Muscle fatigue can decrease the distance of the gait and slow down the gait speed in addition to compromising safety due to the increased risk of falls. Patients with neuropathic pain also report reduced mobility due to pain.[21]

History and Physical Examination

The patient's complaints that accompany impaired mobility provide valuable information and important clues as to the underlying etiologies. Symptoms mediated by sensory and motor nerve dysfunction such as numbness, tingling, pins/needles sensation, and weakness are common manifestations indicative of peripheral neuropathy. Sensory nerve–mediated symptoms can be further classified into positive sensory symptoms such as paresthesia, pain, and pins/needle sensation, and negative sensory symptoms (loss of proprioception, numbness/anesthesia), which are more closely associated with impaired mobility. Negative sensory symptoms become more prominent in advanced sensory neuropathy or ganglionopathy. Autonomic symptoms such as orthostatic hypotension, dryness or excessive sweating, impotence, sphincter disturbance, diarrhea, and constipation may suggest the involvement of small myelinated or unmyelinated fibers. Based on the symptoms, peripheral neuropathy can be classified into motor, sensory, autonomic, or combined neuropathy. An absence of sensory symptoms narrows down the differential diagnoses to motor neuron diseases, motor neuropathies, neuromuscular junction disorders, and myopathies; however, clinicians should be aware of the possibility of concomitant sensory neuropathy with these conditions, which complicates the clinical picture (Fig. 6.1). Determining the location of involvement (especially weakness) provides clues for further differential diagnosis. Involvement of the proximal lower extremities can occur secondary to myopathy, lumbar plexopathy, radiculoplexus-neuropathy

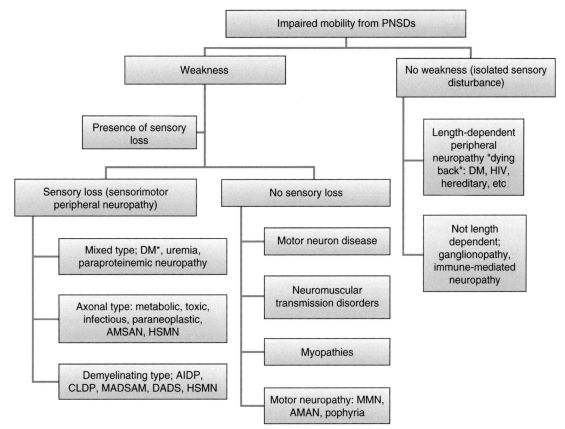

FIG. 6.1 Algorithmic approach to common peripheral nervous system disorders (PNSDs) affecting mobility. *Most common pattern of diabetic peripheral neuropathy. *AIDP*, acute inflammatory demyelinating polyneuropathy; *AMAN*, acute motor axonal neuropathy; *AMSAN*, acute motor sensory axonal neuropathy; *CIDP*, chronic inflammatory demyelinating polyneuropathy; *DADS*, distal acquired demyelinating symmetric neuropathy; *DM*, diabetes mellitus; *HIV*, human immunodeficiency virus; *HSMN*, hereditary sensory motor neuropathy (Charcot-Marie-Tooth disease); *MADSAM*, multifocal acquired demyelinating sensory and motor neuropathy.

(amyotrophy), or radiculopathy. Myopathies commonly involve proximal muscles with difficulty standing from sitting (especially from a lower chair) and dressing (overhead activity), with the exception of several myopathies such as IBM, myotonic dystrophy, and other distal myopathies. Motor neuron disease such as amyotrophic lateral sclerosis can present with asymmetric weakness in the distal extremities that mimics focal neuropathy in the initial stage and progresses to diffuse symmetric weakness. In later-stage mononeuropathy multiplex, the involvement of multiple peripheral nerves in a separate and noncontiguous fashion can mimic diffuse symmetric peripheral neuropathy (confluent mononeuritis multiplex).

Information pertaining to the mode of onset and progression of symptoms is useful to determine the underlying etiologies, with implications for the treatment plan:
- Immediate onset: traumatic neuropathy after identifiable trauma or neuropathy associated with vasculitis in patients with vascular risk factors.
- Acute onset: inflammatory process (such as Guillain-Barré syndrome: acute inflammatory demyelinating neuropathy) over days or weeks. Iatrogenic nerve injury (partial) after an invasive procedure.
- Gradual onset: "dying back neuropathy," symmetric or slowly progressive symptoms from the distal segment (most commonly due to diabetic peripheral

neuropathy), chronic inflammatory demyelinating polyneuropathy, and others.

Rarely, patients with slowly progressive neuropathy such as hereditary sensory motor neuropathy (e.g., Charcot-Marie-Tooth disease) may not notice their symptoms until later in life.

If significant sensory symptoms present in the upper extremity before they present in the lower extremity, sensory neuronopathy (ganglionopathy) should be considered. Common causes of ataxic neuropathy/ganglionopathy include chemotherapy (e.g., vincristine and cisplatin), cobalamin deficiency, pyridoxine (vitamin B6) overdose or deficiency, Sjögren's syndrome, paraproteinemia, and subacute sensory neuropathy, which may be autoimmune or paraneoplastic.[20]

Diurnal variation should alert clinicians to investigate neuromuscular junction disorders, given a relevant clinical context such as facial and/or proximal muscle weakness.

Long-standing diabetes mellitus, which is highly prevalent in older adults, is one of the most common etiologies of "dying back" length-dependent symmetrical neuropathy. Information on any history of systemic disease (e.g., chronic kidney disease, HIV infection, and history of cancer) is valuable for the differential diagnosis, as it may be directly or indirectly attributable (e.g., increasing the risk of peripheral neuropathy) to impaired mobility. Multiple comorbidities are common in the older adult population, which often complicates the picture. Medications should be reviewed with an emphasis on the temporal relationship between the medication and the onset of symptoms. It is important to recognize the typical neuromuscular dysfunction pattern and to evaluate its impact on mobility in association with individual medications (Table 6.1).

Gross deformity (atrophy of the muscle and joint deformity) may indicate significant muscle weakness and secondary imbalance of the agonist/antagonist muscles, which suggests the underlying specific peripheral neuropathy including:

- claw toe deformity secondary to the earlier involvement of foot intrinsic muscles with better preserved foot extrinsic muscles in length-dependent peripheral neuropathy;
- pes cavus with forefoot varus secondary to peroneus brevis/tibialis anterior weakness with better preserved peroneus longus/tibialis posterior muscles.

Development of a tight gastrocnemius with ankle plantarflexion contracture (ankle equinus) is more common in the aging population than most clinicians realize and is highly prevalent in patients with peripheral neuropathy (37.2% vs. 15.3% in a group without peripheral neuropathy).[22] A positive Silfverskiold test involving a loss of ankle dorsiflexion of more than 13 degrees during knee extension from knee flexion indicates gastrocnemius tightness.[23] Palpation of the cutaneous nerve with or without pain along the course of the nerve (Valleix's phenomenon)[24] can be a valuable technique to identify the location of pathology for focal/regional neuropathic pain and can also be useful in nerve conduction studies. Clinicians should be aware of the distant source of neuropathic pain in the distal lower extremity (e.g., saphenous nerve lesion in the knee causing medial ankle and foot pain or soleal tunnel syndrome causing pain in the sole of the foot).

An abnormal gait pattern should be noted as the patient walks in. The posture, speed of gait, asymmetry, and width and length of the steps should be observed, often multiple times in both the frontal (front and behind) and sagittal planes (from the side). In addition, various mobility tests including standing with eye closed, tandem stance/gait, standing on one leg, and heel-and-toe walking can elucidate the degree of mobility impairment and the underlying etiologies.

Neurologic examination including sensory, motor, and deep tendon reflexes is particularly important to diagnose peripheral neuropathy and to delineate its type and severity. Observation of fasciculation and myokymia, although not sufficient to make the diagnosis by itself, can offer useful clues to certain PNSDs. Sensory examination should include modalities mediated by large nerve fibers, such as light touch, proprioception, and vibration thresholds.[25] Vibration thresholds (in the high frequency range) in the distal lower extremity normally decrease with aging, whereas proprioception and light touch decrease to a lesser extent.[26,27] Semiquantitative measurement of vibration sensitivity with a graduated tuning fork (Rydel and Seiffer) can be used as a screening tool with available reference ranges based on age (cutoff of 4.0 [0–8 scale, 0 indicating inability to feel vibration] in ages 41–60 years and 3.5 in ages 61–85).[28,29] However, sensory examination can be challenging because of the variability of perception and reporting from patient to patient. In addition, the cranial nerves/upper motor neuron syndrome, cognition, and cardiopulmonary examinations are important for differential diagnosis and to evaluate any concomitant lesions. Further examination can be conducted based on the clinical impression from the history taking.

Diagnostic Workup for PNSD

The diagnostic study is an extension of the history and physical examination. Based on the clinical impression that is formed, several diagnostic tests can be considered to confirm the diagnosis, evaluate the severity, and elucidate the underlying etiologies. Diagnostic tests should

TABLE 6.1 Medications Implicated in Neuromuscular Dysfunction		
Neuromuscular Dysfunction	**Categories**	**Common Medications**
Peripheral neuropathy	Sensory neuropathy/ neuronopathy	Pyridoxine (vitamin B6) Cisplatin, oxaliplatin, ixabepilone Hydralazine Metronidazole, chloramphenicol, ethambutol Taxol and Taxotere (occasionally sensory and motor neuropathy)
	Sensory and motor	Indomethacin Nitrofurantoin, penicillamine, isoniazid Perhexiline Gold Disulfiram Thalidomide TNF-α antagonists (can cause multifocal motor neuropathy as well)
	Predominantly motor	Dapsone Imipramine Certain sulfonamides
Myopathy		Statin, clofibrate Zidovudine (AZT), daptomycin Imatinib, cyclosporin Emetine Corticosteroid (affecting neuromuscular transmission as well)
Myopathy and neuropathy (myoneuropathy)		Colchicine, amiodarone, chloroquine, penicillamine, phenytoin, and vincristine
Neuromuscular transmission disorder		Aminoglycoside antibiotics, tetracycline, polymyxin, penicillamine Lithium, phenothiazines Magnesium-containing cathartics Procainamide, quinidine/quinine

Data from Weimer LH. Update on medication-induced peripheral neuropathy. *Curr Neurol Neurosci Rep*. 2009;9(1):69–75, Vilholm OJ, Christensen AA, Zedan AH, Itani M. Drug-induced peripheral neuropathy. *Basic Clin Pharmacol Toxicol*. 2014;115(2):185–192, Jones JD, Kirsch HL, Wortmann RL, Pillinger MH. The causes of drug-induced muscle toxicity. *Curr Opin Rheumatol*. 2014;26(6):697–703, Grisold W, Grisold A. Neuromuscular issues in systemic disease. *Curr Neurol Neurosci Rep*. 2015;15(7):48, and Krarup-Hansen A, Helweg-Larsen S, Schmalbruch H, Rørth M, Krarup C. Neuronal involvement in cisplatin neuropathy: prospective clinical and neurophysiological studies. *Brain*. 2007;130(4):1076–1088.

not delay the initial management plan unless there are red flags for serious diagnoses or the nature of the treatment is invasive. Clinicians should be aware of the high prevalence of abnormal imaging findings in asymptomatic older adults, and therefore the findings should be interpreted in the context of the clinical presentation.

Electrodiagnosis

Edx is a useful test to evaluate the peripheral nervous system including anterior horn cells and the distal segments, as well as to evaluate neuromuscular transmission and muscle disorders. As an extension of the history and physical examination, testing and interpretations should be conducted in the clinical context. Edx can confirm the clinical diagnosis and delineate the extent of peripheral neuropathy. It is particularly useful in evaluating subtle motor weakness and fatigue; providing anatomical localization of these motor deficits to root, plexus, peripheral nerve, neuromuscular junction, or muscle pathologies; and in further classifying the lesions as axonal, demyelinating, or combined.

It is important to understand the following limitations of the routine Edx:
- Evaluation of isolated smaller fibers (autonomic nervous system and pain).
- Mild focal proximal lesion or focal proximal sensory lesion (e.g., sensory radiculopathy or mild

plexus/root lesion only involving a focal myelin segment).

- Sensory nerve conduction study in the lower limb in older patients: often unobtainable in an asymptomatic person.

Edx can be useful in the evaluation of ataxia mediated by large sensory fiber dysfunction rather than postural instability secondary to autonomic neuropathy. A normal sensory nerve conduction study of the lower extremities in older adults is useful, as it is against the diagnosis of significant peripheral neuropathy involving large sensory fibers. In addition, the differential diagnosis can be narrowed down to motor system involvement (motor units) or a central nervous system lesion. Motor nerve conduction studies can be useful in localizing focal demyelinating lesions with the findings of a conduction block or conduction slowing across the lesion. Motor nerve conduction slowing/blockage can occur secondary to local entrapment neuropathy (such as the peroneal nerve at the fibular head or the tibial nerve at the tarsal tunnel), multifocal motor neuropathy, or other demyelinating neuropathy (such as chronic inflammatory demyelinating neuropathy or Lewis-Sumner syndrome).[30] The duration and recruitment pattern of motor units can assist in the differentiation of neuropathic (long duration and reduced recruitment pattern) and myopathic (short duration and increased recruitment pattern) processes, with some exceptions (e.g., mixed pattern in IBM or other chronic myopathy or a myopathic pattern in severe/advanced neuropathic disease). Repetitive nerve stimulation (low and high rate) can be useful in the evaluation of neuromuscular transmission disorder with a variability of motor units on needle electromyography (EMG). The amplitude of the combined motor action potential and the motor units (e.g., discrete recruitment pattern or only distant motor units) on needle EMG also provides information on the lesion severity and limited prognostic information. Needle EMG is limited to the evaluation of myopathies that involve type 2 fibers (such as steroid-induced myopathy).

Laboratory test
Common serologic tests to evaluate the etiologies of peripheral neuropathy include blood glucose level, complete blood count, chemistry, urine analysis, thyroid function test, serum and urine protein electrophoresis, erythrocyte sedimentation rate and C-reactive protein for diabetes mellitus, end-stage renal disease, thyroid dysfunction, paraproteinemia (monoclonal gammopathy), inflammatory disease, cancer, etc.

Creatine kinase elevation is common in several myopathies but is often not specific.[31]

Based on the clinical and Edx evaluation, the following additional tests can be ordered:

- Anti-Hu (antineuronal nuclear) Ab, anti-CV2 (collapsin response mediator protein-5), amphiphysin Ab test for paraneoplastic neuropathy.[32]
- Anti-MAG Ab, GM1 Ab, and other gangliosides antibody tests for demyelinating neuropathy.
- HIV Ab test for HIV-associated neuropathy.[33]
- Enzyme-linked immunosorbent assay, IgM, or IgG immunoblots for Lyme disease–related peripheral neuropathy.[34]
- Anti-GQ1b and anti-GAD antibody test for Miller Fisher syndrome.[35]
- Rheumatologic panels for specific rheumatologic disorder.
- Muscle biopsy for certain myopathies.
- Genetic tests in hereditary disorders.

In this stage of the diagnostic workup, appropriate referral to a neuromuscular specialist should occur to permit a more comprehensive evaluation.

Imaging study
In contrast to the essential role of imaging in central nervous system disorders, imaging has been underused in the evaluation of peripheral neuropathy.[36] With the increasing availability of in-office high-resolution ultrasonography, quick and reliable imaging of the peripheral nerve trunks and some branches is possible, with the advantage of wide coverage (particularly useful for multifocal lesions) and dynamic examination. In addition, muscle pathologies (fatty infiltration with denervation, atrophy), underlying structural pathologies surrounding the peripheral nerves, and concomitant musculoskeletal disorders can be evaluated. Magnetic resonance imaging (MRI) is more advantageous for the evaluation of deeply situated or bone-encased nervous structures and offers better soft tissue characterization. MRI techniques that are optimized for nerve imaging include MR neurography, diffusion tractography, and the use of higher-strength magnets. Typically, ultrasonography can be used as a screening tool to detect nervous pathologies as a complement to Edx when it is available, and then MRI can be used when ultrasonography is restricted because of technical limitations.[37]

Rehabilitation Management of Peripheral Neuropathy
Management of peripheral neuropathy focuses on the symptomatic management of clinical manifestations,

as a primary cure is not feasible for most peripheral neuropathies.[38] In some neuropathies, systemic immunomodulation with intravenous immunoglobulin or immunosuppressant medication is effective; therefore, it is important to identify the peripheral neuropathies such as chronic inflammatory demyelinating polyneuropathy, the acute phase of Guillain-Barre syndrome, multifocal motor neuropathy, exacerbated myasthenia gravis, and steroid-resistant inflammatory myopathy[39] and to refer the patient to a neuromuscular specialist.

Rehabilitation includes therapeutic exercise such as strengthening and stretching exercises, evaluation of orthotics, and pain management. Stretching of tight muscles with range-of-motion exercises is commonly used to decrease discomfort and increase joint mobility, and patients should be instructed to perform them at least a few times daily.[40] Early weight-bearing and the early introduction of gait training, even in a patient with severe neuromuscular dysfunction, are essential to achieving optimal rehabilitation outcomes. The early introduction of power wheelchairs and scooters should be discouraged. Gentle, low-impact aerobic exercises, such as walking, swimming, and stationary bicycling, improve cardiovascular performance, increase muscle efficiency, and reduce fatigue. Moderate-resistance exercise (defined by repetitions at <30% of a 1-repetition maximum) can be applied to muscles with antigravity strength and more. High-resistance training does not offer added benefit over moderate-resistance training, and because it can lead to the adverse effect of overwork weakness, it is discouraged. Low-intensity resistance exercise may be indicated if the patient's muscle strength is equal to or lower than the antigravity strength.

Orthotics that are commonly used to improve mobility in patients with peripheral neuropathy include ankle-foot orthotics (AFO), such as posterior leaf spring orthotics (PLSO), to assist ankle dorsiflexion. If the patient needs bilateral orthoses, some ankle joint range should be allowed using articulated AFO or PLSO. Articulated AFO with plantarflexion stop or dorsiflexion stop features may be preferred if partial knee control is desired (e.g., cases of knee recurvatum, knee buckling, or tight gastrocnemius muscle). As a tight shoe can aggravate the pain, the patient should be advised to opt for a roomier shoe. Accommodative devices such as a quarter-inch heel lifts may be helpful for the patients with signs of a tight gastrocnemius-related painful foot condition. Metatarsal pain may be remedied by adding soft metatarsal pads in the roomier footwear. Donut-shaped pads can be applied to alleviate the focal cutaneous nerve irritation from the shoe in addition to using two layers of socks and the roomier footwear.

Symptomatic treatment for neuropathic pain can include gabapentin, pregabalin (calcium channel $\alpha2$ ligand blocker), amitriptyline (tricyclic antidepressant), duloxetine and venlafaxine (selective serotonin-norepinephrine reuptake inhibitors), and others.[41] Clinicians should be well aware of the adverse effects of these medications, and doses should be increased gradually. Opioid analgesics should be reserved for patients who fail both first-line treatment and nonpharmacologic management.[42]

PERIPHERAL VASCULAR DISORDERS
Peripheral Arterial Disease
Peripheral arterial disease (PAD) is most commonly caused by atherosclerosis with progressive obstruction of the arteries by plaque. Other less common etiologies include inflammatory disorders of the arterial walls (vasculitis) or noninflammatory arteriopathies such as fibromuscular dysplasia.[43] The prevalence of PAD is 11%–16% in the population aged 55 years or older. Atherosclerotic PAD is associated with high rates of cardiovascular events and death. Risk factors for PAD are similar to the risk factors for atherosclerosis, with smoking and diabetes being most common. The overall 5-year mortality rate for PAD patients is approximately 15%–30%, more than 75% of which is attributable to cardiovascular causes.[44]

Mobility disability related to peripheral arterial disease
PAD is associated with mobility impairment including poorer standing balance, slower walking speed, and decreased walking distance.[45] Mobility impairment is often associated with feelings of social isolation, a sense of inadequacy, and a perception of being a burden to friends and family in patients with PAD.[46]

History and physical examination
Claudication is one of the most common presenting symptoms accompanying mobility impairment secondary to PAD and/or spinal stenosis. Claudication can be classified into vascular or neurogenic depending on the underlying etiology, with different characteristics (Table 6.2).

Atypical leg pain and a subtle functional decline without leg pain (perhaps the most common) are not uncommon; therefore, clinical suspicion of PAD is critical in patients with unexplained functional decline and impaired mobility. Of those with

TABLE 6.2
Characteristics of Vascular Versus Neurogenic Claudication

	Vascular Claudication	Neurogenic Claudication
Pain type	Tightness, cramping	Vague cramping, aching, burning
Pain location/radiation	Back, buttock, leg, radiation from proximal to distal	Commonly in calf but can be in the ankle or foot, buttock No proximal to distal radiation
Unilateral versus bilateral	Unilateral	Often bilateral
Distance to walk to trigger pain	Fixed	Variable
Triggered/aggravated by	Increased vascular demand/inadequate vascular supply	Lumbar extension/lateral flexion (sitting)
Relieved by	Rest (immediately after stop walking)	Lumbar flexion (lingering pain)
Time to pain relief	Rapid/immediately after stopping walking	Variable, often prolonged
Effect of walking on pain	Pain occurs after fixed amount of exertion	Pain after variable amount of exertion
Walking uphill versus downhill	Symptoms aggravated by walking uphill	Symptoms aggravated by walking downhill
Neurologic examination	Normal	May be abnormal (often subtle and asymmetric)
Pulses	Diminished	Normal

claudication, 20%–25% experience further clinical deterioration over time. However, major amputation is rare and only 1%–3% of patients with intermittent claudication require major amputation in a 5-year period. In the event of severely compromised arterial flow (critical limb ischemia), the patient presents with foot pain at rest that may worsen in the supine position and improve with the leg in a dependent position.

Medical history provides useful clues for the diagnosis. For example, a history of cardiovascular disorders (smoking, hypertension, dyslipidemia, diabetes, etc.) increases the risk of PAD by two to six times, whereas its absence decreases the likelihood of atherosclerotic peripheral arterial disorders.[45]

Undressing a patient is important for the inspection of trophic changes (hair loss, atrophic nail changes), erythema, hyperemia, pallor, and/or wounds (ulcer typically on the toes or on the lateral malleolus), although some of the findings could be observed in older adults without PAD. Elevating the leg immediately followed by lowering the leg can aid differentiating hyperemia (Buerger's sign: hyperemia when the leg is dependent) versus persistent erythema depending on the position of the leg. Palpation of the peripheral pulses (iliac, femoral, popliteal, dorsal pedal, and tibialis posterior arteries) can be challenging but also

helpful to localize the site of stenosis or other vascular pathologies such as aneurysm. Limb temperature can also be measured. A full cardiovascular examination is recommended to identify comorbid cardiovascular disease.

Diagnostic workup
The ankle-brachial index (ABI) is the most commonly used screening test for PAD. The ABI is calculated by the ankle systolic pressure (the higher value of the dorsalis pedis or tibialis posterior artery systolic blood pressure) divided by the brachial systolic pressure with the following interpretation:
- ABI < 0.9: abnormal
- ABI of 0.7–0.89: mild PAD
- ABI of 0.4–0.69: moderate PAD
- ABI of <0.4: severe PAD
- ABI > 1.3: calcified or noncompressible vessels (in patients with diabetes or chronic kidney disease)

Other noninvasive physiologic tests include segmental limb pressures and pulse volume recordings, Doppler tracing, and arterial duplex. Transcutaneous oximetry is used to assess tissue oxygenation in patients with severe PAD to evaluate the healing potential of ischemic wounds.

Computed tomography angiography (CTA) and magnetic resonance angiography (MRA) are highly sensitive and specific tools for PAD. Radiation exposure in CTA, contraindication with some metallic foreign bodies, and the risk of nephrogenic systemic fibrosis in advanced kidney disease in MRA may limit their use. The gold standard imaging study is digital subtraction arteriography; owing to its superior spatial resolution over CTA and MRA, it is often used during endovascular revascularization.

Rehabilitation management of peripheral arterial disease

Modification of risk factors should be implemented immediately. Smoking cessation reduces the progression of PAD to critical limb ischemia in addition to reducing the risk of myocardial infarction and death from vascular causes.[47] Blood pressure management, optimal glucose control, and the lowering of low-density lipoprotein cholesterol are critical in patients with hypertension, diabetes mellitus, or dyslipidemia. Antiplatelet agents such as aspirin (75–325 mg/day) and/or clopidogrel (75 mg/day) are used to decrease cardiovascular risk.

Exercise training is an effective intervention for patients with claudication.[48] The typical exercise protocol includes specific treadmill walking three to five times a week for 3–6 months, with reported improvements in walking distance of 35%–200%. This protocol includes treadmill exercise to elicit a moderate degree of claudication followed by a brief period of rest to resolve the claudication symptom with repetition. Alternatively, a bicycle ergometer can be used. Warming up and cooling down before and after each session is strongly recommended.[49]

Pharmacologic treatment to improve functional capacity[50] includes cilostazol (100 mg, twice daily), a phosphodiesterase inhibitor that was shown to enable modest improvement in walking distance by approximately 25% in the short term. Use of a lipid-lowering agent, atorvastatin (80 mg daily for 12 months), was shown to improve the pain-free walking time but did not result in an increased maximal walking time.[43] Revascularization is rarely indicated for patients with claudication and is reserved only for patients who fail conservative management, patients who have a reasonable likelihood of symptom improvement, or patients with critical limb ischemia. Revascularization strategies should be individualized based on the location of the lesion, anatomical factors, and patients' general medical conditions and preference. Common surgical procedures include endarterectomy for localized disease, but bypass graft is more commonly performed. Endovascular procedures with angioplasty and stenting

are preferred before the surgery if anatomically feasible (aortoiliac disease).

Venous System Disorders

Common chronic venous disorders include varicose veins and chronic venous insufficiency (CVI). CVI is a clinical spectrum ranging from cosmetic problems and edema to severe symptoms including persistent pain and ulceration caused by persistent venous hypertension.[51,52] While varicose veins represent the most common venous disorder, CVI has a more significant impact on mobility in older adults and is generally underrecognized by healthcare providers despite its increasing prevalence.[53,54] Approximately 7 million people in the United States have CVI.[55] Although the underlying mechanism of CVI is not clearly understood, the disorder includes dysfunction of the calf and other lower-limb muscle pump mechanisms leading to impaired venous return, the development of venous hypertension, and distension of capillary walls, eventually leading to insufficient venous valves and the destruction and obstruction of the venous system.

The pumping action of venous blood back to the heart requires well-functioning calf muscles. Calf muscle dysfunction is associated with decreased range of motion of the ankle and often with neuropathy.[56] Calf muscle dysfunction may affect independent mobility[57] in addition to contributing to venous insufficiency. Risk factors include age, sex, obesity, pregnancy, phlebitis, previous leg injury, and a family history of varicose veins.

Clinical presentation

Symptoms of CVI include swelling, restlessness, limb heaviness, fatigue, aching pain, throbbing sensation, burning, tingling, and nocturnal leg cramps.[58] On physical examination, varicose veins, hyperpigmentation (deposits of hemosiderin), stasis dermatitis, atrophic blanche (white scarring at the site of previous ulcerations with a paucity of capillaries), or lipodermatosclerosis can be observed with or without tenderness.

Differential diagnoses of calf pain and tenderness include:
- Deep vein thrombosis
- Arterial ischemic claudication
- Ruptured Baker's cyst
- Radiculopathy
- Tight gastrocnemius

Edema, typically pitting (or less pitting "brawny edema" with a long-standing course), should be assessed, and the limb girth should be measured. A tourniquet test can be done to determine the distribution of venous insufficiency (superficial, deep, or both). In superficial venous insufficiency, the varicose vein will remain collapsed when the patient sits up after the vein is emptied, and a tourniquet is applied in the Trendelenburg position. In deep (or combined) insufficiency, varicose veins will appear.

The diagnosis is largely clinical and based on history and physical examination, but duplex ultrasonography can be used to detect the direction of blood flow and to assess venous reflux and possible venous obstruction. CT and MRI are rarely used to evaluate the proximal veins or neighboring structures for obstruction.[59]

Management

Management includes lifestyle changes including weight loss, leg elevation, and below-knee compressive stocking. Graded compressive stockings at 20 mm Hg (proximally) to 30 mm Hg (distally) alleviate pain and edema. They work best when the patient is ambulatory owing to dynamic stiffness and pressure changes generated by the shift in leg circumference during walking.[60] Higher pressure (30–40 or 40–50 mm Hg) may be indicated in more severe venous insufficiency or with venous ulcers. In addition, compressive stockings provide lower leg cutaneous stimulation, which may improve proprioception and postural stability.[61,62] The use of compression stockings can be challenging in older adults owing to the difficulty of applying them. The Unna boot is a very useful option for the initial management of venous insufficiency. The Unna boot is a special gauze bandage impregnated with glycerine, water, and zinc oxide.[63] Semirigid characteristics make the Unna boot an effective modality to control pain and pitting edema without restricting mobility. Neither of the compressive therapies should be used in patients with active infection until the infection is controlled, and they must be used with caution in patients with congestive heart failure. If there is suspicion of concurrent PAD, noninvasive arterial testing is recommended before compressive therapy. Diuretics and micronized purified flavonoid fractions (diosmin) can be used as an adjunct to compressive therapy in patients with CVI.

CONCLUSION

Symptoms of PNSD and PVD are often perceived by the elderly and their families as part of "getting old." Early recognition and management of PNSD and PVD is important to maximize independence of older adults. High level of suspicion, focused history, and physical examinations are keys for accurate diagnoses. Diagnostic tests are often used to confirm and further localize the pathologies. Successful management of PNSDs and PVDs requires a multidisciplinary approach including modification of risk factors, patient education, therapeutic exercises, home exercise program, and pharmacologic management.

REFERENCES

1. Vasunilashorn S, Coppin AK, Patel KV, et al. Use of the short physical performance battery score to predict loss of ability to walk 400 meters: analysis from the InCHIANTI study. *J Gerontol A Biol Sci Med Sci.* 2009;64(2):223–229.
2. Chung J, Demiris G, Thompson HJ. Instruments to assess mobility limitation in community-dwelling older adults: a systematic review. *J Aging Phys Act.* 2015;23(2):298–313.
3. Iezzoni LI, McCarthy EP, Davis RB, Siebens H. Mobility difficulties are not only a problem of old age. *J Gen Intern Med.* 2001;16(4):235–243.
4. Guralnik JM, Ferrucci L, Simonsick EM, Salive ME, Wallace RB. Lower-extremity function in persons over the age of 70 years as a predictor of subsequent disability. *N Engl J Med.* 1995;332(9):556–561.
5. Kelly-Hayes M, Jette AM, Wolf PA, D'Agostino RB, Odell PM. Functional limitations and disability among elders in the Framingham Study. *Am J Public Health.* 1992;82(6):841–845.
6. van Schie CH. Neuropathy: mobility and quality of life. *Diabetes Metab Res Rev.* 2008;24(suppl 1):S45–S51.
7. Jahn K, Zwergal A, Schniepp R. Gait disturbances in old age: classification, diagnosis, and treatment from a neurological perspective. *Dtsch Ärzteblatt Int.* 2010;107(17):306–316.
8. Ward RE, Caserotti P, Cauley JA, et al. Mobility-related consequences of reduced lower-extremity peripheral nerve function with age: a systematic review. *Aging Dis.* 2016;7(4):466–478.
9. Iezzoni LI, McCarthy EP, Davis RB, Siebens H. Mobility problems and perceptions of disability by self-respondents and proxy respondents. *Med Care.* 2000;38(10):1051–1057.
10. Andrews AW, Chinworth SA, Bourassa M, Garvin M, Benton D, Tanner S. Update on distance and velocity requirements for community ambulation. *J Geriatr Phys Ther.* 2010;33(3):128–134.
11. Gregg EW, Sorlie P, Paulose-Ram R, et al. Prevalence of lower-extremity disease in the US adult population ≥40 years of age with and without diabetes: 1999-2000 national health and nutrition examination survey. *Diabetes Care.* 2004;27(7):1591–1597.
12. Monticelli ML, Beghi E. Chronic symmetric polyneuropathy in the elderly. A field screening investigation in two regions of Italy: background and methods of assessment. The Italian General Practitioner Study Group (IGPSG). *Neuroepidemiology.* 1993;12(2):96–105.
13. Verghese J, Bieri PL, Gellido C, Schaumburg HH, Herskovitz S. Peripheral neuropathy in young-old and old-old patients. *Muscle Nerve.* 2001;24(11):1476–1481.

14. Iwere RB, Hewitt J. Myopathy in older people receiving statin therapy: a systematic review and meta-analysis. *Br J Clin Pharmacol*. 2015;80(3):363–371.

15. Dimachkie MM, Barohn RJ. Inclusion body myositis. *Curr Neurol Neurosci Rep*. 2013;13(1):321.

16. Benveniste O, Guiguet M, Freebody J, et al. Long-term observational study of sporadic inclusion body myositis. *Brain*. 2011;134(Pt 11):3176–3184.

17. Bhardwaj S, Selvarajah S, Schneider EB. Muscular effects of statins in the elderly female: a review. *Clin Interv Aging*. 2013;8:47–59.

18. Ward RE, Boudreau RM, Caserotti P, et al. Sensory and motor peripheral nerve function and incident mobility disability. *J Am Geriatr Soc*. 2014;62(12):2273–2279.

19. Gwathmey KG. Sensory neuronopathies. *Muscle Nerve*. 2016;53(1):8–19.

20. Viswanathan A, Sudarsky L. Balance and gait problems in the elderly. In: Vinken PJ, Bruyn GW, eds. *Handbook of Clinical Neurology*. vol. 103. ; 2012:623–634.

21. O'Connor AB. Neuropathic pain: quality-of-life impact, costs and cost effectiveness of therapy. *Pharmacoeconomics*. 2009;27(2):95–112.

22. Frykberg RG, Bowen J, Hall J, Tallis A, Tierney E, Freeman D. Prevalence of equinus in diabetic versus nondiabetic patients. *J Am Podiatr Med Assoc*. 2012;102(2):84–88.

23. Barouk P, Barouk LS. Clinical diagnosis of gastrocnemius tightness. *Foot Ankle Clin*. 2014;19(4):659–667.

24. Cimino WR. Tarsal tunnel syndrome: review of the literature. *Foot Ankle*. 1990;11(1):47–52.

25. Vinik AI. Clinical practice. Diabetic sensory and motor neuropathy. *N Engl J Med*. 2016;374(15):1455–1464.

26. Benassi G, D'Alessandro R, Gallassi R, Morreale A, Lugaresi E. Neurological examination in subjects over 65 years: an epidemiological survey. *Neuroepidemiology*. 1990; 9(1):27–38.

27. Vrancken AF, Kalmijn S, Brugman F, Rinkel GJ, Notermans NC. The meaning of distal sensory loss and absent ankle reflexes in relation to age: a meta-analysis. *J Neurol*. 2006;253(5):578–589.

28. Martina ISJ, van Koningsveld R, Schmitz PIM, van der Meché FGA, van Doorn PA. Measuring vibration threshold with a graduated tuning fork in normal aging and in patients with polyneuropathy. *J Neurol Neurosurg Psychiatry*. 1998;65(5):743–747.

29. Pestronk A, Florence J, Levine T, et al. Sensory exam with a quantitative tuning fork: rapid, sensitive and predictive of SNAP amplitude. *Neurology*. 2004;62(3):461–464.

30. Van Asseldonk JT, Franssen H, Van den Berg-Vos RM, Wokke JH, Van den Berg LH. Multifocal motor neuropathy. *Lancet Neurol*. 2005;4(5):309–319.

31. Chawla J. Stepwise approach to myopathy in systemic disease. *Front Neurol*. 2011;2:49.

32. Sharp L, Vernino S. Paraneoplastic neuromuscular disorders. *Muscle Nerve*. 2012;46(6):839–840.

33. Robinson-Papp J, Simpson DM. Neuromuscular diseases associated with HIV-1 infection. *Muscle Nerve*. 2009;40(6):1043–1053.

34. Halperin JJ. Lyme disease and the peripheral nervous system. *Muscle Nerve*. 2003;28(2):133–143.

35. Alexopoulos H, Dalakas MC. Immunology of stiff person syndrome and other GAD-associated neurological disorders. *Expert Rev Clin Immunol*. 2013;9(11):1043–1053.

36. Stoll G, Wilder-Smith E, Bendszus M. Imaging of the peripheral nervous system. In: Vinken PJ, Bruyn GW, eds. *Handbook of Clinical Neurology*. vol. 115. ; 2013:137–153.

37. Chhabra A. Peripheral MR neurography: approach to interpretation. *Neuroimaging Clin N Am*. 2014;24(1):79–89.

38. Carter GT. Rehabilitation management of peripheral neuropathy. *Semin Neurol*. 2005;25(2):229–237.

39. Gilardin L, Bayry J, Kaveri SV. Intravenous immunoglobulin as clinical immune-modulating therapy. *Can Med Assoc J*. 2015;187(4):257–264.

40. Abresch RT, Carter GT, Han JJ, McDonald CM. Exercise in neuromuscular diseases. *Phys Med Rehabil Clin North Am*. 2012;23(3):653–673.

41. Kerstman E, Ahn S, Battu S, Tariq S, Grabois M. Neuropathic pain. *Handbook of clinical neurology / edited by PJ Vinken and GW Bruyn*. 2013;110.

42. Baron R, Binder A, Wasner G. Neuropathic pain: diagnosis, pathophysiological mechanisms, and treatment. *Lancet Neurol*. 2010;9(8):807–819.

43. Kullo IJ, Rooke TW. Peripheral artery disease. *N Engl J Med*. 2016;374(9):861–871.

44. Hirsch AT, Haskal ZJ, Hertzer NR, et al. ACC/AHA 2005 practice guidelines for the management of patients with peripheral arterial disease (lower extremity, renal, mesenteric, and abdominal aortic): a collaborative report from the American Association for Vascular Surgery/Society for Vascular Surgery, Society for Cardiovascular Angiography and Interventions, Society for Vascular Medicine and Biology, Society of Interventional Radiology, and the ACC/AHA Task Force on Practice Guidelines (Writing Committee to Develop Guidelines for the Management of Patients with Peripheral Arterial Disease): endorsed by the American Association of Cardiovascular and Pulmonary Rehabilitation; National Heart, Lung, and Blood Institute; Society for Vascular Nursing; TransAtlantic Inter-Society Consensus; and Vascular Disease Foundation. *Circulation*. 2006;113(11):e463–e654.

45. Salameh MJ, Ratchford EV. Update on peripheral arterial disease and claudication rehabilitation. *Phys Med Rehabil Clin North Am*. 2009;20(4):627–656.

46. Treat-Jacobson D, Halverson SL, Ratchford A, Regensteiner JG, Lindquist R, Hirsch AT. A patient-derived perspective of health-related quality of life with peripheral arterial disease. *J Nurs Scholarsh*. 2002;34(1):55–60.

47. Aronow WS. Peripheral arterial disease in the elderly. *Clin Interv Aging*. 2007;2(4):645–654.

48. Stewart KJ, Hiatt WR, Regensteiner JG, Hirsch AT. Exercise training for claudication. *N Engl J Med*. 2002;347(24):1941–1951.

49. Falcone RA, Hirsch AT, Regensteiner JG, et al. Peripheral arterial disease rehabilitation: a review. *J Cardiopulm Rehabil*. 2003;23(3):170–175.

50. Ouriel K. Peripheral arterial disease. *Lancet.* 2001;358 (9289):1257–1264.

51. Eberhardt RT, Raffetto JD. Chronic venous insufficiency. *Circulation.* 2014;130(4):333–346.

52. Raju S, Neglen P. Clinical practice. Chronic venous insufficiency and varicose veins. *N Engl J Med.* 2009;360(22): 2319–2327.

53. Heit JA. Epidemiology of venous thromboembolism. *Nat Rev Cardiol.* 2015;12(8):464–474.

54. Eberhardt RT, Raffetto JD. Chronic venous insufficiency. *Circulation.* 2005;111(18):2398–2409.

55. Weingarten MS. State-of-the-art treatment of chronic venous disease. *Clin Infect Dis.* 2001;32(6):949–954.

56. Yim E, Vivas A, Maderal A, Kirsner RS. Neuropathy and ankle mobility abnormalities in patients with chronic venous disease. *JAMA Dermatol.* 2014;150(4):385–389.

57. Newland MR, Patel AR, Prieto L, Boulton AJ, Pacheco M, Kirsner RS. Neuropathy and gait disturbances in patients with venous disease: a pilot study. *Arch Dermatol.* 2009;145(4):485–486.

58. Hamdan A. Management of varicose veins and venous insufficiency. *JAMA.* 2012;308(24):2612–2621.

59. Meissner MH, Gloviczki P, Bergan J, et al. Primary chronic venous disorders. *J Vasc Surg.* 2007;46(6, supplement): S54–S67.

60. Sundaresan S, Migden MR, Silapunt S. Stasis dermatitis: pathophysiology, evaluation, and management. *Am J Clin Dermatol.* 2017;18(3).

61. Espeit L, Pavailler S, Lapole T. Effects of compression stockings on ankle muscle H-reflexes during standing. *Muscle Nerve.* 2017;55(4):596–598.

62. Michael JS, Dogramaci SN, Steel KA, Graham KS. What is the effect of compression garments on a balance task in female athletes? *Gait Posture.* 2014;39(2):804–809.

63. Luz BSR, Araujo CS, Atzingen DANCV, Mendonça ARdA, Mesquita Filho M, de Medeiros ML. Evaluating the effectiveness of the customized Unna boot when treating patients with venous ulcers. *An Bras Dermatol.* 2013;88(1):41–49.

64. Weimer LH. Update on medication-induced peripheral neuropathy. *Curr Neurol Neurosci Rep.* 2009;9(1):69–75.

65. Vilholm OJ, Christensen AA, Zedan AH, Itani M. Drug-induced peripheral neuropathy. *Basic Clin Pharmacol Toxicol.* 2014;115(2):185–192.

66. Jones JD, Kirsch HL, Wortmann RL, Pillinger MH. The causes of drug-induced muscle toxicity. *Curr Opin Rheumatol.* 2014;26(6):697–703.

67. Grisold W, Grisold A. Neuromuscular issues in systemic disease. *Curr Neurol Neurosci Rep.* 2015;15(7):48.

68. Krarup-Hansen A, Helweg-Larsen S, Schmalbruch H, Rørth M, Krarup C. Neuronal involvement in cisplatin neuropathy: prospective clinical and neurophysiological studies. *Brain.* 2007;130(4):1076–1088.

CHAPTER 7

Arthritis and Joint Replacement

PETER J. MOLEY, MD • ERIC K. HOLDER, MD

INTRODUCTION

In this chapter, we present a comprehensive general overview of osteoarthritis with special attention to osteoarthritis as it pertains to the hip. We discuss the epidemiology, etiology, pathogenesis, recommended grading systems, treatment paradigms progressing from "conservative" measures to joint replacement techniques, postoperative care, and surgical outcomes relevant to the hip. The knee joint is often referenced as a point of comparison, as there is frequent overlap in the literature regarding the hip and the knee.

Throughout the chapter, there are references made to the knee interspersed within the main text, as well as high-yield "Knee OA Clinical Pearls" noted separately. Historically, much of our methodology for hip osteoarthritis care has mimicked treatment algorithms formulated based on investigations of the knee. However, as our understanding of hip pathology has advanced, hip osteoarthritis care has developed its own identity. This is a vast and rapidly evolving subject matter. Thus, we hope to provide you with the most pertinent scientific and clinical pearls in an interactive, interesting, and succinct manner.

GENERAL OVERVIEW OF OSTEOARTHRITIS EPIDEMIOLOGY

According to the most recent data from the Centers for Disease Control and Prevention, osteoarthritis affects over 30 million adults in the United States (US).[1] Primary osteoarthritis ranks high among the most common causes of pain and disability in the elderly population. In fact, it is the most common form of arthritis. However, there is pronounced variability among people with regards to the age of onset, disease progression, associated pain, and functional limitations. The underlying cause precipitating the osteoarthritic cascade is also variable. Therefore, it is plausible to think of osteoarthritis as a spectrum of disease of variable phenotypic presentations rather than a singular disease process. Notable risk factors that predispose an individual to osteoarthritis are history of joint injury (posttraumatic), older age, metabolically associated conditions (obesity), genetics, gender, and iatrogenic (postsurgical) and anatomic factors. As a point of reference, we discuss the roles each of these risk factors play in the development of hip osteoarthritis.

PATHOGENESIS OF OSTEOARTHRITIS

Historically, osteoarthritis has been dismissed as a normal and expected component of the natural course of aging. Frequently, it is colloquially referred to simply as "wear and tear," falling under the category of degenerative joint disease. However, with an increased interest in reducing morbidity and adding life to years and not simply years to life in an aging population, there has been considerable research dedicated to furthering our understanding of not only the factors that predispose to osteoarthritis but also the actual underlying pathophysiologic mechanisms that drive joint tissue destruction in osteoarthritis. With our ever-evolving knowledge and understanding of the pathogenesis of osteoarthritis, it has become clear that it is a complex, sophisticated process, and simply referring to it as "wear and tear" is quite the understatement.

Inflammation and Primary Osteoarthritis

There are several factors that contribute to the pathogenesis of osteoarthritis, and it is now well established that proinflammatory mediators play an important role. The interplay among proinflammatory mediators, proteases, and biomechanical factors is an active area of investigation.[2] Traditionally, an inflammatory arthropathy is diagnosed in part by the leukocyte count within the affected joint tissue and synovial fluid. In this sense, classic cellular inflammation is not a significant feature of osteoarthritis.[2] Generally, the leukocyte count found within an osteoarthritic joint aspirate is low and rarely surpasses 2000 white blood cells per milliliter.[2] However, in the inflammatory arthropathies (i.e., rheumatoid arthritis, ankylosing spondylitis), it is generally expected that the leukocyte count of synovial fluid aspirate will exceed 2000 white blood cells per milliliter.[2] There may be cases where the synovial inflammatory cell count is equivocal, and the importance of a comprehensive clinical history and diagnostic evaluation cannot be understated in determining the primary arthritic process. A discussion of the inflammatory arthropathies is beyond the scope of this chapter, and our discussion remains focused on osteoarthritis.

To understand the inflammatory component of osteoarthritis, we must look at the molecular level, where there is a fascinating interplay between cytokines and chemokines acting as proinflammatory mediators[2,3] (Box 7.1). These proinflammatory mediators play an integral role in the signaling pathway that leads to the activation of proteolytic enzymes (proteases). Once activated, these proteases function to break down the extracellular matrix joint tissue.[2,4] Although this is still an area of active investigation, it is postulated that excessive force or abnormal joint contact leads to an innate immune response, whereby the joint tissue upregulates proinflammatory factors and proteases further mediating destruction.[2–4]

When signaled by activated proinflammatory mediators, proteases begin the process of hydrolytic degradation of cartilage extracellular matrix proteins. Several proteases have been implicated, including serine proteases, cysteine proteases (i.e., cathepsin K), and matrix metalloproteinases (MMPs).[9] Specifically, ADAMTS-4 (adistintegrin and metalloproteinase with thrombospondin motifs) and ADAMTS-5, and MMP-13 play a significant role in the breakdown of aggrecan and type II collagen, respectively.[9,10] Aggrecan (also known as cartilage-specific proteoglycan core protein or chondroitin sulfate proteoglycan 1) is a large, high-molecular-weight proteoglycan that plays a crucial role in cartilage function and resiliency.[2] Type II collagen is the most abundant collagen found in cartilage. As one can imagine, there is considerable interest in formulating disease-modifying therapies targeted at inhibiting the activation of proteases that degrade aggrecan and type II collagen.[2,10]

Individual Joint Components and Primary Osteoarthritis

The order in which joint tissue undergoes destructive changes is variable and is determined in a large part by the predisposing etiology. The primary generators for the development of osteoarthritis may be compartmentalized into:

1. Age associated,
2. Injury induced (posttraumatic),
3. Iatrogenic (postsurgical),

BOX 7.1

Potential Proinflammatory Mediators That May Play a Role in the Inflammatory Cascade, Resulting in Osteoarthritis

Proinflammatory Mediators of Investigation

Cytokine interleukin (IL)-1 "catabolin"

Tumor necrosis factor-α

Transforming growth factor-α

IL-6

IL-7

IL-8

Oncostatin M

Growth-related oncogene-α

Chemokine (C—C motif) ligand (CCL19)

Macrophage inflammatory protein-1β

Macrophage chemotactic protein-1

Interferon-induced protein-10

Monokine induced by interferon

Alarmins (S100 proteins)

Damage-associated molecular patterns

Complement activation

Data from Loeser RF. *Pathogenesis of Osteoarthritis*. https://www.uptodate.com/contents/pathogenesis-of-osteoarthritis; Liu-Bryan R, Terkeltaub R. Emerging regulators of the inflammatory process in osteoarthritis. *Nat Rev Rheumatol*. 2015;11(1):35–44; Liu-Bryan R, Terkeltaub R. The growing array of innate inflammatory ignition switches in osteoarthritis. *Arthritis Rheum*. 2012;64(7):2055–2058; Loeser RF, Goldring SR, Scanzello CR, Goldring MB. Osteoarthritis: a disease of the joint as an organ. *Arthritis Rheum*. 2012;64(6):1697–1707; Sohn DH, Sokolove J, Sharpe O, et al. Plasma proteins present in osteoarthritic synovial fluid can stimulate cytokine production via Toll-like receptor 4. *Arthritis Res Ther*. 2012;14(1):R7; Little CB, Fosang AJ. Is cartilage matrix breakdown an appropriate therapeutic target in osteoarthritis–insights from studies of aggrecan and collagen proteolysis? *Curr Drug Targets*. 2010;11(5):561–575; and Wang Q, Rozelle AL, Lepus CM, et al. Identification of a central role for complement in osteoarthritis. *Nat Med*. 2011;17(12):1674–1679.

4. Metabolically associated (obesity), and
5. Anatomically or genetically predisposed.

There is often frequent overlap among these categories. Regardless of the underlying etiology, as osteoarthritis progresses to end stage, it affects the entire joint to varying degrees. Thus, it is important that we review the manner in which the osteoarthritic cascade affects each individual component of the joint, including the articular cartilage, synovium, adjacent bone, meniscus, and extraarticular soft tissues.

The joint space articular cartilage is frequently referred to as the "shock absorber," because of its ability to reduce the transference of forces felt by the subchondral components of the joint. Although this may be partially accurate, its primary function is to provide a smooth, articulating surface to allow for the efficient gliding motion of the joint. It is composed of a tightly woven collagen network, which provides tensile strength and contains hydrophilic proteoglycans. Frequently, the earliest evidence of pathoanatomy in osteoarthritis involves the articular cartilage, as noted by fibrillations in focal areas of the joint subject to the greatest load.[2] Once the integrity of the articular cartilage is compromised, the collagen network unwinds on a microscopic level, allowing the influx of water drawn to the hydrophilic proteoglycans; consequently, the cartilage expands.[2] Chondrocytes are the only cell type found within the cartilage and function to maintain the cartilage matrix. When damage to the cartilage occurs, chondrocytes upregulate their activity, and it is believed that some of the cells undergo a phenotypic transformation to a hypertrophic chondrocyte producing type X collagen and proteases, such as MMP-13. The activation of proteases results in further destruction of collagen via a proinflammatory signaling pathway. This results in a destructive feedback loop whereby chondrocyte activity is once again upregulated, leading to the production of more cytokines and proteases.[2]

Synovium is a form of connective tissue that lines the inner capsular surface of diarthrodial joints and is responsible for the production of synovial fluid. Synovial fluid is necessary to maintain a low-friction state within the joint space and acts as a lubricant. Hyaluronic acid (HA) is a component of the synovial fluid that is important for maintaining its viscosity. In the osteoarthritic cascade, most individuals demonstrate some degree of synovial membrane inflammation (synovitis) with or without synovial hypertrophy.[11,12] Synovitis can be quite painful. It may also further the degeneration of cartilage through the production of proinflammatory factors, such as damage-associated molecular patterns.[3,5] However, synovitis is not considered to be the primary instigating factor in osteoarthritis.

The subchondral bone, along with the periarticular musculature, is responsible for bearing most of the joint load. When excessive shear and load are placed upon the subchondral bone, thickening (bony sclerosis) develops as a result of the enhanced production of improperly mineralized collagen[2] (Fig. 7.1). In addition, bone spurs (osteophytes) develop at joint margins (Fig. 7.2A and B). These osteophytes frequently develop at the insertion

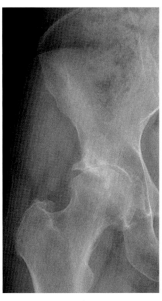

FIG. 7.1 Anteroposterior (AP) right hip with crest view. Demonstrates osteoarthritic changes notable for bone-on-bone apposition in the right hip. There is subchondral sclerosis and cystic changes. Of note, osseous structures about the right hip are relatively osteoporotic, attributed in part to disuse.

points of various muscles, tendons, and ligaments. In advanced disease, bony cysts may also be visualized, although bony erosions would be an atypical finding in primary osteoarthritis. In addition, with advanced imaging modalities such as magnetic resonance imaging, bony marrow lesions indicative of localized bony edema, necrosis, and fibrosis are often visualized in areas subjected to the greatest mechanical stress.[2,13]

Additional soft tissue structures that are important to discuss include the menisci (knee), labrum (hip), ligaments, joint capsule, periarticular muscles, and nerves. Each of these structures plays an important role in maintaining the stability and promoting proper joint mechanics in the hip and knee. In addition to the subchondral bone and periarticular musculature, the menisci play a prominent load-bearing role in the knee. It has long been established that physiologic biomechanical loading is required for joint tissue homeostasis. In the elderly population, it is common for tears to be visualized within the surrounding ligaments, labrum, and menisci, often without a prior known traumatic event. Meniscal tears can be an origin for proinflammatory mediators[14] and an obvious source of mechanical instability, igniting the degenerative

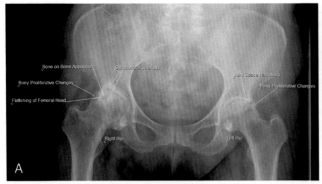
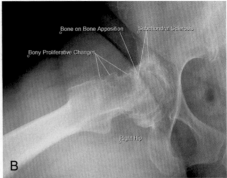

FIG. 7.2 **(A)** AP pelvis with crest and **(B)** elongated frog-leg lateral right hip view. Severe hip osteoarthritis, right greater than left. There is flattening of the superolateral aspect of the right femoral head attributed to chronic impaction with subchondral sclerosis and lucencies. There are bony proliferative changes (osteophytes) lateral to both acetabulae.

osteoarthritic cascade. Similarly, labral tears, muscle imbalances, muscle weakness, or nerve injury can result in instability, which greatly alters the joint biomechanical homeostasis, thus generating enhanced shear stress and load and igniting the osteoarthritic cascade.

Now that we have created a solid foundational understanding of osteoarthritis, we will take a closer look at osteoarthritis and its management as it pertains to the hip (*and knee*) (Fig. 7.3A and B).

HIP OSTEOARTHRITIS
Epidemiology
The estimated overall prevalence of radiographic hip osteoarthritis in persons 45 years or older is 27.6%, of which 9.7% of individuals are estimated to be symptomatic.[15] Generally, women are affected more so than men.[1,15] The reported prevalence of hip osteoarthritis in the literature varies greatly depending on the characteristics of the cohort and the definition of osteoarthritis applied (self-reported, radiologic, or clinical criteria).[16] There is almost a 10% lifetime risk of undergoing a total hip replacement for advanced osteoarthritis.[17,18] Within the US from 1992 to 2011, the rate of total hip replacements increased by 119% from 139.9 to 306.6 per 100,000 persons.[19] In 2009, the estimated costs as a result of hospital expenditures for total hip replacements in the US were $13.7 billion.[20] With rapidly evolving advances in medical care and a trend toward increasing life expectancy, it is inevitable that the prevalence of surgery in middle-aged to elderly adults with hip osteoarthritis will only continue to increase. Dr. Michael Leunig and Dr. Reinhold Ganz, renowned orthopedic experts in hip surgery, wisely stated the

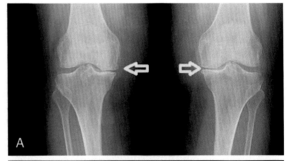
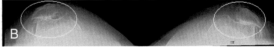

FIG. 7.3 **(A)** AP view of bilateral knees demonstrating osteoarthritis preferentially affecting the medial compartments with loss of the normal valgus alignment (yellow arrows). **(B)** Merchant view of bilateral knees. Circles demonstrate severe bilateral patellofemoral osteoarthritis.

following in their editorial comments regarding the 2014 International Hip Society Proceedings: "Total hip replacement is currently one of the most successful procedures surgeons perform. While this operation works well for patients 65 years of age and older, patients under the age of 50 do not appear to do as well. Avoiding, or at least delaying, the occurrence of osteoarthritis in the younger age group could make a substantial difference in the lives of our younger patients."[21] The role of the musculoskeletal specialist in identifying those patients who would be best served by joint replacement is crucial to optimizing surgical outcomes and healthcare expenditure.

Knee OA Clinical Pearl: In 2009, there were 620,192 US hospital discharges associated with total knee joint replacements, corresponding to $28.5 billion dollars in expenditures. From 2000 to 2006, total knee replacement procedures performed increased by 58%, from 5.5 to 8.7 procedures performed per 1000 Medicare beneficiaries.[20]

Anatomy and Biomechanics of the Hip

Thus far, we have discussed the basic anatomic makeup of a diarthrodial joint, the pathogenesis of osteoarthritis, and its effects on each individual joint component. Now, we further describe the intraarticular and extraarticular components of the hip and their biomechanical function. Through the "layered concept/approach," we illustrate an algorithmic approach to understanding functional hip anatomy.[22]

The four-layer approach was originally described by Kelly et al. as a systematic means of discerning which hip-related structures are the source of pathology and/or pain.[22] It was fundamentally formatted as a means to investigate the young, painful, nonarthritic hip, which historically has been figuratively regarded as a black box, proving to be a diagnostic quandary, even for the astute clinician. Although this approach was not originally described as an assessment tool for the less diagnostically perplexing elderly osteoarthritic hip, it remains a useful paradigm for methodically evaluating the hip, regardless of age or pathology. It involves compartmentalizing functional hip anatomy into osteochondral, inert, contractile, and neuromechanical layers.

Layer I is the osteochondral layer, which is formed by the pelvis, acetabulum, and femur. In the normal hip, this layer demonstrates normal joint congruence and normal osteoarticular kinematics, which is greatly altered in the osteoarthritic hip.[22] Abnormalities within this layer have been classified into three categories: static overload, dynamic impingement, and dynamic instability. Several factors may result in static overload, including anterior or lateral acetabular undercoverage (dysplasia), femoral anteversion, or femoral valgus.[22] Dynamic impingement may result from femoroacetabular impingement (FAI), femoral retroversion, or femoral varus. Dynamic instability may occur when the functional range-of-motion demands exceed the normal motion parameters, resulting in the potential for subluxation and intraarticular joint damage.

Layer II is described as the "inert" layer and is composed of the labrum, joint capsule, ligamentous complex, and ligamentum teres.[22] These structures work in

cohort to maintain the static stability of the hip joint. If the static stability of the joint is compromised, further degeneration is likely to occur, eventually inciting the osteoarthritic cascade.

Layer III is described as the "contractile" layer of the hip and hemipelvis.[22] This layer is composed of the entire hemipelvis musculature, which extends from the lumbosacral musculature to the pelvic floor. Through muscular balance, layer III is responsible for promoting dynamic stability of not only the hip but also the pelvis and trunk. Likewise, loss of hip motion, as seen in osteoarthritis, may hinder motion throughout the entire kinetic chain, predisposing to injury elsewhere.

Layer IV is described as the "neurokinetic" layer and is composed of the thoracolumbar plexus, lumbopelvic tissue, and lower extremity structures.[22] This layer provides innervation to most of the hemipelvis musculature, facilitates neuromechanical control and feedback, initiates physiologic muscular activation patterns, and controls neuromuscular proprioception. In addition, this layer is crucial to orienting posture and position of the pelvis over the femur. It is of upmost importance to understand how the constituents of the osseous, inert, contractile, and neuromechanical layers work in unison to promote normal hip mechanics. Clearly, if there is an insult to any one of the four layers that is not addressed in an appropriate and timely manner, it is only a matter of time before the degenerative cascade begins and osteoarthritis ensues. We next investigate the effects of hip joint pathomorphologies.

Hip Joint Pathomorphologies

In our general overview of osteoarthritis, we described the theoretical interplay between supraphysiologic forces caused by abnormal joint contact that result in an innate immune response, whereby joint tissue upregulates proinflammatory factors and proteases that further mediate destruction. This is an area of active investigation. It is fair to say that the literature regarding the hip is rapidly evolving. It was once believed that most hip osteoarthritis were idiopathic. In the last 15–20 years, we have made tremendous strides in understanding hip osteoarthritis and its link with subtle developmental hip pathomorphologies that result in prearthritic hip disease and eventually osteoarthritis.[17,23,24]

The two areas of particular interest are FAI and developmental dysplasia of the hip (DDH). Developmental hip conditions, such as slipped capital femoral epiphysis and Legg-Calve-Perthes disease, have also been linked to FAI morphology but are believed to make up a small minority of hips with FAI.[17] It is not yet well understood why certain individuals with FAI morphology become symptomatic, given that only a fraction of individuals with FAI morphology become symptomatic. It is theorized that symptomatic FAI develops because of labral and chondral injury that occurs secondary to bony impingement.[25,26] Symptoms are often described as groin or buttock pain that is made worse with physical activity and is often associated with loss of end range of hip motion.

Nonoperative and operative hip preservation care has grown exponentially, with the goal being to curtail the onset of the osteoarthritic cascade and the need for hip joint replacement surgery later in life. Hip preservation care has become a subspecialty within orthopedic surgery with great promise. With this knowledge, there is consensus agreement among musculoskeletal practitioners that hip pathomorphology is a dominant player in hip osteoarthritis pathophysiology, supported by thorough, well-studied mechanistic evidence.[23,24]

Femoroacetabular impingement syndrome

The notion of hip "impingement" is not a new phenomenon but has actually been described in the literature dating back to at least 1936 by Smith-Petersen.[27,28] In 1965, Murray described a minor anatomic abnormality, which he termed the "tilt deformity."[24,29,30] He described the tilt deformity as a medial angulation of the femoral head in relation to the femoral neck and illustrated an association with the later development of osteoarthritis of the hip.[29,30] The insightful findings of Murray inspired many, and further investigation into this theory was championed by the likes of Harris and colleagues in the US and Solomon and colleagues in South Africa.[24,31–40] In the early 2000s, Ganz and colleagues described the concept of FAI and its association with osteoarthritis in further detail and also described a new surgical technique to treat the disorder.[28,41,42] The literature provided by Ganz and the incorporation of arthroscopic surgery in the early 2000s resulted in an upsurge of interest in the diagnosis and treatment of FAI and a tremendous growth in the literature.[24,28]

Two types of FAI have been characterized: the cam-type morphology and the pincer-type morphology. However, it is not uncommon to observe combined deformities.[41]

Cam-type morphology. The cam-type morphology is caused by a loss of offset between the head and neck of the femur, resulting in an "outside-in" delamination of the acetabulum.[24] "Offset" refers to the contour of the head-neck junction, which should be concave as opposed to flat or convex (a prominence); this is referred to as a cam-type deformity[28,43] (Fig. 7.4). The loss of

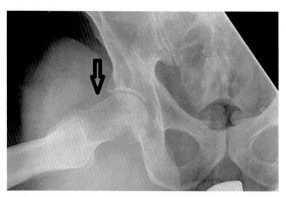

FIG. 7.4 AP pelvis with crest view (reformatted with pelvis cropped). The black arrow demonstrates mild joint space narrowing with bony prominence of the head-neck junction, indicative of cam-type morphology.

femoral neck offset usually occurs anterolaterally. It has been documented that FAI can occur anywhere within the joint, although it tends to occur anterolaterally and is produced by internal rotation of the femur while in flexion.[24] This occurs as a result of abnormal contact between the cam lesion and acetabulum, resulting in cartilage injury. As the area of cartilage injury extends, the femoral head resettles within the defect, resulting in joint space narrowing (JSN). In addition, the cam lesion abuts the anterosuperior labrum of the hip. The summative result is separation of the acetabular cartilage from the labrum and delamination of the acetabular cartilage from the subchondral bone.[17,24,44] Over time, subchondral cysts develop within the femoral head or near the head-neck junction because of the chronic effects of impingement of the femoral head against the acetabulum.[24,45] This deformity tends to be more prevalent in young athletic males.[24,39] Hips with cam FAI tend to fail over time as a result of anterosuperior osteoarthritis.[24]

Pincer-type morphology. The pincer-type morphology describes overcoverage of the femoral head by the acetabulum (Fig. 7.5). This results in linear impact of the acetabular rim against the femoral head-neck junction, which is normal in morphology in an isolated pincer-type deformity. The area of impact tends to be anterior.[24] Unlike the isolated cam lesion, the first structure to fail in the pincer-type deformity tends to be the labrum anterosuperiorly.[24,28,46] Over time, bone apposition develops on the bony rim next to the labrum, extending the margins of the labrum and enhancing the impingement and secondary labral degeneration.[24] Likewise, the acetabular cartilage in

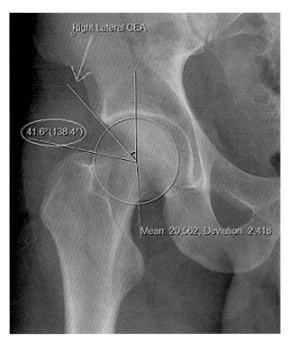

FIG. 7.5 AP pelvis with crest view (reformatted with pelvis cropped). The lateral center-edge angle (also known as the center-edge angle of Wiberg) is used to assess the superolateral coverage of the femoral head by the acetabulum.[43] Values greater than 36 degrees may indicate overcoverage of the femoral head (pincer-type morphology).[47]

proximity to the degenerated labrum begins to break down, and the focal area of impact on the femoral neck undergoes callus formation and ulcerations of the periosteum. Late in the disease, the posteroinferior femoral head cartilage/acetabular cartilage wears down as well, which is referred to as a "contrecoup lesion."[44] This deformity is more often seen in active women between the ages of 30 and 40 years. Hips with pincer FAI tend to fail over time as a result of posteroinferior or central osteoarthritis.[24]

Management of femoroacetabular impingement syndrome. In 2016, an international, multidisciplinary group of experts was convened at the University of Warwick to format a consensus statement on the diagnosis and management of patients with FAI syndrome.[17,28] The panel defined FAI syndrome as a "motion-related clinical disorder of the hip with a triad of symptoms, clinical signs and imaging findings. It represents symptomatic premature contact between the proximal femur and the acetabulum."[17,28] The key point is that symptoms must be present to diagnose FAI syndrome, with the primary symptom being pain, which is often motion or position related.[28,42] In addition, patients with FAI may also report catching, locking, clicking, stiffness, or give-way. Otherwise, isolated pathomorphology in the asymptomatic patient should be referred to as cam or pincer morphology.[17,28]

The appropriate management of the heterogeneous patient population with FAI syndrome requires the availability of all three of these resources.[28]

The goal of treatment for FAI syndrome is to alleviate pain and functional limitations in the short term and to potentially curtail the development or progression of osteoarthritis in the long term. Treatment strategies typically fall into three categories: conservative care, rehabilitation, and surgery.[17,28] It is recommended that joint preserving surgery is considered before the development of hip osteoarthritis or in very mild cases of hip osteoarthritis, as these individuals tend to obtain greater symptomatic benefit from the procedure than those with advanced hip osteoarthritis.[17,53] Although there has been considerable research to date regarding hip preservation care, there is currently no high-level evidence supporting a definitive treatment choice for FAI syndrome[28,48,50] (Table 7.1). There is no definitive evidence that treating individuals with cam or pincer morphology will reduce their risk of developing FAI syndrome or osteoarthritis in the long term. There is sufficient evidence that an association does exist between cam morphology and hip osteoarthritis.[28,54–57] However, whether an association exists between pincer morphology and hip osteoarthritis is not as clearly defined.[28] Lastly, as hip preservation care is still in its infancy, there are no long-term prospective outcome studies to determine whether treatment of FAI syndrome alters the development of osteoarthritis later in life. There are several ongoing randomized clinical trials comparing conservative, rehabilitation, and surgical care options, with study outcomes expected to be published within the next few years.[28]

Developmental dysplasia of the hip
DDH refers to an underdeveloped, shallow, or deformed (that may also be improperly oriented) acetabulum resulting in decreased acetabular coverage of the femoral head[17,40,58,59] (Figs. 7.6 and 7.7). DDH predisposes the labrum and articular cartilage to abnormal contact forces, resulting in early degeneration of the hip. It is recognized as a major cause of osteoarthritis in the young adult. Studies suggest that acetabular dysplasia can lead to secondary osteoarthritis in 25%–50% of patients by the age of 52 years.[40,58,59] The young adult

TABLE 7.1
Conservative, Rehabilitation, or Surgical Approaches for Treating Femoroacetabular Impingement (FAI) Syndrome

Treatment	Purpose	Outcomes
Conservative care	• Patient education • Activity modification • Lifestyle modification • Nonsteroidal antiinflammatory drugs • Intraarticular steroid injection • Close follow-up	• There are no reports of the outcomes that conservative care alone has on symptoms of FAI syndrome[28]
Structured physical therapy program	• Hip stability assessment, treatment, and education • Neuromuscular control • Functional movement pattern assessment and treatment • Lumbosacral range of motion	• Physical therapy components have not been well tested, and there is variation in treatment provided per institution and therapist • Physical therapy may be associated with improvement for at least 2 years[28,48,49]
Surgery (arthroscopic or open)	• Goal is to correct hip morphology to allow for impingement-free motion • Debride cam lesion • Trim and/or reorient acetabulum in pincer lesion. • ±Correct femoral torsion • ±Adjust femoral neck angle • Resect, repair, and reconstruct labrum or cartilage if needed	• More studies have been published regarding surgical outcomes, but there are issues regarding poor design and sample size, and thus risk for bias • Studies indicate that there may be improvement in symptoms for up to at least 5–10 years[28,50–52]

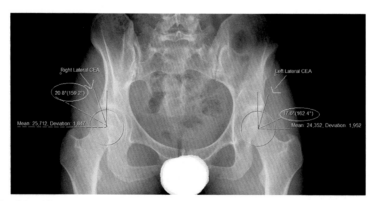

FIG. 7.6 AP pelvis with crests. There is bilateral uncoverage of both femoral heads (dysplasia) with respect to shallow acetabulae. The lateral center-edge angle is used to assess the superolateral coverage of the femoral head by the acetabulum. Values less than 25 degrees may indicate inadequate coverage of the femoral head (dysplasia).[43]

patient often reports pain in the hip region, owing to overload of the acetabular rim (frequently anterosuperiorly), which is referred to as acetabular rim syndrome[17,58] (Fig. 7.8). The patient often describes this pain as sudden, sharp, localized to the groin region associated with mechanical overload, and increasing in severity and frequency over time.[58] The young adult patient with DDH may also report snapping, locking, and clicking, which can be attributed to intraarticular (i.e., labral tear) and extraarticular processes (i.e., snapping psoas tendon). A sensation of instability is also quite common.

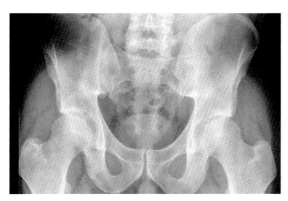

FIG. 7.7 Anteroposterior view of pelvis with crest. There is lateral uncoverage of both femoral heads (dysplasia) with bilateral hip joint space narrowing. In addition, subtle features of underlying cam-type morphology are present. Of note, this patient is 48 years old, and the osteoarthritic cascade has already begun.

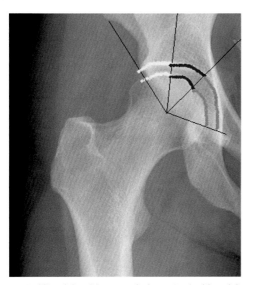

FIG. 7.8 AP pelvis with crests (reformatted with pelvis cropped). Representation of areas of joint space narrowing. Yellow: superior/lateral joint space; blue: axial joint space; orange: medial/inferior joint space. The joint space is well maintained in this image.

As with FAI syndrome, hip-preserving surgical techniques have been formulated to treat DDH. Once the diagnosis of dysplasia is made in the symptomatic patient, it should be determined whether the patient is an appropriate candidate for hip-preserving surgery. The patient should be fully educated on the indications, potential benefits, risks, and literature regarding outcomes. The surgery most commonly recommended to treat this condition is known as Bernese periacetabular osteotomy.[58,60] Patients with no or minimal osteoarthritis are the most appropriate candidates for this surgery, and the goals are to alleviate pain, restore function, and curtail the development or progression of osteoarthritis of the hip.

ASSOCIATED RISK FACTORS FOR HIP OSTEOARTHRITIS

Gender

Female sex has often been conferred as a risk factor for the development of osteoarthritis in other joints, although the relationship between gender and hip osteoarthritis is less clear, with conflicting study results. A large meta-analysis review of nine studies involving more than 14,000 participants determined that there were no significant sex differences in the severity of hip osteoarthritis. There was a higher incidence risk of hip osteoarthritis for women but no significant gender differences for the prevalence of hip osteoarthritis.[61] The Framingham Osteoarthritis Study found a higher prevalence of radiographic hip osteoarthritis in men than in women. However, there was no significant difference in the prevalence of symptomatic hip osteoarthritis in men compared with women.[62]

> **Knee OA Clinical Pearl**: *Studies demonstrate that knee osteoarthritis is significantly more prevalent in women as compared with men.*[16]

Genetics and Ethnicity

Genetic factors have been well established as predisposing factors for the development of hip osteoarthritis. A classic twin study, formulated to determine the genetic contribution to radiographic hip osteoarthritis in women, determined that genetic factors play a significant role in the development of osteoarthritis of the hip in women, accounting for up to 60% of the risk.[63] The heritability estimates reduced slightly when potential confounders such as age, hip bone density, and body mass index (BMI) were considered.[63] As noted previously, FAI has been established as a potential precursor to the development of osteoarthritis. Pollard et al. compared 96 siblings of 64 patients treated for primary impingement with a screening protocol for clinically and radiologic evidence of cam and pincer deformities and osteoarthritis.[64] It was determined that the siblings of patients with a cam deformity had a relative risk of 2.8 of having the same deformity, and the siblings of patients with a pincer deformity had a relative risk of 2.0 of having the same deformity. Likewise, bilateral deformity occurred more often in the siblings compared with controls.[64] Pelt et al. determined that the relative risk of undergoing total hip arthroscopy for osteoarthritis was increased in first-degree, second-degree, and third-degree relatives.[65] One study discussing the genetic epidemiologic scope of hip and knee osteoarthritis reported that the heritable component for primary osteoarthritis may account for 50% of susceptibility. Thus far, at least 18 osteoarthritis-associated genetic loci have been established.[66] Further studies are required to determine the exact genes, genetic mutations, and associated diagnostic biomarkers that are necessary for the accurate screening of osteoarthritis before disease manifestation and the creation of targeted therapeutic disease protocols.[66]

There is believed to be a genetic variation in the prevalence of hip osteoarthritis based on ethnicity. One such example is a study conducted by Nevitt and colleagues comparing the prevalence of osteoarthritis of the hip among elderly persons in the US and China.[67] It was determined that the crude prevalence of radiographic hip osteoarthritis in Chinese adults (60–89 years old) was 0.9% in women and 1.1% in men, and this did not increase with age. Chinese women had a lower age-standardized prevalence of radiographic hip osteoarthritis when compared with Caucasian women, and Chinese men had a lower prevalence of radiographic hip osteoarthritis when compared with age-matched Caucasian men, summating to an 80%–90% less frequent presentation of hip osteoarthritis in Chinese study subjects compared with Caucasian study subjects.[67] In a large community-based cohort study, which included both African Americans (AA) and Caucasians, it was determined that AA and Caucasians exhibited similar baseline frequencies of radiographic hip osteoarthritis, although differences in baseline hip radiographic features were noted.[68] After 6 years of follow-up, AA had increased pain and disability, whereas Caucasians had more radiographic hip osteoarthritis.[68] It was deemed plausible that the worsening of disability in AAs was due to an unmet need for hip osteoarthritis management in this population.

Dietary Factors

The literature regarding the association of dietary factors with osteoarthritis is not definitive, with studies demonstrating conflicting results and lacking high-quality evidence.[17,69] Many vitamins and minerals have been implicated as being potentially protective against the development, progression, or minimization of osteoarthritis. These include vitamins D, K, C, and E and selenium.[17,69–71] For example, vitamin D has been proved to be very important in maintaining bone health and bone metabolism. In a study evaluating serum vitamin D and incident changes of radiographic hip osteoarthritis, it was determined that the risk of incident hip osteoarthritis (defined as definite JSN) was increased for subjects who were in the lowest (8–22 ng/mL) or middle tertiles (23–29 ng/mL) for 25-hydroxy (OH) vitamin D compared with subjects in the highest tertile (30–72 ng/mL).[70] However, vitamin D levels were not associated with the development of definite osteophytes or new disease.[70] A recently published meta-analysis evaluating the relationship between 25-(OH) vitamin D serum levels and osteoarthritis determined that epidemiologic studies do not provide any clear evidence of an independent association between 25-(OH) vitamin D serum levels and hip osteoarthritis.[71] Similar conflicting results have been published regarding the other aforementioned dietary factors.[17,69]

Obesity

It has long been an established mantra within musculoskeletal medicine that obesity is a modifiable risk factor for the development or progression of osteoarthritis, especially in the weight-bearing joints. The evidence in the literature regarding the effects of obesity on hip osteoarthritis is not as clearly defined as the effects of obesity on the development of knee osteoarthritis.[69,72–74] However, the evidence suggests that obesity promotes the development of hip osteoarthritis through both biomechanical factors and an upregulation of proinflammatory mediators.[17] Studies have demonstrated a correlation between BMI and bilateral hip osteoarthritis.[72,75] In one study evaluating 568 women who underwent total hip replacement because of primary osteoarthritis, a higher BMI was associated with an increased risk of hip replacement. Women with a BMI equal to or greater than 35 kg/m^2 had a twofold increased risk of hip replacement owing to osteoarthritis compared with those with a BMI less than 22 kg/m^2.[76] In a large systematic review and meta-analysis evaluating 14 epidemiologic studies, it was determined that BMI was strongly associated with an increase in the risk of hip osteoarthritis, which did not vary by sex, study design, or osteoarthritis definition.[77] Each 5-unit increase in BMI was associated with an 11% increase in the risk of hip osteoarthritis.[77] Contrarily, an epidemiologic study with 10 years' follow-up determined that a high BMI was significantly associated with knee osteoarthritis and hand osteoarthritis but not with hip osteoarthritis.[74] The association between obesity and hip osteoarthritis requires refinement, and further investigation will prove useful in better understanding this association.

> *Knee OA Clinical Pearl: The AAOS Treatment of Osteo-arthritis of the Knee Evidence-Based Guideline, 2nd Edi-tion (2013), recommends weight loss for patients with symptomatic osteoarthritis of the knee and a BMI ≥25 kg/ m²; moderate-level evidence.[78]*

Age

Older age is undeniably one of the strongest risk factors for osteoarthritis in all joints. It is multifactorial and likely related to the cumulative exposure to risk factors and biologic decline, such as cellular senescence, decreasing chondrocyte density resulting in cartilage thinning, weakening perimusculature support and diminishing proprioceptive feedback.[17,69,76,79–82] The net effect is disequilibrium between joint synthesis and degradation, promoting the osteoarthritic cascade.

Occupation

It is believed that frequent high-impact activity through occupation or long-term exposure to high-impact sports predisposes an individual to the development of osteoarthritis of the hip (as well as other joints). The mechanism is due to long-term biomechanical stress resulting in shear forces and enhanced load, igniting the osteoarthritic cascade. Epidemiologic studies have demonstrated a strong correlation between hip osteoarthritis and heavy manual labor.[83–85] A particularly high risk has been documented in farmers.[83,84] A study reviewing the literature cross-referencing hip osteoarthritis and heavy lifting, including farming, construction work, and climbing stairs, concluded that moderate to strong evidence exists for a relationship between heavy lifting and hip osteoarthritis.[84] Specifically, burdens had to be at least 10–20 kg for 10–20 years to demonstrate a definitively increased risk for hip osteoarthritis. It was noted that the risk of hip osteoarthritis doubled after 10 years of farming. However, the evidence of a relationship between hip osteoarthritis and construction workers was limited, and there was insufficient evidence demonstrating a correlation between climbing stairs or ladders and hip osteoarthritis.[84] Similarly, an earlier study demonstrated a direct correlation between hip osteoarthritis and the duration and heaviness of occupational lifting. This study also demonstrated a pattern implicating a causal relationship between frequent stair climbing and hip osteoarthritis.[85]

It has also been noted that athletes participating in high-impact sports have a higher risk of developing hip osteoarthritis. Several mechanisms that generally revolve around two concepts have been proposed. The first concept is that high-impact biomechanical joint loading and shear stress leads to osteoarthritis; a similar mechanism is observed in heavy manual laborers. The second concept relates to the higher prevalence of the cam-type morphology, which may develop during the crucial adolescent years, while osseous development is still occurring and the youth is participating in frequent cutting, rotational, and high-impact activity through sports. It is believed that frequent exposure to these forces through sporting activity during this critical period of development results in a repetitive insult to the proximal femoral physis, resulting in the cam-type morphology.[17,24,29,30,39,86]

Overall, although long-term participation in heavy-duty manual labor or high-impact sports has been shown to predispose a person to hip osteoarthritis, epidemiologic evidence is lacking to support the belief that exercise or physical activity has a detrimental effect on the hip in the general population.[17]

CLINICAL DIAGNOSTIC CRITERIA FOR HIP AND KNEE OSTEOARTHRITIS

In 1981, the American Rheumatism Association (now known as the American College of Rheumatology [ACR]) requested that the Diagnostic and Therapeutic Criteria Committee establish a subcommittee focused on the development of criteria for classification of osteoarthritis.[87] Altman and colleagues published criteria for the classification of osteoarthritis of the knee first in 1986 and subsequently the hip in 1991.[87,88] These studies rank among the most commonly cited articles in the musculoskeletal medical literature and remain relevant. During the initial study of the knee, it was believed that no single set of criteria could satisfy all circumstances to which the criteria for knee osteoarthritis would be applied. Thus, the subcommittee designed distinct sets of classification criteria that can be used depending on the circumstances and tools that the diagnostician has available (Table 7.2). The investigators determined that the presence of osteophytes seemed to best differentiate osteoarthritis from non-osteoarthritis-mediated knee pathology.[87]

In 1991, ACR created the criteria for the classification of osteoarthritis of the hip and determined that clinical criteria without a radiographic evaluation were fairly sensitive but not particularly specific (Table 7.3).[17,88] Notably, reduced internal rotation and hip flexion were of significant clinical importance. Similar to previous studies, pain was noted to be the major symptom in hip osteoarthritis, although the distribution of pain and characteristics of physical activities inducing pain

TABLE 7.2
American Rheumatism Association Criteria for the Classification and Reporting of Knee Osteoarthritis

Clinical + Laboratory	Clinical + Radiographic	ClinicalΦ
Knee pain **and** (at least 5 of 9): • Age >50 years • Stiffness <30 min • Crepitus • Bony enlargement • Bony tenderness • No palpable warmth • ESR <40 mm/h • RF <1:40 • SF OA *92% Sensitive* *75% Specific*	Knee pain, osteophytes, **and** (at least 1 of 3): • Age >50 years • Stiffness <30 min • Crepitus *91% Sensitive* *86% Specific*	Knee pain **and** (at least 3 of 6): • Age >50 years • Stiffness <30 min • Crepitus • Bony enlargement • Bony tenderness • No palpable warmth *95% Sensitive* *69% Specific*

ESR, erythrocyte sedimentation rate; *RF*, rheumatoid factor; *SF OA*, synovial fluid signs of osteoarthritis (clear, viscous, or white blood cell count <2000 cells/mm³); *Φ*, option for clinical category would be 4 of 6, noted to be 84% sensitive and 89% specific.
Adapted from Altman R, Asch E, Bloch D, et al. Development of criteria for the classification and reporting of osteoarthritis. Classification of osteoarthritis of the knee. Diagnostic and Therapeutic Criteria Committee of the American Rheumatism Association. *Arthritis Rheum.* 1986;29(8):1047; with permission.

TABLE 7.3
American College of Rheumatology Criteria for the Classification and Reporting of Hip Osteoarthritis[87]

Clinical Criteria Group I	Clinical Criteria Group II	Clinical + Radiographic Criteria
Hip pain **and** Hip internal rotation <15 degrees **and** ESR ≤45 mm/h (If ESR is not available, replace with hip flexion ≤115 degrees)	Hip pain **and** Hip internal rotation ≥15 degrees **and** Pain on hip internal rotation **and** Morning stiffness of the hip ≤60 min **and** Age >50 years	Hip pain **and** at least two of the features below: ESR <20 mm/h Radiographic femoral and/or acetabular osteophytes Radiographic joint space narrowing (superior, axial, and/or medial)

ESR, erythrocyte sedimentation rate.

were inconsistent among patients with hip osteoarthritis and did not differ significantly from patients with hip pain from other causes.[87] Among radiographic features, it was determined that osteophytes were the feature that best delineated patients with hip osteoarthritis from those with hip pain due to other causes.[87]

GRADING OSTEOARTHRITIS OF THE HIP AND KNEE

Several grading systems have been generated to describe the severity of osteoarthritis based on radiologic criteria. Hip osteoarthritis is often evaluated by overall global visual qualitative assessment tools[89–91] or by analyzing the joint space width (JSW)[90,92–95] (Tables 7.4–7.5; Box 7.2; Table 7.6). Most commonly, the Tönnis and Heinecke classification system and Kellgren and Lawrence classification are used to grade hip osteoarthritis,

TABLE 7.4
Tönnis and Heinecke Classification

Grade	Characteristics
0	No signs of osteoarthritis
1	Slight narrowing of joint space, slight lipping at joint margin, slight sclerosis of femoral head or acetabulum
2	Small cysts in femoral head or acetabulum, increasing narrowing of joint spine, moderate loss of sphericity of femoral head
3	Large cysts, severe narrowing or obliteration of joint space, severe deformity of femoral head, avascular necrosis

From Tönnis D, Heinecke A. Acetabular and femoral anteversion: relationship with osteoarthritis of the hip. *J Bone Joint Surg Am.* 1999;81(12):1747–1770; with permission.

TABLE 7.5
Kellgren and Lawrence Classification

Grade	Characteristics
None (0)	Definite absence of x-ray changes of osteoarthrosis
Doubtful (1)	Doubtful joint space narrowing (JSN) and possible osteophytic lipping
Minimal (2)	Definite osteophytes and possible JSN on anteroposterior weight bearing radiograph
Moderate (3)	Multiple osteophytes, definite JSN, sclerosis, possible bony deformity
Severe (4)	Large osteophytes, marked JSN, severe sclerosis, and definite bony deformity

Originally studied as a grading tool for the hand, wrist, spine, hip, and knee. Currently, it is more commonly used to grade osteoarthritis of the hip and knee.
Data from Kellgren JH, Lawrence JS. Radiological assessment of osteo-arthrosis. *Ann Rheum Dis*. 1957;16(4):494–502s and O'Brien WM. In: Lawrence JS, ed. *Rheumatism in Populations*. London: William Heinemann Medical Books; 1977:572 pp. *Arthritis Rheum*. 1978;21(3):398.

BOX 7.2
Radiologic Indices of Hip Osteoarthritis Compared by Croft et al. to Determine the Best Definition of the Disease for Epidemiologic Purposes

Lateral joint space

Superior joint space

Medial joint space

Minimal joint space

Maximum thickness of subchondral sclerosis

Size of the largest osteophyte

Overall qualitative assessment (**Refer to** Table 7.6)

From Croft P, Cooper C, Wickham C, et al. Defining osteoarthritis of the hip for epidemiologic studies. *Am J Epidemiol*. 1990;132(3):514–522; with permission.

TABLE 7.6
Overall Qualitative Assessment Tool for Hip Osteoarthritis Formatted by Croft et al.

Grade 0	No changes of osteoarthritis
Grade 1	Osteophytosis only
Grade 2	Joint space narrowing (JSN) only
Grade 3	Two of osteophytosis, JSN, subchondral sclerosis, and cyst formation
Grade 4	Three of osteophytosis, JSN, subchondral sclerosis, and cyst formation
Grade 5	As in grade 4, but with deformity of the femoral head

From Croft P, Cooper C, Wickham C, et al. Defining osteoarthritis of the hip for epidemiologic studies. *Am J Epidemiol*. 1990;132(3):514–522; with permission.

whereas knee osteoarthritis is most commonly graded with the Kellgren and Lawrence classification system (Tables 7.3–7.5). Regardless of the grading assessment tool, it is important that intraobserver and interobserver agreement is maintained. Often within an institution, it is recommended that all musculoskeletal practitioners are trained to use the same grading system, so that there is strong intraobserver and interobserver reliability. The

global visual assessment tools have been criticized for being somewhat subjective with nebulous distinctions between grades that are often open to the interpretation of the examiner.

In the often cited 1990 Croft et al. study, the authors compared seven radiologic indices of hip osteoarthritis in an effort to determine the best definition of the disease for epidemiologic purposes (Box 7.2; Table 7.6). In a subset of 759 men, minimal joint space and thickness of the subchondral sclerosis were the radiologic characteristics that were most predicative of hip pain.[90] Minimal joint space is defined as the shortest distance from the margin of the femoral head to the acetabulum.[90] Lastly, Croft et al. concluded that "minimal joint space is a simple, repeatable index of osteoarthritis of the hip which relates to other radiologic features of the disease and to symptoms and is suitable for use in epidemiologic studies. None of the other radiologic indices that we examined performed as well by these criteria"[90] (Box 7.2). Thus, minimal joint space demonstrated the best intraobserver and interobserver repeatability. A major limitation of this study was that it included only men, aged 60–75 years old.[90]

In 2004, Jacobsen et al. conducted a large cohort study of 3807 subjects (1448 men and 2359 women) and determined that the average minimum JSW was narrower in women than in men.[95] In addition, they determined that regardless of sex, the minimum JSW decreased after the fourth decade of life, but even more so in women.[95] Lastly, when the cutoff value of 2.0 mm for JSW was used, regardless of other radiologic features of osteoarthritis, the prevalence of hip osteoarthritis ranged from 4.4% to 5.3% in participants older than

60 years, and a minimum JSW less than 2.0 mm held the strongest association with self-reported hip pain.[95] In a study comparing the minimum JSW method, Kellgren and Lawrence grading system, and Croft grading system, Terjesen et al. determined that the minimum JSW method (defined in this study as less than 2.0 mm) was the simplest, most reliable, and reproducible classification when grading hip osteoarthritis in patients with DDH.[93]

In everyday practice, there is often discordance between symptoms and imaging findings. It is not uncommon for patients with evidence of osteoarthritis by radiologic criteria to be asymptomatic and for patients complaining of joint pain to lack radiologic evidence of osteoarthritis.[96] Thus, a fundamental understanding of the anatomy and biomechanics of the hip, along with the clinical and radiographic diagnostic criteria, is crucial to direct care. Lastly, it is worth mentioning that magnetic resonance imaging is more helpful than radiographs for detecting early structural changes of osteoarthritis.

CARING FOR THE ELDERLY OSTEOARTHRITIC HIP AND KNEE JOINT

Osteoarthritis in the elderly is an onerous burden for the elderly patient who was once highly functional, active, and independent. Thus, the perceptive practitioner should be aware of the physical and psychological encumbrance this places on the elderly patient seeking his/her counsel. A crucial part of the clinical evaluation should be focused on assessing for confounding psychosocial factors, including mood disorders, sleep disturbances, family, relationship, or employment stressors. A comprehensive, holistic approach to managing the patient should be formatted, taking into account the patient's comorbidities, social support, activities of daily living, and functional goals.

Historically, clinical guidelines for the management of hip and knee osteoarthritis have been combined, attributable to a lack of research specific to the hip. The literature specific to knee osteoarthritis has been more robust, possibly because of the higher prevalence of knee osteoarthritis and greater ease with which the knee joint can be evaluated and accessed for clinical interventions.[17,97,98] Although there is overlap, based on our discussion of the spectral pathogenesis of osteoarthritis and pathomorphologies specific to the hip, it is clear that this generalized grouping of care is fundamentally flawed. As eloquently stated by Hunter and

colleagues, "This is despite the growing consensus that osteoarthritis is not a single disease affecting the joints, but rather a number of distinct conditions, each with unique etiological factors and possible treatments, which share a common final pathway."[17]

Patient Education on Osteoarthritis

A crucial component of the treatment algorithm for elderly patients with osteoarthritis is to lay the groundwork through patient education. Considerable effort should be made to explain the underlying pathology causing their symptoms through an individualized patient-centered approach using concise and easy-to-understand terminology. There are several different delivery modes that can be used, including a discussion with the physician or physical therapist involved in the patient's care, written handouts, self-management programs, support groups, and approved websites.[16,99] It is important that the patient plays an active rather a passive role in the care plan, incorporating a shared decision-making paradigm based on preferences and goals. The current standard of care for patients with symptomatic osteoarthritis involves activity and lifestyle modifications, assistive devices as deemed appropriate, physical therapy, oral and topical medications, and intraarticular injections. If the symptoms remain refractory to conservative measures, then surgical intervention may be necessary.[16,17,53,69,99]

Activity and Lifestyle Modification

The conservative management of osteoarthritis is aimed at preserving the remaining joint integrity, providing pain relief and maintaining the patient's overall functionality. With that being stated, weight loss and exercise have long been considered as cornerstone pillars in the nonpharmacologic management of joint osteoarthritis.[16,17,69,97–104] Weight loss is generally recommended for those with lower limb osteoarthritis who are classified as overweight or obese by a BMI criteria of $>25 \, kg/m^2$.[16,97,100] Historically, the recommendations regarding the benefits of weight loss and exercise for osteoarthritis have been based on research dedicated to the knee and have been assumed to be adaptable to the hip.[16,98,99] In general, the research on conservative care of patients with hip osteoarthritis is lacking high-quality evidence.[16,97–104]

However, as one may intuitively expect, the recent literature demonstrates preliminary evidence that improvements in self-reported physical function and pain of overweight or obese patients with hip osteoarthritis can be achieved through the combination of exercise, weight loss, and dietary modifications.[99] However, this study is considered preliminary, and there are no randomized trials of weight loss interventions in individuals with hip osteoarthritis.[16] Similarly, although exercise is widely recommended in guidelines for the treatment of hip osteoarthritis, the studies are limited and demonstrate a small to moderate benefit in minimizing pain and improving function. In contrast, the literature for the knee is more robust and convincing.[16,17,99,102–104]

A randomized study evaluated the efficacy of exercise therapy and patient education versus patient education alone (control) on the 6-year survival of the mild to moderate symptomatic osteoarthritic hip.[104] Patients ($n = 109$) were randomized evenly to exercise/patient education and control groups (patient education). It was determined that only 22 of 55 patients in the exercise/patient education group compared with 31 of 54 patients in the patient education group underwent total hip replacement. The median time to total hip replacement was 3.5 years in the control group versus 5.4 years in the exercise/patient education group. There were no significant differences in pain or stiffness between groups, although the exercise therapy group reported better hip function before the end of the study or before undergoing total hip replacement. The author noted that this could indicate that hip function may play a bigger role than hip pain in delaying the need to undergo total hip replacement.[104] The exercise therapy program was designed specifically for individuals with hip osteoarthritis and involved supervised sessions at least once weekly for 3 months, as well as home exercises 2–3 times a week. However, along with other limitations, no data were obtained on the continuation of the exercise therapy program after 12 weeks.[104]

Further investigation is necessary to conclusively determine the long-term effects of exercise and weight loss as conservative measures for managing hip osteoarthritis and postponing hip replacement.[99] Further specifications regarding the type, frequency, mode of delivery (i.e., land or aqua based), and length of exercise regimens are required.[16] Regardless, the Ottawa Panel guidelines recommend that weight loss in overweight or obese patients should be considered before instituting weight-bearing exercises to avoid further joint destruction.[16,101] Overall, it is recommended that the exercise, dietary, and weight loss programs should be specific to the unique requirements of each patient.

Physical Therapy Program

An integral part of the care paradigm for the osteoarthritic hip or knee is the determination of the utility of enrolling a patient in a physical therapy program to enhance function and overall well-being. Aerobic and strengthening exercises are the most frequently reported interventions in the nonoperative management of hip or knee osteoarthritis.[98,105] A structured therapy program in the geriatric patient with hip or knee osteoarthritis is of particular importance, as comorbidities frequently play a confounding role in adherence and tolerance to exercise. In addition, the challenge of formulating a therapy program to stimulate improvements in pain, stiffness, and functionality without inducing pain and motivating the patient to maintain long-term adherence to the program can prove to be formidable.

Surprisingly, before 2010, it has been argued that no exercise programs formatted specifically for hip osteoarthritis were found in the literature.[98] A targeted assessment of the patient's range of motion, strength, endurance, motor control, and function should be completed during the initial clinical encounter before prescribing a physical therapy program.[106,107] In general, a target therapeutic exercise program for hip or knee osteoarthritis should include warm-up, strength training, functional exercises, and flexibility/stretching. The frequency, total number of visits, and participatory precautions should be noted, along with the patients' comorbidities and functional and pain limitations.[98]

The warm-up should be individualized based on the patient but frequently involves light walking on a treadmill or the use of a stationery or recumbent bike. If walking is tolerated, special attention should be paid to the gait mechanics, including symmetry and cadence, with an assessment for improvements with assistive devices if needed. In the warm-up, manual therapy and modalities should be used at the discretion of the physical therapist, based on the individual needs of the patient. Strength training has numerous potential benefits. Case-control studies have demonstrated decreased muscle strength and muscle hypotrophy in patients with hip osteoarthritis.[108,109] As expected, randomized controlled trials have shown benefits from strengthening and functional exercises in both the young and elderly.[98] Strengthening exercises for both the core musculature and the hip periarticular supporting musculature should be incorporated as hip muscle activation during the performance of core exercises.[98,108]

Functional therapeutic exercises that imitate the individualistic demands of the patient's daily activities should also be incorporated. One goal of the therapy program is to increase the degree of difficulty of the functional exercises by adding dynamic movements, reducing the base of support, and/or potentially increasing the range through which a movement is performed.[110] The stretching/flexibility program should involve passive relaxed motions that are mechanically initiated by the physical therapist, as well as patient-initiated active static and dynamic stretches.[98] It is important that the therapist is attune to range-of-motion limitations that are truly musculature and not structural (i.e., hip ball and socket configuration), as this is integral to increasing functional range of motion without exacerbating pain related to underlying osteoarthritis.

There are several caveats that should be mentioned in regards to hip osteoarthritis and physical therapy. First, within the musculoskeletal community, there is some contention as to the value of physical therapy in the management of hip osteoarthritis.[17,111-114] Some investigators have debated that therapy offers minimal benefit beyond that expected of a self-guided exercise program.[17,112] Bennell and colleagues completed a randomized, placebo-controlled, participant-and-assessor-blinded study comparing physical therapy–led management with sham therapy and did not find differences in pain or function between groups.[114] In contrast, several studies have demonstrated an increased survival time of the native hip, improved physical function, and reduced pain in patients receiving exercise therapy.[103,104]

Furthermore, the optimal exercise dosage (i.e., number of exercise sets, repetitions, and duration of each session and therapy program) for patients with hip osteoarthritis is not clear, with limited studies comparing exercise regimen parameters.[112] The current best available evidence from several randomized controlled trials and systematic reviews have demonstrated that manual therapies (i.e., joint manipulation and mobilization techniques, muscle stretching, soft tissue massage) are unlikely to provide any additional benefit as an adjunct treatment to an exercise program in patients with hip and knee osteoarthritis in terms of improving physical function, range of motion, and participant-assessed improvement.[17,111-113] Further high-quality research is required to definitively state which subgroup of patients with hip osteoarthritis will respond best to physical therapy, as well as the optimal therapy approach, timing, frequency, and duration.

> **Knee OA Clinical Pearl:** AAOS Treatment of Osteoarthritis of the Knee Evidence-Based Guideline, 2nd Edition *(2013), strongly recommends that patients with symptomatic knee osteoarthritis participate in self-management programs, strengthening, low-impact aerobic exercises, and neuromuscular education, as well as engage in physical activity consistent with national guidelines. They were unable to provide a recommendation for or against manual therapy or modalities.*[78]

Assistive Devices: The Formidable Cane

The cane is interlaced in the history of mankind. The staff was illustrated in the Egyptian tombs of the Sixth Dynasty (2830 BC).[115] Historically, the cane was a symbol of style and nobility. As the population has aged over time, the cane has become associated with debility and diminished vitality. However, Blount's statements in his sentinel article published in 1956 ("Don't Throw Away The Cane") remain pertinent and valuable. He keenly stated, "Gradually, we are coming to look upon eye glasses, hearing devices, and dentures as welcome aids to gracious living rather than as the stigmata of senility. They should be accepted as components of a richer life. The cane, too, should be restored to favor as a means of preventing fatigue and a halting gait, rather than maligned as a sign of deterioration."[115]

An antalgic (limping) gait, which is often associated with a lurch, is fatiguing, frequently places undo strain on the lumbar spine, and may result in undo pressure on the femoral head (up to four times the body weight), potentiating further deterioration of the hip.[115] The use of a cane in the opposite hand of the arthritic hip (i.e., right hand, left hip) reduces the forces across the hip and decreases the pull required of the ipsilateral hip abductor muscles (i.e., left hip) needed to support the body weight in a single-support (i.e., left leg) stance phase.[115,116] Thus, the cane should be advanced with the affected limb in what is referred to as a three-point gait pattern.[116] A cane is capable of offloading up to 20% of the patient's body weight from the affected limb.[116]

The cane is an effective, supportive device and proprioceptive aid that has the potential to prolong the lifespan of the native osteoarthritic hip while enhancing well-being and functionality. An informed discussion with the patient regarding the utility of the cane should be held, and this discussion should include a realistic assessment of the patient's current limitations, degree of osteoarthritis, pain, comorbidities, and functional goals, as a cane may not be the appropriate adjunct in every case. The goal is to provide the patient with all the information and tools needed to be an active participant in their care plan.

> **Knee OA Clinical Pearl:** AAOS Treatment of Osteo-arthritis of the Knee Evidence-Based Guideline, 2nd Edition (2013), was unable to provide a recommenda-tion for or against a valgus-directing force brace (medial compartment unloader). Similarly, based on moderate evidence, the committee could not suggest that lateral wedge insoles be used for patients with symptomatic medial compartment osteoarthritis of the knee.[78]

Pharmacologic Management

Historically, pharmacologic management of osteoar-thritis has been palliative and focused on symptomatic relief. Alternatively, there have been several disease-mod-ifying osteoarthritic agents that have demonstrated great promise in preclinical trials but unfortunately have not demonstrated the same promise in clinical studies.[17] A brief overview of the more commonly used pharmaco-logic treatments is provided. To date, few trials have been performed in patients with hip osteoarthritis. Often, patients with hip osteoarthritis are treated in a manner similar to patients with knee osteoarthritis.[97]

The authors of this chapter recommend referring to clinical guidelines created by the American Academy of Orthopaedic Surgeons (AAOS), ACR, Osteoarthritis Research Society International, and National Institute for Health and Care Excellence "Osteoarthritis: Care and Management in Adults" for the most up-to-date infor-mation regarding recommendations in osteoarthritis treatment. When considering medical management of patients with osteoarthritis, there is not one singular "cookbook" algorithmic approach to care. Each patient should undergo an individualized assessment based upon the patient's functional level, pain, comorbidities, values, and goals. Thus, the guidelines should be used as a tool and are not intended to be absolute, as there is variability in patient symptoms and responses to treat-ments provided. Please refer to Box 7.3 and Table 7.7 for a summary of the ACR and AAOS recommendations regarding the management of hip osteoarthritis. Please also refer to "Knee OA Clinical Pearls" for a summary of high-yield recommendations regarding the manage-ment of knee osteoarthritis by the ACR and AAOS.

Supplements

"Supplement" is often used interchangeably with "nutraceuticals," which is a term that originated

---

> **BOX 7.3**
> **American College of Rheumatology (ACR) 2012 Recommendations for Pharmacologic Management of Hip Osteoarthritis**
>
> **ACR Pharmacologic Recommendations for Hip Osteoarthritis Management (2012)**
>
> Conditionally recommend the following:
> - Acetaminophen
> - Oral nonsteroidal anti-inflammatory drugs (NSAIDs)
> - Intraarticular corticosteroid injections
> - Tramadol
>
> Conditionally do *NOT* recommend the following:
> - Chondroitin sulfate
> - Glucosamine
>
> No recommendations regarding:
> - Topical NSAIDs
> - Intraarticular hyaluronate injections
> - Duloxetine
> - Opioid analgesics
>
> Please note that these are the most current published recommendations by the ACR and are based on the evi-dence available through the end of 2010. Please refer to the ACR website (http://www.rheumatology.org/) peri-odically for any revisions or updates. The information in this table may predate many of the studies referenced within this chapter.

Adapted from Hochberg MC, Altman RD, April KT, et al. Ameri-can College of Rheumatology 2012 recommendations for the use of nonpharmacologic and pharmacologic therapies in osteoar-thritis of the hand, hip, and knee. *Arthritis Care Res (Hoboken)*. 2012;64(4):471; with permission.

---

from "nutrition" and "pharmaceutical" and essentially describes "a food that has health benefits including the prevention and/or treatment of a disease."[117] Frequently described supplements for osteoarthritis include glu-cosamine sulfate, chondroitin, diacerein, avocado, soybean unsaponifiables, and turmeric.[17,117–119] The literature regarding the efficacy of these supplements in the treatment of osteoarthritis is highly heteroge-neous, in part because of variations in study param-eters, sponsorship bias, lack of adequate long-term follow-up time, and the subjectivity of measuring pain as a primary outcome. However, based on the body of literature, it is fair to say that there is no definitive evidence that supplements alter the natural progression of osteoarthritis. However, they generally have a low side-effect profile and are well tolerated. In certain cases, some of the supplements have dem-onstrated benefit in reducing pain and enhancing function.[118]

TABLE 7.7

Excerpts of Recommendations From the 2017 American Academy of Orthopaedic Surgeons (AAOS) Management of Osteoarthritis of the Hip Evidence-Based Clinical Practice Guidelines

AAOS Evidence-Based Clinical Practice Guideline for Management of Osteoarthritis of the Hip (2017)	Recommendations
Nonnarcotic management	**Strong** evidence **supports** nonsteroidal anti-inflammatory drugs in improving short-term pain, function, or both in patients with symptomatic osteoarthritis of the hip
Glucosamine sulfate	**Moderate** evidence **does not support** the use of glucosamine sulfate because it does not perform better than placebo for improving function, reducing stiffness, and decreasing pain for patients with symptomatic osteoarthritis of the hip
Intraarticular corticosteroids	**Strong** evidence **supports** the use of intraarticular corticosteroids to improve function and reduce pain in the short term for patients with symptomatic osteoarthritis of the hip
Intraarticular hyaluronic acid (HA)	**Strong** evidence **does not support** the use of intraarticular HA because it does not perform better than placebo for function, stiffness, and pain in patients with symptomatic osteoarthritis of the hip
Physical therapy as a conservative treatment	**Strong** evidence **supports** the use of physical therapy as a treatment to improve function and reduce pain for patients with osteoarthritis of the hip and mild to moderate symptoms
Preoperative physical therapy	**Limited** evidence **supports** the use of preoperative physical therapy to improve early function in patients with symptomatic osteoarthritis of the hip following total hip arthroplasty
Special note: biological injectables	There were **no high-quality** randomized controlled trials comparing the performance of intraarticular injections of stem cells or prolotherapy with placebo at the time these guidelines were prepared. Three studies[139–141] compared intraarticular injections of platelet-rich plasma (PRP) with HA or a combination of PRP or HA, but there were no high-quality studies comparing PRP with placebo for inclusion in this analysis

Endorsed by the Pediatric Orthopaedic Society of North America (POSNA), American Physical Therapy Association (APTA), and the American College of Radiology (ACR).

Data from American Academy of Orthopaedic Surgeons Board of Directors. *Management of Osteoarthritis of the Hip: Evidence-Based Clinical Practice Guideline*; 2017. Available at: https://www.aaos.org/uploadedFiles/PreProduction/Quality/Guidelines_and_Reviews/OA%20Hip%20C PG_5.22.17.pdf.

> **Knee OA Clinical Pearl:** The ACR (2012) conditionally recommends that practitioners avoid using nutritional supplements (i.e., chondroitin sulfate, glucosamine).[97] AAOS Treatment of Osteoarthritis of the Knee Evidence-Based Guideline, 2nd Edition (2013), strongly does **not** recommend using glucosamine and chondroitin for patients with symptomatic osteoarthritis of the knee.[78]

Acetaminophen

For safety reasons, guidelines frequently recommend the prescription of acetaminophen as the first-line pharmacologic agent for the treatment of osteoarthritic conditions.[97,120,121] However, this is highly controversial, as several studies have demonstrated limited effects of acetaminophen when compared with placebo in osteoarthritis.[120–124] There is high-quality evidence that acetaminophen has a significant but small short-term benefit in patients with hip or knee osteoarthritis when compared with placebo.[120] Also, high-quality evidence demonstrates that frequent acetaminophen use increases the risk of having abnormal values on liver function tests, although the clinical relevance of this is unclear.[120] The ACR conditionally recommends that patients with hip osteoarthritis use acetaminophen.[97] If acetaminophen is used, the authors of this chapter recommend using the lowest effective dose for the shortest time frame possible for pain relief. As per the US Food and Drug Administration, the maximum daily dose recommended is 4000 mg.[97,120]

Knee OA Clinical Pearl: The ACR (2012) conditionally recommends that practitioners use acetaminophen in patients with symptomatic knee osteoarthritis.[97] AAOS Treatment of Osteoarthritis of the Knee Evidence-Based Guideline, 2nd Edition (2013), was unable to provide recommendations for or against the use of acetaminophen for symptomatic knee osteoarthritis.[78]

Nonsteroidal Antiinflammatory Medications

Nonsteroidal antiinflammatory drugs (NSAIDs) are generally considered to be the main form of treatment for osteoarthritis [(124)]. In the US, approximately 65% of patients with osteoarthritis are prescribed NSAIDs as the pharmacologic agent of choice.[124] NSAIDs have been well studied and validated for the symptomatic relief of osteoarthritis.[17,121-125] However, only certain NSAIDs have consistently demonstrated clinically substantiated benefit in osteoarthritic pain.[124] Regardless, when choosing prescribed NSAIDs, a careful risk versus benefit analysis should be contemplated. In the geriatric population in particular, the patient's comorbidities and current medications should be meticulously evaluated before selecting the NSAID of choice, as there are variations in side-effect profiles. Regardless, in light of the well-established cardiovascular, renal, and gastrointestinal adverse effects of NSAIDs, they should be prescribed only as needed for short, limited time frames using the minimally effective dose with detailed instructions provided to the patient regarding the optimal method of intake (i.e., with food and water). In addition, the patient should be educated on potential side effects of the medication. Lastly, NSAIDs can be administered orally or topically. Topical NSAIDs have been proved to be beneficial in relief of knee osteoarthritis, but there are no recommendations for their use in hip osteoarthritis because of the depth of the hip joint.[17,97,126]

Alternative Oral Agents

In patients who fail to demonstrate an adequate response to initial therapy options, alternative options may be considered. Duloxetine is a centrally acting selective norepinephrine and serotonin reuptake inhibitor that has demonstrated efficacy in osteoarthritis-related knee pain.[127-129] One published study that included a very small subset of patients with hip osteoarthritis along with a much larger cohort of patients with knee osteoarthritis also demonstrated favorable results of duloxetine for the management of chronic pain due to osteoarthritis.[129] Further studies dedicated to evaluating the efficacy of duloxetine in alleviating hip osteoarthritis pain are necessary.

If all other measures fail or are contraindicated, tramadol is a weak opioid that may be considered for judicious use. However, careful evaluation of the side-effect profile should be made and discussed with the patient.[17,97] As noted in the ACR 2012 recommendations, tramadol is considered separate from other opioids because of its central analgesic effect, which "is thought to be mediated not only by a weak opioid receptor agonist effect but also through modulation of serotonin and norepinephrine levels."[129] Opioids are otherwise not generally recommended for the treatment of knee or hip osteoarthritis, as the adverse effects frequently outweigh the benefit in the geriatric population.[17]

Knee OA Clinical Pearl: AAOS Treatment of Osteoarthritis of the Knee Evidence-Based Guideline, 2nd Edition (2013), was unable to provide a recommendation for or against the use of opioids or pain patches for symptomatic knee osteoarthritis.[78]

Intraarticular Injections

Intraarticular injection options for osteoarthritis are an area of much interest because of the direct action within the joint and relative lack of systemic effects.[129-132] Injection options are usually considered in patients who fail to experience relief with nonpharmacologic and oral pharmacologic treatment measures. Often, these patients are not quite yet eligible for a joint replacement because of various factors or are eligible but choose to defer. Regardless, the authors of this chapter recommend that all hip intraarticular injections be performed under either ultrasound or fluoroscopic guidance.

Corticosteroid Injections. International guidelines are in favor of intraarticular steroid injections (IASIs) in the management of hip osteoarthritis, although these recommendations have generally been assumed to be applicable based on studies of knee osteoarthritis.[129] Historically, there have been studies demonstrating the transient efficacy of corticosteroids in knee osteoarthritis, and the ACR guidelines conditionally recommend that healthcare providers use knee IASIs as a treatment option.[96] However, the recent literature regarding the use of IASIs in knee osteoarthritis has been conflicting, raising concerns regarding the risk versus benefit of IASIs for the knee (refer to the following *Knee OA Clinical Pearl* for further details).

A large systematic review of the literature suggested that "hip IASI may be efficacious in delivering short term but clinically significant, pain reduction in those with hip osteoarthritis, and may also lead to transient improvement in function."[129] However, it is important to restate that the number of studies performed in patients with symptomatic hip osteoarthritis are few, and the quality of evidence is relatively poor, with few participants overall in comparison to studies of the knee.[129] Therefore, it is possible to "overestimate treatment effect size or report significant effect when none is present."[129] Once more, in the studies evaluated, most of the participants were awaiting or candidates for total hip replacement, indicating severe end-stage hip osteoarthritis. Thus, these results cannot be generalized to patients with a lesser grade of hip osteoarthritis.[129] Further studies are required to determine the ideal candidates, evaluate the best steroid preparation and dose, and confirm both the efficacy and safety of IASIs in the management of hip osteoarthritis.[129,132]

> **Knee OA Clinical Pearl:** A recent randomized, placebo-controlled, double-blinded 2-year trial of an intraarticular injection of 40 mg triamcinolone every 3 months versus saline for symptomatic knee osteoarthritis with ultrasound features of synovitis was conducted in 140 patients. Intraarticular triamcinolone injections resulted in significantly greater cartilage volume loss than saline, and there was no significant difference in knee pain between groups.[130] These results contradicted a previous smaller, but highly cited, study that found no difference in the rate of radiographic joint space loss with a detected benefit on knee pain.[131] AAOS Treatment of Osteoarthritis of the Knee Evidence-Based Guideline, 2nd Edition (2013), was unable to provide recommendations for or against the use of IASIs for symptomatic knee osteoarthritis.[78]

Hyaluronans. Endogenous hyaluronan (HA, also known as hyaluronic acid) is described as a linear, large glycosaminoglycan found in synovial fluid and is made in the lining layer cells of the joint. It is sequestered from the joint through the lymphatic circulation and is broken down by hepatic endothelial cells.[132] Its primary function is to provide lubrication, viscoelasticity, and tissue hydration. It maintains protein homeostasis by acting as an osmotic buffer, thus preventing large fluid shifts.[132] Commercial HA was first isolated from roosters' combs and umbilical cord tissue in the 1960s for the treatment of arthritis and use in ophthalmic surgery.[132]

The rationale for "viscosupplementation" is to replace the properties lost by a reduction in intrinsic HA production and quality that occurs with osteoarthritis.[132] Although considerable effort has been dedicated to investigating the method by which HA exerts its potential therapeutic benefit, it remains unclear and significant evidence for "restoration of rheological properties is lacking."[132] Simply stated, it is believed that two stages may be involved: an initial mechanical stage and a secondary physiologic stage. The benefit for the initial mechanical stage is believed to be due to the injected HA restoring elastoviscosity, thus providing lubrication and shock-absorbing capabilities of the synovial fluid. The physiologic benefit refers to the longer sustained benefit of injected HA that persists beyond the residence time (hours to days) of HA, which is largely based on preclinical studies.[132] Overall, the literature regarding the efficacy of HA for hip osteoarthritis demonstrates large heterogeneity and is conflicting.[132-137] Currently, clinical guidelines do not recommend HA injections for the management of hip osteoarthritis.[17,97,132,138]

> **Knee OA Clinical Pearl:** The ACR (2012) recommendations regarding the pharmacologic management of knee osteoarthritis state "we have no recommendations regarding the use of intraarticular hyaluronates" (along with duloxetine and opioid analgesics).[97] The AAOS Treatment of Osteoarthritis of the Knee Evidence-Based Guideline, 2nd Edition (2013), could not recommend using HA for patients with symptomatic osteoarthritis of the knee.[78]

Biologic Injectables. The literature regarding the use of cellular-based therapies, such as platelet-rich plasma (PRP) and mesenchymal stem cells (MSCs), to treat hip osteoarthritis is very limited, and it is too early to make any definitive conclusion regarding efficacy and outcomes.[139-142] By comparison, there have been several prospective, randomized controlled clinical studies evaluating biological interventions for knee osteoarthritis and symptom modulation, some of which have shown some benefits.[142-153] However, there is large heterogeneity in treatment protocols, biologic injectate preparation, study length, severity of knee osteoarthritis treated, baseline patient characteristics, control groups used, and primary outcomes measured, making it difficult to formulate a consensus statement.[142-153] As a result, there is no US Food and Drug Administration (FDA)-licensed or FDA-approved biological therapy or procedure that halts the degenerative cascade of osteoarthritic joints.[143] In general, results have demonstrated that PRP use is safe and that bone marrow aspirate concentrate is a safe and feasible source of MSCs.[141-152] Both treatments may have the *potential* to provide symptomatic benefit for osteoarthritis in at least the short term.[142,143]

Further high-quality studies are necessary to determine the optimal patient population, biologic preparation protocols, and mechanism of action before clinical efficacy and cost-effectiveness can be fully recognized.[142,154] An expert consensus statement on the minimum reporting requirements for clinical studies evaluating PRP and MSCs was published in an attempt to address the limitations in reporting of scientific data critical to outcomes and to create more stringent study parameters to improve research regarding biologics.[154]

> **Knee OA Clinical Pearl**: The ACR (2012) guidelines regarding pharmacologic management of knee osteoarthritis did not make any recommendations regarding biologics.[97] This is understandable, as the overwhelming majority of randomized controlled clinical studies investigating biologics (PRP, MSCs for knee osteoarthritis) occurred after the publication date. Likewise, the AAOS Treatment of OA of the Knee Evidence-Based Guideline, 2nd Edition (2013), was unable to provide recommendations for or against growth factor injections and/or PRP for patients with symptomatic osteoarthritis of the knee.[78]

TOTAL JOINT REPLACEMENT (ARTHROPLASTY)

In the patient with severe osteoarthritis that remains painful, functionally limiting, and refractory to all conservative measures, total joint replacement surgery should be considered.[155] Total hip replacement has evolved from a procedure with poor outcomes reserved for the most debilitated patients to one of the most successful orthopedic surgeries available.[17,21,156,157] Studies in the US and United Kingdom show greater than 95% implant survivorship at the 10-year follow-up and greater than 80% implant survivorship at the 25-year follow-up.[157-159] Approximately 65% of total hip replacements occur in patients 65 years and older.[157]

Incidence and Prevalence

The overall incidence of joint replacement procedures is quite high, with over 1 million total hip and total knee replacement procedures performed annually in

TABLE 7.8
Estimated Prevalence of Total Hip (THR) and Total Knee Replacements (TKR) by Age in 2010

Age	US Prevalence of THR (%)	US Prevalence of TKR (%)
50 years old	0.58	0.68
60 years old	1.49	2.92
70 years old	3.25	7.29
80 years old	5.26	10.38
90 years old	5.87	8.48

Please note these data do not include individuals who have undergone joint replacement techniques other than total hip or knee replacement (i.e., partial hip or partial knee replacement).
Adapted from Maradit Kremers H, Larson DR, Crowson CS, et al. Prevalence of total hip and knee replacement in the United States. *J Bone Joint Surg Am*. 2015;97(17):1387; with permission.

the US.[156] As of 2010, it is estimated that the prevalence of total hip replacements and total knee replacements among the entire US population was 0.83% and 1.52%, respectively.[156] This equates to 2% of the US population living with a total hip or total knee replacement, corresponding to an estimated 7 million people, of which 620,000 underwent both procedures.[156] For both procedures, the prevalence is noted to increase with age and more steadily for total knee replacements than for total hip replacements (Table 7.8). For both procedures, the prevalence is higher in women than in men.[156] Given the overall success of hip and knee replacement procedures in improving quality of life and functionality, it is anticipated that the incidence and prevalence rates of total hip and knee replacement procedures will continue to increase in the years to come (Figs. 7.9–7.11).

Hip Arthroplasty Patient and Implant Selection

Optimal surgical outcomes are maximized through careful patient selection. Obesity, advanced age, and medical comorbidities are not absolute contraindications, although a careful risk-to-benefit assessment should be considered.[78,138,157] According to the 2017 AAOS hip clinical practice guidelines, moderate-strength evidence supports that when obese patients are compared with nonobese patients with symptomatic osteoarthritis of the hip, they may achieve lower absolute outcome scores but have a similar level of patient satisfaction and relative improvement in pain and function after total hip replacement. Moderate-strength evidence also suggests that increased age is associated with lower

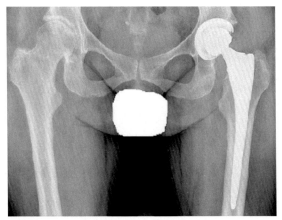

FIG. 7.9 AP with crests view (reformatted with crests cropped) image of noncemented left hip total replacement in anatomic alignment. There is also joint space narrowing and minimal osteophytes of the right hip.

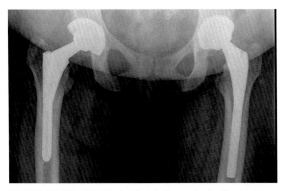

FIG. 7.10 AP with crests view (reformatted with crests cropped) status post-anatomically aligned left and right total hip replacement with noncemented femoral and acetabular components.

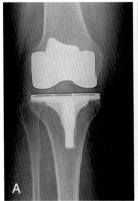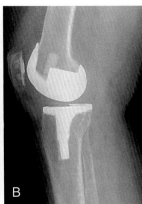

FIG. 7.11 **(A)** AP and **(B)** lateral views status post-total right knee replacement.

function and quality of life in patients with hip osteoarthritis undergoing total hip replacement. Lastly, moderate-strength evidence demonstrates that mental health disorders, such as depression, anxiety, and psychosis, are associated with decreased function, pain relief, and quality of life status post-total hip replacement.[138]

A comprehensive assessment of the patient is required to identify which implant design or surgical techniques will provide the best benefit. There are several bearing surfaces available, including metal on polyethylene, metal on metal, ceramic on ceramic, and metal on ceramic, and there are also resurfacing techniques.[157,160,161] However, each of the bearing surfaces has certain associated benefits and risks (i.e.,

polyethylene wear, metallic wear debris resulting in increased serum levels of chromium and cobalt, fracture of the ceramic components).[157,160] Cemented or noncemented components (or a hybrid of the two) may be used for total hip replacement. Cementless stems are more commonly used and with good results. In the US, 60%–90% of total hip replacement procedures use cementless stems.[157] One of the theoretical benefits of cementless fixation is remodeling of the bone-implant interface.[157] Resurfacing is considered to be a bone-conserving option that is most often recommended for younger, active patients, and its use is controversial. It is technically more demanding, with a potentially increased risk of aseptic loosening and revision surgery compared with total hip replacement.[157,162]

Currently, AAOS guidelines indicate that moderate-strength evidence supports no clinically significant differences in patient-oriented outcomes related to the surgical approach for patients undergoing total hip replacement for symptomatic osteoarthritis.[138] National registries have revolutionized our ability to assess patient outcomes, surgical techniques, and implant survivorship on a national and global scale.[157]

Total Hip Replacement Complications
Although total hip replacement surgery is usually quite successful, complications may occur. Despite advances in total hip replacement surgical techniques and implant designs, revision rates have remained unchanged over the past several decades.[157] The most common reasons for revision surgery are instability (22%), mechanical loosening (20%), infection (15%), implant failure (10%), osteolysis (7%), and

TABLE 7.9 Excerpts of Recommendations From the Evidence-Based Clinical Practice Guidelines for Surgical Management of Knee Osteoarthritis	
American Academy of Orthopaedic Surgeons Evidence-Based Clinical Practice Guidelines for Surgical Management of Knee Osteoarthritis (2015)	**Recommendations**
Obesity	**Strong** evidence **supports** that obese patients have less improvement in outcomes with total knee arthroplasty (TKA)
Preoperative physical therapy	**Limited** evidence **supports** that supervised exercise before TKA might improve pain and physical function after surgery
Polyethylene tibial component	**Strong** evidence **supports** use of either all-polyethylene or modular tibial components in knee arthroplasty (KA), because of no difference in outcomes
Cemented versus cementless tibial components	**Strong** evidence **supports** the use of tibial component fixation that is cemented or cementless in TKA because of similar functional outcomes and rates of complications and reoperations
Cemented femoral and tibial components versus cementless femoral and tibial components	**Moderate** evidence **supports** the use of either cemented femoral and tibial components or cementless femoral and tibial components in KA because of similar rates of complications and reoperations
Continuous passive motion (CPM)	**Strong** evidence **supports** that CPM after KA does not improve outcomes
Postoperative mobilization and length of stay	**Strong** evidence **supports** that rehabilitation started on the day of the TKA reduces length of hospital stay
Postoperative mobilization and pain/function	**Moderate** evidence **supports** that rehabilitation started on the day of the TKA compared with rehabilitation started on postoperative day 1 reduces pain and improves function
Early-stage supervised exercise program and function and pain	**Moderate** evidence **supports** that a supervised exercise program during the first 2 months after TKA improves physical function. Limited evidence supports a decrease in pain.

Supported by the American Society of Anesthesiologists. Endorsed by The Knee Society, American Association of Hip and Knee Surgeons, American College of Radiology, Arthroscopy Association of North America, and AGS Geriatric Healthcare Professionals. Please refer to the AAOS guidelines for a complete list of recommendations. Overall, the AAOS guidelines and recommendations regarding knee osteoarthritis are more comprehensive than those provided for the hip.

Data from American Academy of Orthopaedic Surgeons Board of Directors. *Surgical Management of Osteoarthritis of the Knee: Evidence-Based Clinical Practice Guideline*; 2015. Available at: https://www.aaos.org/uploadedFiles/PreProduction/Quality/Guidelines_and_Reviews/ guidelines/SMOAK%20CPG_4.22.2016.pdf.

periprosthetic fracture (6%). The most common causes of failure after revision include infection (30%), instability (25%), and loosening (19%).[157]

Limited-strength evidence supports that patients who are obese or use tobacco products are at an increased risk for complications after total hip replacement.[138] Also, limited-strength evidence supports an association between increased age and mortality risk in patients with symptomatic hip osteoarthritis receiving total hip replacement.[138] Regardless, moderate-level evidence supports the use of postoperative physical therapy. It is generally believed that

postoperative physical therapy may improve early function to a greater extent than no physical therapy management.[138] Please refer to Table 7.9 for data regarding total knee replacement guidelines for comparison (Table 7.9).

Total Hip Replacement Survivorship

Regardless of the prosthetic component used, the survivorship of the artificial hip is quite good. There have been several revisions and upgrades in surgical technique and implant design over the years. It is believed that patients can expect their prosthesis to last well over 20 years.[157] Although complications may occur, the great majority of patients do not experience these complications.[157]

FUTURE CONSIDERATIONS

The science of joint preservation care is rapidly evolving. It is likely inevitable that the trend toward shifting the care paradigm from palliative management of end-stage osteoarthritis toward a focus on the earliest stages of the condition's precursors will continue to be fine tuned. In just the last 15–20 years, there have been considerable advances in our understanding of the role that abnormal hip morphology, specifically FAI and DDH, plays in developing hip osteoarthritis later in life. Hip arthroscopy is increasingly used to correct joint pathomorphologies in hopes of curtailing the osteoarthritic cascade. However, further clinical trials and long-term, prospective, observational studies remain crucial for us to truly understand the efficacy of hip arthroscopy versus conservative care measures in curtailing hip osteoarthritis risk. Hip and knee total joint replacements have proved to be highly successful surgeries, and it is to be expected that surgical techniques and componentry will only continue to improve.

The literature regarding the use of biologic treatment options in knee osteoarthritis is rapidly expanding, and similar studies are increasingly being formatted for the hip. Recently and for the first time, a consensus statement on the minimum reporting requirements for clinical studies evaluating PRP and MSCs has been created, and it is anticipated that the consensus parameters will only improve the quality of research into biologics. It is also likely that further research into the role genetics plays in the development of osteoarthritis will continue with the formulation of gene-specific targeted treatments.

REFERENCES

1. *Osteoarthritis Fact Sheet.* https://www.cdc.gov/arthritis/basics/osteoarthritis.htm.
2. Loeser RF. *Pathogenesis of Osteoarthritis.* https://www.uptodate.com/contents/pathogenesis-of-osteoarthritis.
3. Liu-Bryan R, Terkeltaub R. Emerging regulators of the inflammatory process in osteoarthritis. *Nat Rev Rheumatol.* 2015;11(1):35–44.
4. Liu-Bryan R, Terkeltaub R. The growing array of innate inflammatory ignition switches in osteoarthritis. *Arthritis Rheum.* 2012;64(7):2055–2058.
5. Loeser RF, Goldring SR, Scanzello CR, Goldring MB. Osteoarthritis: a disease of the joint as an organ. *Arthritis Rheum.* 2012;64(6):1697–1707.
6. Sohn DH, Sokolove J, Sharpe O, et al. Plasma proteins present in osteoarthritic synovial fluid can stimulate cytokine production via Toll-like receptor 4. *Arthritis Res Ther.* 2012;14(1):R7.
7. Little CB, Fosang AJ. Is cartilage matrix breakdown an appropriate therapeutic target in osteoarthritis–insights from studies of aggrecan and collagen proteolysis? *Curr Drug Targets.* 2010;11(5):561–575.
8. Wang Q, Rozelle AL, Lepus CM, et al. Identification of a central role for complement in osteoarthritis. *Nat Med.* 2011;17(12):1674–1679.
9. Troeberg L, Nagase H. Proteases involved in cartilage matrix degradation in osteoarthritis. *Biochim Biophys Acta.* 2012;1824(1):133–145.
10. Tonge DP, Pearson MJ, Jones SW. The hallmarks of osteoarthritis and the potential to develop personalised disease-modifying pharmacological therapeutics. *Osteoarthr Cartil.* 2014;22(5):609–621.
11. Loeuille D, Chary-Valckenaere I, Champigneulle J, et al. Macroscopic and microscopic features of synovial membrane inflammation in the osteoarthritic knee: correlating magnetic resonance imaging findings with disease severity. *Arthritis Rheum.* 2005;52(11):3492–3501.
12. Baker K, Grainger A, Niu J, et al. Relation of synovitis to knee pain using contrast-enhanced MRIs. *Ann Rheum Dis.* 2010;69(10):1779–1783.
13. Taljanovic MS, Graham AR, Benjamin JB, et al. Bone marrow edema pattern in advanced hip osteoarthritis: quantitative assessment with magnetic resonance imaging and correlation with clinical examination, radiographic findings, and histopathology. *Skeletal Radiol.* 2008;37(5):423–431.
14. Brophy RH, Rai MF, Zhang Z, Torgomyan A, Sandell LJ. Molecular analysis of age and sex-related gene expression in meniscal tears with and without a concomitant anterior cruciate ligament tear. *J Bone Joint Surg Am.* 2012;94(5):385–393.
15. Jordan JM, Helmick CG, Renner JB, et al. Prevalence of hip symptoms and radiographic and symptomatic hip osteoarthritis in African Americans and Caucasians: the Johnston county osteoarthritis project. *J Rheumatol.* 2009;36(4):809–815.
16. Bennell K. Physiotherapy management of hip osteoarthritis. *J Physiother.* 2013;59(3):145–157.
17. Murphy NJ, Eyles JP, Hunter DJ. Hip osteoarthritis: etiopathogenesis and implications for management. *Adv Ther.* 2016;33(11):1921–1946.
18. Culliford DJ, Maskell J, Kiran A, et al. The lifetime risk of total hip and knee arthroplasty: results from the UK general practice research database. *Osteoarthr Cartil.* 2012;20(6):519–524.
19. Helmick CG. *Arthritis.* http://www.boneandjointburden.org/2013-report/iv-arthritis/iv.
20. Murphy L, Helmick CG. The impact of osteoarthritis in the United States: a population-health perspective. *Am J Nurs.* 2012;112(3 suppl 1):S13–S19.

21. Leunig M, Ganz R. Editorial comment: 2014 international hip society proceedings. *Clin Orthop Relat Res.* 2015;473(12):3714–3715.
22. Poultsides LA, Bedi A, Kelly BT. An algorithmic approach to mechanical hip pain. *HSS J.* 2012;8(3):213–224.
23. Clohisy JC, Callaghan JJ. Editorial comment: 2015 International Hip Society proceedings. *Clin Orthop Relat Res.* 2016;474(10):2112–2114.
24. Ganz R, Leunig M, Leunig-Ganz K, Harris WH. The etiology of osteoarthritis of the hip: an integrated mechanical concept. *Clin Orthop Relat Res.* 2008;466(2):264–272.
25. Kuhns BD, Weber AE, Levy DM, Wuerz TH. The natural history of femoroacetabular impingement. *Front Surg.* 2015;2:58.
26. Tibor LM, Leunig M. The pathoanatomy and arthroscopic management of femoroacetabular impingement. *Bone Joint Res.* 2012;1(10):245–257.
27. Smith-Petersen MN. The classic: treatment of malum coxae senilis, old slipped upper femoral epiphysis, intrapelvic protrusion of the acetabulum, and coxa plana by means of acetabuloplasty. 1936. *Clin Orthop Relat Res.* 2009;467(3):608–615.
28. Griffin DR, Dickenson EJ, O'Donnell J, et al. The Warwick Agreement on femoroacetabular impingement syndrome (FAI syndrome): an international consensus statement. *Br J Sports Med.* 2016;50(19):1169–1176.
29. Murray RO. The aetiology of primary osteoarthritis of the hip. *Br J Radiol.* 1965;38(455):810–824.
30. Murray RO, Duncan C. Athletic activity in adolescence as an etiological factor in degenerative hip disease. *J Bone Joint Surg Br.* 1971;53(3):406–419.
31. Solomon L. Patterns of osteoarthritis of the hip. *J Bone Joint Surg Br.* 1976;58(2):176–183.
32. Solomon L. Geographical and anatomical patterns of osteoarthritis. *Br J Rheumatol.* 1984;23(3):177–180.
33. Solomon L. Studies on the pathogenesis of osteoarthritis of the hip. *Trans Coll Med South Afr.* 1981:104–124.
34. Solomon L, Beighton P. Osteoarthrosis of the hip and its relationship to pre-existing in an African population. *J Bone Joint Surg Br.* 1973;55:216–217.
35. Solomon L, Schnitzler CM, Browett JP. Osteoarthritis of the hip: the patient behind the disease. *Ann Rheum Dis.* 1982;41(2):118–125.
36. Harris WH. Etiology of osteoarthritis of the hip. *Clin Orthop Relat Res.* 1986;(213):20–33.
37. Harris WH. Primary osteoarthritis of the hip: a vanishing diagnosis. *J Rheumatol.* 1983;(suppl 9):64.
38. Harris WH, Bourne RB, Oh I. Intra-articular acetabular labrum: a possible etiological factor in certain cases of osteoarthritis of the hip. *J Bone Joint Surg Am.* 1979;61(4):510–514.
39. Stulberg SD. Unrecognized childhood hip disease: a major cause of idiopathic osteoarthritis of the hip. In: *Paper Presented at: The Hip: Proceedings of the Third Open Scientific Meeting of the Hip Society.* 1975. St. Louis, MO.
40. Stulberg SD, Harris WH. Acetabular dysplasia, development of osteoarthritis of the hip. In: *Paper Presented at: The Hip: Proceedings of the Second Open Scientific Session of the Hip Society.* 1974. St. Louis, MO.
41. Ganz R, Gill TJ, Gautier E, Ganz K, Krugel N, Berlemann U. Surgical dislocation of the adult hip a technique with full access to the femoral head and acetabulum without the risk of avascular necrosis. *J Bone Joint Surg Br.* 2001;83(8):1119–1124.
42. Ganz R, Parvizi J, Beck M, Leunig M, Notzli H, Siebenrock KA. Femoroacetabular impingement: a cause for osteoarthritis of the hip. *Clin Orthop Relat Res.* 2003;(417):112–120.
43. Clohisy JC, Carlisle JC, Beaule PE, et al. A systematic approach to the plain radiographic evaluation of the young adult hip. *J Bone Joint Surg Am.* 2008;90(suppl 4):47–66.
44. Beck M, Kalhor M, Leunig M, Ganz R. Hip morphology influences the pattern of damage to the acetabular cartilage: femoroacetabular impingement as a cause of early osteoarthritis of the hip. *J Bone Joint Surg Br.* 2005;87(7):1012–1018.
45. Leunig M, Beck M, Kalhor M, Kim YJ, Werlen S, Ganz R. Fibrocystic changes at anterosuperior femoral neck: prevalence in hips with femoroacetabular impingement. *Radiology.* 2005;236(1):237–246.
46. Werlen S, Leunig M, Ganz R. Magnetic resonance arthrography of the hip in femoroacetabular impingement: technique and findings. *Oper Tech Orthop.* 2005;15(3):191–203.
47. Hunt D, Prather H, Harris Hayes M, Clohisy JC. Clinical outcomes analysis of conservative and surgical treatment of patients with clinical indications of prearthritic, intra-articular hip disorders. *PM R.* 2012;4(7):479–487.
48. Wall PD, Fernandez M, Griffin DR, Foster NE. Nonoperative treatment for femoroacetabular impingement: a systematic review of the literature. *PM R.* 2013;5(5):418–426.
49. Emara K, Samir W, Motasem el H, Ghafar KA. Conservative treatment for mild femoroacetabular impingement. *J Orthop Surg (Hong Kong).* 2011;19(1):41–45.
50. Wall PD, Brown JS, Parsons N, Buchbinder R, Costa ML, Griffin D. Surgery for treating hip impingement (femoroacetabular impingement). *Cochrane Database Syst Rev.* 2014;(9):Cd010796.
51. Palmer DH, Ganesh V, Comfort T, Tatman P. Midterm outcomes in patients with cam femoroacetabular impingement treated arthroscopically. *Arthroscopy.* 2012;28(11):1671–1681.
52. Steppacher SD, Anwander H, Zurmuhle CA, Tannast M, Siebenrock KA. Eighty percent of patients with surgical hip dislocation for femoroacetabular impingement have a good clinical result without osteoarthritis progression at 10 years. *Clin Orthop Relat Res.* 2015;473(4):1333–1341.
53. Kemp JL, MacDonald D, Collins NJ, Hatton AL, Crossley KM. Hip arthroscopy in the setting of hip osteoarthritis: systematic review of outcomes and progression to hip arthroplasty. *Clin Orthop Relat Res.* 2015;473(3):1055–1073.

54. Agricola R, Heijboer MP, Bierma-Zeinstra SM, Verhaar JA, Weinans H, Waarsing JH. Cam impingement causes osteoarthritis of the hip: a nationwide prospective cohort study (CHECK). *Ann Rheum Dis.* 2013;72(6):918–923.

55. Agricola R, Waarsing JH, Arden NK, et al. Cam impingement of the hip: a risk factor for hip osteoarthritis. *Nat Rev Rheumatol.* 2013;9(10):630–634.

56. Thomas GE, Palmer AJ, Batra RN, et al. Subclinical deformities of the hip are significant predictors of radiographic osteoarthritis and joint replacement in women. A 20 year longitudinal cohort study. *Osteoarthr Cartil.* 2014;22(10):1504–1510.

57. Saberi Hosnijeh F, Zuiderwijk M, Versteeg M, et al. The shape of the hip joint as a risk factor for osteoarthritis. *Osteoarthr Cartil.* 2016;24:S21–S22.

58. Garbuz DS, Masri BA, Haddad F, Duncan CP. Clinical and radiographic assessment of the young adult with symptomatic hip dysplasia. *Clin Orthop Relat Res.* 2004;(418):18–22.

59. Cooperman DR, Wallensten R, Stulberg SD. Acetabular dysplasia in the adult. *Clin Orthop Relat Res.* 1983;(175):79–85.

60. Ganz R, Klaue K, Vinh TS, Mast JW. A new periacetabular osteotomy for the treatment of hip dysplasias. Technique and preliminary results. *Clin Orthop Relat Res.* 1988;(232):26–36.

61. Srikanth VK, Fryer JL, Zhai G, Winzenberg TM, Hosmer D, Jones G. A meta-analysis of sex differences prevalence, incidence and severity of osteoarthritis. *Osteoarthr Cartil.* 2005;13(9):769–781.

62. Kim C, Linsenmeyer KD, Vlad SC, et al. Prevalence of radiographic and symptomatic hip osteoarthritis in an urban United States community: the Framingham osteoarthritis study. *Arthritis Rheumatol.* 2014;66(11):3013–3017.

63. MacGregor AJ, Antoniades L, Matson M, Andrew T, Spector TD. The genetic contribution to radiographic hip osteoarthritis in women: results of a classic twin study. *Arthritis Rheum.* 2000;43(11):2410–2416.

64. Pollard TC, Villar RN, Norton MR, et al. Genetic influences in the aetiology of femoroacetabular impingement: a sibling study. *J Bone Joint Surg Br.* 2010;92(2):209–216.

65. Pelt CE, Erickson JA, Peters CL, Anderson MB, Cannon-Albright L. A heritable predisposition to osteoarthritis of the hip. *J Arthroplast.* 2015;30(9 suppl):125–129.

66. Zengini E, Finan C, Wilkinson JM. The genetic epidemiological landscape of hip and knee osteoarthritis: where are we now and where are we going? *J Rheumatol.* 2016;43(2):260–266.

67. Nevitt MC, Xu L, Zhang Y, et al. Very low prevalence of hip osteoarthritis among Chinese elderly in Beijing, China, compared with whites in the United States: the Beijing osteoarthritis study. *Arthritis Rheum.* 2002;46(7):1773–1779.

68. Foley B, Cleveland RJ, Renner JB, Jordan JM, Nelson AE. Racial differences in associations between baseline patterns of radiographic osteoarthritis and multiple definitions of progression of hip osteoarthritis: the Johnston County Osteoarthritis Project. *Arthritis Res Ther.* 2015;17:366.

69. Zhang Y, Jordan JM. Epidemiology of osteoarthritis. *Clin Geriatr Med.* 2010;26(3):355–369.

70. Lane NE, Gore LR, Cummings SR, et al. Serum vitamin D levels and incident changes of radiographic hip osteoarthritis: a longitudinal study. Study of Osteoporotic Fractures Research Group. *Arthritis Rheum.* 1999;42(5):854–860.

71. Bergink AP, Zillikens MC, Van Leeuwen JP, Hofman A, Uitterlinden AG, van Meurs JB. 25-Hydroxyvitamin D and osteoarthritis: a meta-analysis including new data. *Semin Arthritis Rheum.* 2016;45(5):539–546.

72. Tepper S, Hochberg MC. Factors associated with hip osteoarthritis: data from the first national health and nutrition examination survey (NHANES-I). *Am J Epidemiol.* 1993;137(10):1081–1088.

73. van Saase JL, Vandenbroucke JP, van Romunde LK, Valkenburg HA. Osteoarthritis and obesity in the general population. A relationship calling for an explanation. *J Rheumatol.* 1988;15(7):1152–1158.

74. Grotle M, Hagen KB, Natvig B, Dahl FA, Kvien TK. Obesity and osteoarthritis in knee, hip and/or hand: an epidemiological study in the general population with 10 years follow-up. *BMC Musculoskelet Disord.* 2008;9:132.

75. Heliovaara M, Makela M, Impivaara O, Knekt P, Aromaa A, Sievers K. Association of overweight, trauma and workload with coxarthrosis. A health survey of 7,217 persons. *Acta Orthop Scand.* 1993;64(5):513–518.

76. Karlson EW, Mandl LA, Aweh GN, Sangha O, Liang MH, Grodstein F. Total hip replacement due to osteoarthritis: the importance of age, obesity, and other modifiable risk factors. *Am J Med.* 2003;114(2):93–98.

77. Jiang L, Rong J, Wang Y, et al. The relationship between body mass index and hip osteoarthritis: a systematic review and meta-analysis. *Joint Bone Spine.* 2011;78(2):150–155.

78. *Treatment of Osteoarthritis of the Knee: Evidence-Based Guidelines.* 2nd ed. 2013. https://www.aaos.org/research/guidelines/TreatmentofOsteoarthritisoftheKneeGuideline.pdf.

79. Martin JA, Buckwalter JA. The role of chondrocyte senescence in the pathogenesis of osteoarthritis and in limiting cartilage repair. *J Bone Joint Surg Am.* 2003;85-A (suppl 2):106–110.

80. Vignon E, Arlot M, Patricot LM, Vignon G. The cell density of human femoral head cartilage. *Clin Orthop Relat Res.* 1976;(121):303–308.

81. Buckwalter JA, Roughley PJ, Rosenberg LC. Age-related changes in cartilage proteoglycans: quantitative electron microscopic studies. *Microsc Res Tech.* 1994;28(5):398–408.

82. Loeser RF. Age-related changes in the musculoskeletal system and the development of osteoarthritis. *Clin Geriatr Med.* 2010;26(3):371–386.

83. Harris EC, Coggon D. HIP osteoarthritis and work. *Best Pract Res Clin Rheumatol.* 2015;29(3):462–482.

84. Jensen LK. Hip osteoarthritis: influence of work with heavy lifting, climbing stairs or ladders, or combining kneeling/squatting with heavy lifting. *Occup Environ Med.* 2008;65(1):6–19.

85. Coggon D, Kellingray S, Inskip H, Croft P, Campbell L, Cooper C. Osteoarthritis of the hip and occupational lifting. *Am J Epidemiol.* 1998;147(6):523–528.

86. Packer JD, Safran MR. The etiology of primary femoroacetabular impingement: genetics or acquired deformity? *J Hip Preserv Surg.* 2015;2(3):249–257.

87. Altman R, Alarcon G, Appelrouth D, et al. The American College of Rheumatology criteria for the classification and reporting of osteoarthritis of the hip. *Arthritis Rheum.* 1991;34(5):505–514.

88. Altman R, Asch E, Bloch D, et al. Development of criteria for the classification and reporting of osteoarthritis. Classification of osteoarthritis of the knee. Diagnostic and therapeutic criteria Committee of the American Rheumatism Association. *Arthritis Rheum.* 1986;29(8):1039–1049.

89. Kellgren JH, Lawrence JS. Radiological assessment of osteo-arthrosis. *Ann Rheum Dis.* 1957;16(4):494–502.

90. Croft P, Cooper C, Wickham C, Coggon D. Defining osteoarthritis of the hip for epidemiologic studies. *Am J Epidemiol.* 1990;132(3):514–522.

91. Tönnis D, Heinecke A. Acetabular and femoral anteversion: relationship with osteoarthritis of the hip. *J Bone Joint Surg Am.* 1999;81(12):1747–1770.

92. Jacobsen S, Sonne-Holm S. Hip dysplasia: a significant risk factor for the development of hip osteoarthritis. A cross-sectional survey. *Rheumatology (Oxford).* 2005;44(2):211–218.

93. Terjesen T, Gunderson RB. Radiographic evaluation of osteoarthritis of the hip: an inter-observer study of 61 hips treated for late-detected developmental hip dislocation. *Acta Orthop.* 2012;83(2):185–189.

94. O'Brien WM. In: Lawrence JS, ed. *Rheumatism in Populations.* London: William Heinemann Medical Books; 1977. 572 pp. *Arthritis Rheum.* 1978;21(3):398–398.

95. Jacobsen S, Sonne-Holm S, Soballe K, Gebuhr P, Lund B. Radiographic case definitions and prevalence of osteoarthrosis of the hip: a survey of 4 151 subjects in the Osteoarthritis Substudy of the Copenhagen City Heart Study. *Acta Orthop Scand.* 2004;75(6):713–720.

96. Pereira D, Peleteiro B, Araujo J, Branco J, Santos RA, Ramos E. The effect of osteoarthritis definition on prevalence and incidence estimates: a systematic review. *Osteoarthr Cartil.* 2011;19(11):1270–1285.

97. Hochberg MC, Altman RD, April KT, et al. American College of Rheumatology 2012 recommendations for the use of nonpharmacologic and pharmacologic therapies in osteoarthritis of the hand, hip, and knee. *Arthritis Care Res (Hoboken).* 2012;64(4):465–474.

98. Fernandes L, Storheim K, Nordsletten L, Risberg MA. Development of a therapeutic exercise program for patients with osteoarthritis of the hip. *Phys Ther.* 2010;90(4):592–601.

99. Paans N, van den Akker-Scheek I, Dilling RG, et al. Effect of exercise and weight loss in people who have hip osteoarthritis and are overweight or obese: a prospective cohort study. *Phys Ther.* 2013;93(2):137–146.

100. Zhang W, Doherty M, Arden N, et al. EULAR evidence based recommendations for the management of hip osteoarthritis: report of a task force of the EULAR Standing Committee for International Clinical Studies Including Therapeutics (ESCISIT). *Ann Rheum Dis.* 2005;64(5):669–681.

101. Brosseau L, Wells GA, Tugwell P, et al. Ottawa Panel evidence-based clinical practice guidelines for the management of osteoarthritis in adults who are obese or overweight. *Phys Ther.* 2011;91(6):843–861.

102. Fransen M, McConnell S, Harmer AR, Van der Esch M, Simic M, Bennell KL. Exercise for osteoarthritis of the knee. *Cochrane Database Syst Rev.* 2015;1:Cd004376.

103. Fransen M, McConnell S, Hernandez-Molina G, Reichenbach S. Exercise for osteoarthritis of the hip. *Cochrane Database Syst Rev.* 2014;(4):Cd007912.

104. Svege I, Nordsletten L, Fernandes L, Risberg MA. Exercise therapy may postpone total hip replacement surgery in patients with hip osteoarthritis: a long-term follow-up of a randomised trial. *Ann Rheum Dis.* 2015;74(1):164–169.

105. Zhang W, Moskowitz RW, Nuki G, et al. OARSI recommendations for the management of hip and knee osteoarthritis, part I: critical appraisal of existing treatment guidelines and systematic review of current research evidence. *Osteoarthr Cartil.* 2007;15(9):981–1000.

106. Malanga GA, Aydin SM, Holder EK, Petrin Z. Functional therapeutic and core strengthening. In: Seidenberg Md FFRPH, Bowen Md FCRCJD, King Md DJ, eds. *The Hip and Pelvis in Sports Medicine and Primary Care.* Cham: Springer International Publishing; 2017:185–214.

107. Waldhelm A, Li L. Endurance tests are the most reliable core stability related measurements. *J Sport Health Sci.* 2012;1(2):121–128.

108. Arokoski JP, Kankaanpaa M, Valta T, et al. Back and hip extensor muscle function during therapeutic exercises. *Arch Phys Med Rehabil.* 1999;80(7):842–850.

109. Rasch A, Bystrom AH, Dalen N, Berg HE. Reduced muscle radiological density, cross-sectional area, and strength of major hip and knee muscles in 22 patients with hip osteoarthritis. *Acta Orthop.* 2007;78(4):505–510.

110. Chodzko-Zajko WJ, Proctor DN, Fiatarone Singh MA, et al. American College of Sports Medicine position stand. Exercise and physical activity for older adults. *Med Sci Sports Exerc.* 2009;41(7):1510–1530.

111. French HP, Cusack T, Brennan A, et al. Exercise and manual physiotherapy arthritis research trial (EMPART) for osteoarthritis of the hip: a multicenter randomized controlled trial. *Arch Phys Med Rehabil.* 2013;94(2):302–314.

112. Bennell KL, Buchbinder R, Hinman RS. Physical therapies in the management of osteoarthritis: current state of the evidence. *Curr Opin Rheumatol.* 2015;27(3):304–311.

113. Wang Q, Wang TT, Qi XF, et al. Manual therapy for hip osteoarthritis: a systematic review and meta-analysis. *Pain Physician.* 2015;18(6):E1005–E1020.

114. Bennell KL, Egerton T, Martin J, et al. Effect of physical therapy on pain and function in patients with hip osteoarthritis: a randomized clinical trial. *JAMA.* 2014;311(19):1987–1997.

115. Blount WP. Don't throw away the cane. *J Bone Joint Surg Am.* 1956;38-a(3):695–708.

116. Shatzer M. *Physical Medicine and Rehabilitation Pocketpedia.* Wolters Kluwer Health; 2012.

117. Kalra EK. Nutraceutical–definition and introduction. *AAPS Pharm Sci.* 2003;5(3):E25.

118. Percope de Andrade MA, Campos TV, Abreu ESGM. Supplementary methods in the nonsurgical treatment of osteoarthritis. *Arthroscopy.* 2015;31(4):785–792.

119. Clegg DO, Reda DJ, Harris CL, et al. Glucosamine, chondroitin sulfate, and the two in combination for painful knee osteoarthritis. *N Engl J Med.* 2006;354(8):795–808.

120. Machado GC, Maher CG, Ferreira PH, et al. Efficacy and safety of paracetamol for spinal pain and osteoarthritis: systematic review and meta-analysis of randomised placebo controlled trials. *BMJ.* 2015;350:h1225.

121. Zhang W, Jones A, Doherty M. Does paracetamol (acetaminophen) reduce the pain of osteoarthritis? A meta-analysis of randomised controlled trials. *Ann Rheum Dis.* 2004;63(8):901–907.

122. Towheed TE, Maxwell L, Judd MG, Catton M, Hochberg MC, Wells G. Acetaminophen for osteoarthritis. *Cochrane Database Syst Rev.* 2006;(1):Cd004257.

123. Zhang W, Nuki G, Moskowitz RW, et al. OARSI recommendations for the management of hip and knee osteoarthritis: part III: changes in evidence following systematic cumulative update of research published through January 2009. *Osteoarthr Cartil.* 2010;18(4):476–499.

124. da Costa BR, Reichenbach S, Keller N, et al. Effectiveness of non-steroidal anti-inflammatory drugs for the treatment of pain in knee and hip osteoarthritis: a network meta-analysis. *Lancet.* 2016;387(10033):2093–2105.

125. Gore M, Tai KS, Sadosky A, Leslie D, Stacey BR. Use and costs of prescription medications and alternative treatments in patients with osteoarthritis and chronic low back pain in community-based settings. *Pain Pract.* 2012;12(7):550–560.

126. Derry S, Conaghan P, Da Silva JA, Wiffen PJ, Moore RA. Topical NSAIDs for chronic musculoskeletal pain in adults. *Cochrane Database Syst Rev.* 2016;4:Cd007400.

127. Chappell AS, Ossanna MJ, Liu-Seifert H, et al. Duloxetine, a centrally acting analgesic, in the treatment of patients with osteoarthritis knee pain: a 13-week, randomized, placebo-controlled trial. *Pain.* 2009;146(3):253–260.

128. Chappell AS, Desaiah D, Liu-Seifert H, et al. A double-blind, randomized, placebo-controlled study of the efficacy and safety of duloxetine for the treatment of chronic pain due to osteoarthritis of the knee. *Pain Pract.* 2011;11(1):33–41.

129. McCabe PS, Maricar N, Parkes MJ, Felson DT, O'Neill TW. The efficacy of intra-articular steroids in hip osteoarthritis: a systematic review. *Osteoarthr Cartil.* 2016;24(9):1509–1517.

130. McAlindon TE, LaValley MP, Harvey WF, et al. Effect of intra-articular triamcinolone vs saline on knee cartilage volume and pain in patients with knee osteoarthritis: a randomized clinical trial. *JAMA.* 2017;317(19):1967–1975.

131. Raynauld JP, Buckland-Wright C, Ward R, et al. Safety and efficacy of long-term intraarticular steroid injections in osteoarthritis of the knee: a randomized, double-blind, placebo-controlled trial. *Arthritis Rheum.* 2003;48(2):370–377.

132. National Clinical Guideline C. *National Institute for Health and Clinical Excellence: Guidance. Osteoarthritis: Care and Management in Adults.* London: National Institute for Health and Care Excellence (UK); 2014. Copyright (c) National Clinical Guideline Centre, 2014.

133. Rivera F. Single intra-articular injection of high molecular weight hyaluronic acid for hip osteoarthritis. *J Orthop Traumatol.* 2016;17(1):21–26.

134. Qvistgaard E, Christensen R, Torp-Pedersen S, Bliddal H. Intra-articular treatment of hip osteoarthritis: a randomized trial of hyaluronic acid, corticosteroid, and isotonic saline. *Osteoarthr Cartil.* 2006;14(2):163–170.

135. Atchia I, Kane D, Reed MR, Isaacs JD, Birrell F. Efficacy of a single ultrasound-guided injection for the treatment of hip osteoarthritis. *Ann Rheum Dis.* 2011;70(1):110–116.

136. Migliore A, Granata M, Tormenta S, et al. Hip viscosupplementation under ultra-sound guidance reduces NSAID consumption in symptomatic hip osteoarthritis patients in a long follow-up. Data from Italian registry. *Eur Rev Med Pharmacol Sci.* 2011;15(1):25–34.

137. Lieberman JR, Engstrom SM, Solovyova O, Au C, Grady JJ. Is intra-articular hyaluronic acid effective in treating osteoarthritis of the hip joint? *J Arthroplast.* 2015;30(3):507–511.

138. *Management of Osteoarthritis of the Hip: Evidence-Based Guidelines.* 2nd ed. 2017. https://www.aaos.org/Quality/Clinical_Practice_Guidelines/Clinical_Practice_Guidelines.

139. Battaglia M, Guaraldi F, Vannini F, et al. Platelet-rich plasma (PRP) intra-articular ultrasound-guided injections as a possible treatment for hip osteoarthritis: a pilot study. *Clin Exp Rheumatol.* 2011;29(4):754.

140. Battaglia M, Guaraldi F, Vannini F, et al. Efficacy of ultrasound-guided intra-articular injections of platelet-rich plasma versus hyaluronic acid for hip osteoarthritis. *Orthopedics.* 2013;36(12):e1501–e1508.

141. Dallari D, Stagni C, Rani N, et al. Ultrasound-guided injection of platelet-rich plasma and hyaluronic acid, separately and in combination, for hip osteoarthritis: a randomized controlled study. *Am J Sports Med.* 2016;44(3):664–671.

142. Bennell KL, Hunter DJ, Paterson KL. Platelet-rich plasma for the management of hip and knee osteoarthritis. *Curr Rheumatol Rep.* 2017;19(5):24.

143. Shapiro SA, Kazmerchak SE, Heckman MG, Zubair AC, O'Connor MI. A prospective, single-blind, placebo-controlled trial of bone marrow aspirate concentrate for knee osteoarthritis. *Am J Sports Med.* 2017;45(1):82–90.

144. Cerza F, Carni S, Carcangiu A, et al. Comparison between hyaluronic acid and platelet-rich plasma, intra-articular infiltration in the treatment of gonarthrosis. *Am J Sports Med.* 2012;40(12):2822–2827.

145. Riboh JC, Saltzman BM, Yanke AB, Fortier L, Cole BJ. Effect of leukocyte concentration on the efficacy of platelet-rich plasma in the treatment of knee osteoarthritis. *Am J Sports Med.* 2016;44(3):792–800.

146. Filardo G, Di Matteo B, Di Martino A, et al. Platelet-rich plasma intra-articular knee injections show no superiority versus viscosupplementation: a randomized controlled trial. *Am J Sports Med.* 2015;43(7):1575–1582.

147. Cole BJ, Karas V, Hussey K, Pilz K, Fortier LA. Hyaluronic acid versus platelet-rich plasma: a prospective, double-blind randomized controlled trial comparing clinical outcomes and effects on intra-articular biology for the treatment of knee osteoarthritis. *Am J Sports Med.* 2017;45(2):339–346.

148. Hart R, Safi A, Komzak M, Jajtner P, Puskeiler M, Hartova P. Platelet-rich plasma in patients with tibiofemoral cartilage degeneration. *Arch Orthop Trauma Surg.* 2013;133(9):1295–1301.

149. Patel S, Dhillon MS, Aggarwal S, Marwaha N, Jain A. Treatment with platelet-rich plasma is more effective than placebo for knee osteoarthritis: a prospective, double-blind, randomized trial. *Am J Sports Med.* 2013;41(2):356–364.

150. Campbell KA, Saltzman BM, Mascarenhas R, et al. Does intra-articular platelet-rich plasma injection provide clinically superior outcomes compared with other therapies in the treatment of knee osteoarthritis? A systematic review of overlapping meta-analyses. *Arthroscopy.* 2015;31(11):2213–2221.

151. Sanchez M, Fiz N, Azofra J, et al. A randomized clinical trial evaluating plasma rich in growth factors (PRGF-Endoret) versus hyaluronic acid in the short-term treatment of symptomatic knee osteoarthritis. *Arthroscopy.* 2012;28(8):1070–1078.

152. Simental-Mendia M, Vilchez-Cavazos JF, Pena-Martinez VM, Said-Fernandez S, Lara-Arias J, Martinez-Rodriguez HG. Leukocyte-poor platelet-rich plasma is more effective than the conventional therapy with acetaminophen for the treatment of early knee osteoarthritis. *Arch Orthop Trauma Surg.* 2016;136(12):1723–1732.

153. Smith PA. Intra-articular autologous conditioned plasma injections provide safe and efficacious treatment for knee osteoarthritis: an FDA-sanctioned, randomized, double-blind, placebo-controlled clinical trial. *Am J Sports Med.* 2016;44(4):884–891.

154. Murray IR, Geeslin AG, Goudie EB, Petrigliano FA, LaPrade RF. Minimum information for studies evaluating biologics in orthopaedics (MIBO): platelet-rich plasma and mesenchymal stem cells. *J Bone Joint Surg Am.* 2017;99(10):809–819.

155. Dieppe PA, Lohmander LS. Pathogenesis and management of pain in osteoarthritis. *Lancet.* 2005;365:965–973.

156. Maradit Kremers H, Larson DR, Crowson CS, et al. Prevalence of total hip and knee replacement in the United States. *J Bone Joint Surg Am.* 2015;97(17):1386–1397.

157. Pivec R, Johnson AJ, Mears SC, Mont MA. Hip arthroplasty. *Lancet.* 2012;380(9855):1768–1777.

158. Kurtz S, Ong K, Lau E, Mowat F, Halpern M. Projections of primary and revision hip and knee arthroplasty in the United States from 2005 to 2030. *J Bone Joint Surg Am.* 2007;89(4):780–785.

159. *National Joint Registry for England and Wales. 7th Annual Report.* 2010.

160. Varnum C. Outcomes of different bearings in total hip arthroplasty – implant survival, revision causes, and patient-reported outcome. *Dan Med J.* 2017;64(3).

161. Keurentjes JC, Pijls BG, Van Tol FR, et al. Which implant should we use for primary total hip replacement? A systematic review and meta-analysis. *J Bone Joint Surg Am.* 2014;96(suppl 1):79–97.

162. Smith TO, Nichols R, Donell ST, Hing CB. The clinical and radiological outcomes of hip resurfacing versus total hip arthroplasty: a meta-analysis and systematic review. *Acta Orthop.* 2010;81(6):684–695.

163. *Surgical Management of Osteoarthritis of the Knee: Evidence-Based Clinical Practice Guidelines.* 2015. https://www.aaos.org/uploadedFiles/PreProduction/Quality/Guidelines_and_Reviews/guidelines/SMOAK%20CPG_4.22.2016.pdf.

CHAPTER 8

Prevention of Hospital-Acquired Deconditioning

DER-SHENG HAN, MD, PHD • SHIH-CHING CHEN, MD, PHD

EPIDEMIOLOGY AND EFFECT OF DECONDITIONING

Unnecessary bed rest often occurs in hospitals or institutions, resulting in deconditioning.[1] The diagnosis of debility (deconditioning) is coded as R53.81 in the International Statistical Classification of Diseases and Related Health Problems, 10th revision (ICD-10).[2] The concept of deconditioning has been discussed in many articles, and synonyms for the term include debility, generalized weakness, asthenia, and immobilization syndrome. What does the above definition of functional decline refer to? Functional status represents the ability to perform basic activities of daily living (ADLs), such as bathing, dressing, transferring from bed to chair, using the toilet, and sphincter control. It is estimated that 34%–50% of older adult patients experience functional decline in at least one basic ADL during hospitalization.[3] Prevalent losses occurred in the ability to perform bathing and dressing skills, and the onset of decline occurs as early as day 3 of the hospital stay.[4] Those patients with hospital-associated deconditioning have a higher risk of mortality and nursing home institutionalization. It is absolutely important for healthcare workers to pay attention proactively to avoid unnecessary bed rest.

The causes of deconditioning are multifactorial and include a low premorbid functional status, immobility, iatrogenic complications, generalized inflammation, compromised nutrition, anemia, pain, sleep deprivation, fatigue, and depression.[5]

Immobility results in adverse consequences in multiple organ systems (Table 8.1). In the musculoskeletal system, it results in a decline in strength/endurance, muscle atrophy, and decreases in metabolism and oxygen utilization rate. In the circulatory system, immobility results in a decrease in functional capacity (including cardiac output and workload), orthostatic hypotension, and deep vein thrombosis. Osteoporosis is one of the complications of immobility.[6]

IMPACT OF BED REST AND IMMOBILITY

Musculoskeletal System

There are three main effects of bed rest on the musculoskeletal system:

1. sarcopenia (muscle atrophy and weakness)
2. joint contracture
3. osteoporosis

Sarcopenia

Activity-related sarcopenia resulting from bed rest, deconditioning, or zero-gravity conditions is one type of secondary sarcopenia. According to the diagnostic criteria proposed by the European Working Group on Sarcopenia in Older People, sarcopenia is defined as low muscle mass plus low muscle strength or low physical performance. Low grip strength is deemed as low muscle strength, and usual gait speed is employed for physical function evaluation.[7] The muscle mass can be easily measured with bioimpedance analyzer or dual-energy X-ray absorptiometry (DXA). The DXA cutoff value for low muscle mass is below $7.23\,kg/m^2$ for the male and $5.67\,kg/m^2$ for the female.[8] The cause of activity-related sarcopenia is multifactorial, including decreased cardiovascular function, muscle atrophy, and motor neuron loss. Berg et al.[9] carried out a classic study on young healthy men and found that after 6 weeks of bed rest, maximum voluntary isometric and concentric knee extensor torque was decreased by 25%–30% and the cross-sectional area of the quadriceps femoris muscle was decreased by 14%. The decline in muscle strength was more significant than the decrease in the cross-sectional area of muscles, showing that changes in neural control efficiency or neurotransmitter secretion and other factors can similarly cause a decline in muscle strength. Another study on young healthy men found that bed rest for 29 days resulted in a 10% decrease in the volume of the quadriceps femoris muscle and a 16% decrease in the volume of the gastrocnemius/soleus muscle complex.[10] Immobility and muscle disuse cause muscle atrophy, which leads to weakness

TABLE 8.1
Complications of Immobility

System	Complication
Musculoskeletal	Sarcopenia (muscle atrophy and weakness), joint contracture, osteoporosis, hypercalcemia
Circulatory and respiratory	Body fluid accumulation, orthostatic hypotension, decreased cardiac output, deep vein thrombosis, impaired lung function, pneumonia
Metabolic and endocrine	Electrolyte imbalance, glucose intolerance, endocrine dysfunction, hyperparathyroidism
Others	Urolithiasis, urinary tract infection, low appetite, constipation, sensation deprivation, anxiety/depression, confusion, impaired cognition, balance, and coordination disorders

and functional defects. A study in the elderly found that 10 days of bed rest caused a decrease in muscle protein synthesis, total lean mass, and appendicular lean mass. The effects observed were more severe than the effects found in young people who had 28 days of bed rest.[11] Early termination of immobility can reduce the length of stay, expense, and incidence of complications due to immobility.

Overall, under conditions of complete rest, the decrease in muscle mass in the first 2 days is not significant but accelerates in the following 10 days, with large decreases on days 8–10, followed by even further decreases. Approximately 10%–15% of muscle strength will be lost per week (1%–3% per day). After 3–5 weeks, only half of the original muscle strength remains. Muscle atrophy is mainly caused by a decrease in protein synthesis rather than an increase in degradation. Myostatin, a negative muscle growth regulator, expresses more actively in catabolic state. The serum myostatin peptide concentration increased during immobilization and in the patient receiving hemodialysis.[12,13] Although collagen synthesis also decreases, the speed of this decrease is relatively slower, and therefore there is a comparative increase in the collagen ratio. In normal urine, creatinine levels are low, but in an immobile and zero-gravitational environment, creatinine excretion increases.

Histologic changes accompany muscle weakness, but it is seldom performed in a clinical scenario. After 4 weeks of immobility, muscle mass decreases by 69%. The average cross-sectional area of type II muscle fibers

(responsible for rapid movement) decreases by 46%, while the average cross-sectional area of type I muscle fibers (responsible for slow movement) decreases by 69%. At the same time, the size and number of mitochondria decrease, leading to decreases in aerobic respiration.[14]

Regarding metabolism, the main source of energy at rest is derived from carbohydrates and fat, and nitrogen loss increases during immobility. The main cause is decreased muscular activity, resulting in decreased protein synthesis and consequently in a decrease in blood proteins. This is exacerbated by poor appetite, poor gastrointestinal absorption of proteins, constipation, and other digestive tract factors. During immobility, a normal human loses 2 g of nitrogen daily, whereas a malnourished patient loses 12 g daily, and a patient with a long bone fracture loses 8 g daily. On day 5 or 6 of bed rest, nitrogen loss is increased, reaching the highest amount in week 2. The nitrogen loss is accompanied by decreases in muscle blood flow, metabolic activity, and muscle endurance.[15]

The main reason for decreased muscle endurance is decreased oxidative enzyme activity in the muscles, resulting in decreased oxygen utilization efficiency and lactic acid tolerance in the blood, followed by changes in the size and shape of the end plate. In addition, decreases in intramuscular glycogen storage and lipid utilization and changes in the function of acetylcholine receptors also result in decreased muscle endurance.

As the relative concentration of collagen increases, muscle tightness and myogenic contracture occurs, which particularly affects type I fibers in the lower limbs. When the quadriceps femoris muscle is continuously in a state of contraction, large histochemical changes occur in the vastus intermedius muscle consisting mainly of type I muscle fibers. When muscles are maintained in a shortened state, muscle fibers lose 40% of their sarcomeres, and decrease in serially connected sarcomeres results in a shortening of length at rest. Stretching exercises for just half an hour a day prevents sarcomere loss, showing that stretching is an important factor for maintaining function. The rate of muscle atrophy varies according to the muscle, with the quadriceps femoris muscle, hip joint extensors, and back extensors undergoing rapid atrophy, further decreasing walking tolerance and inducing back pain.[16]

Joint Contracture

Contracture refers to a clinical condition caused by restriction of passive or active range of motion (ROM) in joints, muscles, or soft tissues. Reasons for the restricted ROM include joint pain, paresis, and fibrosis,

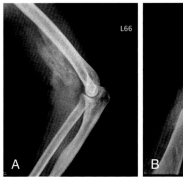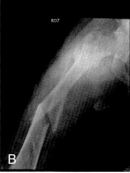

FIG. 8.1 **(A)** Elbow joint and **(B)** hip joint heterotopic ossification in the nursing home residents.

but the most important single factor is lack of joint movement. Other contracture-inducing factors include inappropriate limb positioning, length of immobility, preexisting etiology, peri-joint edema, hematoma, and ischemia.

Connective tissue is a complicated and dynamic structure. This tissue is important for structure stability and movement, and external mechanical stress will result in changes to connective tissue. When damage or inflammation occurs in connective tissue, the damaged area will be repaired, and reassembly will be carried out according to the strength and direction of stretching exercises. Collagen is the most abundant protein in the body, and the synthesis and decomposition of collagen occurs in dynamic balance. Trauma, inflammation, ischemia, and degeneration increase collagen synthesis. When compounded by lack of stretching, this results in fibrosis, which affects normal function. Collagen in muscles can fix muscle fibers, and its synthesis increases with activity and increased stretching but decreases because of immobility. The main cause of myogenic contracture is shortening of the sarcolemma and muscle fiber length.[17]

Heterotopic ossification refers to an abnormal pathologic condition of bone accumulation in soft tissue. This is most commonly observed after joint surgery (especially hip joints), trauma, and spinal cord injury, and in patients with a central nervous system injury. The cause for this disease is unknown but may involve local metabolism, blood flow changes, and abnormalities in systemic calcium metabolism (Fig. 8.1). Preventive care measures mainly include getting off bed rest early. Treatment must maintain joint ROM, and surgical resection can be carried out only if the ossification process is complete. A larger area of bone accumulation will result if the surgery is performed too early.[18]

The main clinical effects of contracture are decreased mobility, ADL dependence, and increased difficulty with respect to skin care. Hip joint flexion contracture restricts hip joint extension, affects gait, and increases energy consumption by 60% during ambulation. From a biophysical perspective, hip joint flexion contracture causes hamstring muscle shortening, which further results in knee joint and ankle joint contracture. Ankle joint plantarflexion contracture will prevent heel strike during the gait cycle and increase walking energy consumption. Hip joint extension contracture is rarely seen but causes difficulty in using a wheelchair. Knee joint flexion contracture will cause difficulty in getting in and out of cars. Multiple joint contractures will hinder positioning in the bed, standing, mobility, perineal hygiene, and skin care.

Complete assessment of contracture is helpful to design a treatment plan. The main points of complete assessment are:
1. analyzing the causes of contracture and identifying the actual contracture location and
2. carefully measuring passive and active ROM.

When passive and active ROM differs, there is a need to distinguish whether muscle weakness or an increase in spasticity is present, since rapid joint movement can induce spasticity. Nerve blockade can be used to assist in determination if there is no other way of distinguishing between these conditions.

Osteoporosis

Bone mass increases because of stress loading and decreases because of zero gravitation or low muscle activity. Normal bone mass begins to decrease around the ages of 31–50 years and accelerates 5–7 years after menopause. Because of low physical activity, patients with spinal cord injury have significant bone loss. Immobility results in decreased bone density. Osteoporosis is defined as T-score below –2.5 when compared with young healthy women.[19] The cause of this type of osteoporosis is increased osteoclast activity, resulting in obvious calcium and hydroxyproline loss of cancellous bone in the epiphyses and metaphyses of long bones and an increase in the excretion of calcium in the urine and stool.[20] After 12 weeks of bed rest, bone density is reduced by almost 50%. The causes of bone absorption are unclear, and osteopenia is a risk factor of hip joint fracture. In addition, under non-weight-bearing conditions, bone mineralization becomes poorer, easily resulting in fractures. In osteopenia, because of immobility, bone mineralization continues to decrease for 5–8 weeks, even after resumption of activity.

CIRCULATORY AND RESPIRATORY SYSTEM

Effects on the Circulatory System

Every 2 days of immobility results in an increase in the resting heart rate of one beat per minute, leading to tachycardia. Stroke volume decreases by 15% (possibly caused by a decrease in blood volume) after 2 weeks of bed rest. Although heart rate is increased, cardiac output decreases under normal workload conditions. The resting heart rate increases 10–12 beats after 3 weeks of bed rest. Walking on a 10% slope for half an hour at 5.6 km/h will increase heart rate by a further 35–45 beats than the normal response if an individual is subjected to a 3-week bed rest before the exercise. Increased peripheral vessel resistance will cause an increase in systolic pressure, whereas cardiac ejection and refill time are both decreased, resulting in a decreased stroke volume and a further decrease in total work capacity.[21]

Immobility can also cause body fluid redistribution. Under normal circumstances, 20% of blood volume is in the arteries, 5% is in the capillaries, and 75% is in the veins. Compared with the sitting or standing position, when a person is lying down, 500 mL of blood will rush to the thoracic cavity and heart rate will decrease, increasing cardiac output by 24%. During bed rest, the most significant decrease in blood volume occurs on day 14. As the decrease in plasma volume is more significant than the decrease in red blood cells, this causes increased blood viscosity and an increased tendency to cause thromboembolism. Plasma volume will decrease by 5% after a day of bed rest and it will further decrease by 10% after 6 days and by 20% after 14 days. Performing exercises can decrease the loss in plasma volume in normal people.[22]

Effects on the Respiratory System

Respiratory system complications induced by immobility can be lethal. The primary changes include (1) a supine position restricting thoracic cage movement and (2) gravitation-induced changes in perfusion as lying down increases venous pressure and pulmonary perfusion. When changing from a standing to a supine position, vital capacity decreases by 2% and total lung capacity decreases by 7%. After prolonged bed rest, vital capacity and total lung capacity decrease by 25%–50%, with probable mechanisms, including decreased diaphragmatic excursion, decreased rib cage ROM, and fast and shallow breathing.[23]

A decrease in gaseous exchange and an increase in perfusion will cause significant arteriovenous shunting. This can easily result in alveolar atelectasis and pneumonia if accompanied by a decrease in secretion discharge ability in the upper lungs (due to weaknesses in the abdominal muscles or ciliary dysfunction causing a decrease in coughing ability).

Orthostatic Hypotension

After a few days of bed rest in normal humans, 500 mL of blood will flow from the thoracic cavity to the lower limbs once they stand up and ankle venous pressure increases from 15 to 120 cm H_2O. Decreases in intravascular volume, changes in the compliance of venous walls, and intravenous retention will cause a decreased stroke volume and cardiac output, resulting in a decrease in systolic blood pressure. Under normal circumstances, activation of the sympathetic nervous system will increase the heart rate and maintain blood pressure stability and prevent decreases in blood pressure. After bed rest, normal sympathetic nervous responses cannot be induced, resulting in orthostatic hypotension.

Orthostatic hypotension is defined as a decrease in systolic pressure by 20 mmHg or a decrease in diastolic blood pressure by 10 mmHg within 3 min in a standing posture compared with a lying position.[24] The presentation includes dizziness, light-headedness, vertigo, and a burning sensation in the lower extremities. Patients with a history of heart disease may even experience angina because of insufficient coronary circulation. This regulatory mechanism is totally lost in normal humans who were bedridden for 3 weeks, and complete recovery requires 20–72 days (even longer in the elderly). Patients with quadriplegia are more prone to orthostatic hypotension.[25]

Deep Vein Thrombosis

Immobility clearly results in venous stasis and increases coagulation. The probability of thrombosis is increased if vascular wall injury is present. Paresis, bed rest, and trauma increase the risk of deep vein thrombosis. The probability of stroke patients developing deep vein thrombosis in the ipsilateral side is 10 times that of the contralateral side. The risk of thrombosis in patients who are unable to walk is five times that of patients who can walk 50 ft. Deep vein thrombosis readily occurs in the first week of immobility. Thrombi are often hidden in deep veins, with the most common site of occurrence being the calf vein, and 20% will extend up to the knee and thigh veins, of which half of them will result in a life-threatening pulmonary embolism. Blood stasis causes embolus formation, resulting in platelet aggregation and thrombosis. The risk factors of blood stasis are decreased calf muscle contraction strength for venous return, recent surgery, old age, obesity, heart failure, and other coagulation-prone conditions, such as cancer or high blood viscosity.[26]

Deep vein thrombosis may be lethal. First-line medical staff should observe clinical symptoms, such as edema, tenderness, erythema, and venous dilation. The presentation of deep vein thrombosis is similar to cellulitis, and it is not easy to distinguish between the two. Pulmonary embolism is a serious complication. It is difficult to diagnose, and the symptoms include dyspnea, tachycardia, bradypnea, and chest pain. Diagnosis requires sampling arterial blood gas, a radionuclide breathing scan, and angiography.

The commonly used clinical diagnostic tools include:

1. Doppler ultrasonography, which is highly accurate and the most commonly used;
2. radionuclide venous scan, which has high sensitivity and specificity with respect to large blood vessels but cannot detect calf emboli; and
3. angiography, which is considered the gold standard; however, its utilization is limited because of high invasiveness, time consumption, and low accessibility.

METABOLIC AND ENDOCRINE SYSTEM

Immobility induces changes in body composition. Total lean mass decreases and is substituted by fat mass, and bone mass insufficiency is observed. Low total lean mass further results in a low metabolic rate, decreased maximal oxygen consumption, and impaired musculoskeletal function.

Immobility results in a sodium, calcium, potassium, and phosphate ion imbalance. Bed rest leads to hyponatremia and diuresis. The symptoms of hyponatremia include drowsiness, confusion, disorientation, poor appetite, and even convulsion. The elderly are especially vulnerable. In the first few weeks of bed rest, potassium levels may also decrease, but this rarely results in serious complications.[27]

Abnormal glucose tolerance appears on the third day of immobility, and tissue glucose uptake decreases by 50% after 14 days, which worsens with increasing length of bed rest. This form of abnormal glucose tolerance can show improvement with isotonic exercises in large muscle groups, but isometric exercise is ineffective.[28] This form of abnormal glucose tolerance is not due to insufficient insulin but increased insulin resistance. Therefore, hyperglycemia or hyperinsulinemia could be due to the decrease in the quantity or affinity of insulin receptors or changes in the downstream receptor of target organs.

After bed rest, parathyroid hormone levels increase, causing hypercalcemia of unknown etiology. Other accompanying endocrine changes include increased urine cortisol levels, a decreased ACTH response in the adrenal glands, increased blood hydrocortisone levels, and decreased norepinephrine levels. Bed rest for 1 month will increase ACTH levels threefold, which requires 20 days of exercise to return to normal. In addition, total cholesterol levels do not increase.[29]

OTHER ORGAN SYSTEMS

Immobility clearly results in bladder or kidney stone and urinary tract infection. The etiology of stone formation is hypercalciuria, hyperphosphaturia, and high postvoid residue (the main cause of which is difficulty in urination in the supine position). Kidney stones cause bacterial growth and affect the efficacy of antibiotics. Stimulation of the bladder mucosa predisposes the patient to infections. Urea-decomposing bacteria can alkalinize urine and further precipitate calcium and magnesium ions.[30] Functional incontinence is an inability to reach the toilet in time because of the difficulties caused by physical or mental illness. Bed rest–induced delirium or immobility is the common cause.[31]

Bed rest decreases intestinal peristalsis, lowers appetite, and decreases blood protein levels, resulting in malnutrition. Food intake in the supine position will increase the time taken for food to pass through the digestive system, whereas a standing posture can increase esophageal peristalsis speed and shorten the time of esophageal expansion; therefore, increasing the height at the head of the bed can prevent and treat gastroesophageal reflux.[32]

The etiologies of constipation include (1) immobility increasing adrenal gland activity, inhibiting peristalsis, and increasing sphincter contractility; (2) dehydration and desiccation of stool; and (3) the stool pan causing awkwardness, resulting in patients not defecating.

Social isolation results in emotional disorders and anxiety. Combined with immobility, social isolation results in disorientation to person, time, and place; confusion and delusion; and even pain, hostility, insomnia, depression, and irritability. Bed rest and isolation for 2 weeks can incur the abovementioned symptoms. These symptoms further affect functional status and independence, resulting in a vicious cycle. The balance and coordination disorders caused by immobility could be caused by changes in nervous control rather than muscle weakness.[33]

Cognitive function may deteriorate with hospitalization. Up to 50%–60% of hospitalized older adults may develop delirium during hospitalization. Delirium is described further in detail in Chapter 13, Geriatric Psychiatric and Cognitive Disorders: Depression, Dementia, and Delirium.

ASSESSMENT

Comprehensive geriatric assessment (CGA) is used to create a plan of care for hospitalized elderly patients. A specific goal of the CGA is early identification of elder care needs to provide interventions to minimize high-risk events including deconditioning. A CGA should include assessment of ADL and instrumental ADL performance, as well as assessment of cognition, vision and hearing, social support, and psychologic well-being. A number of geriatric assessment tools can be used to make initial and ongoing evaluations of hospitalized elderly patients.[34]

PREVENTION OF COMPLICATION OF BED REST IN ACUTE HOSPITALIZATION

For the hospitalized patients, general conditions deteriorate not only caused by diseases but also by consequential effects of diseases and subsequent limitation of activities. All of the following aspects require attention and comprehensive intervention to prevent hospital-acquired deconditioning. At the acute stage of hospitalization, it is most important to prevent complications including pneumonia, urinary tract infection, joint contracture, pressure ulcer, orthostatic hypotension, and deep vein thrombosis.

Pneumonia

Breathing exercise should be instructed for the cases before surgery related with the chest or abdomen, or for cases with pulmonary disorders. Chest percussion and posture drainage should be applied once pneumonia is noted. Proper food texture and specific swallowing skills to prevent aspiration should be considered for the subjects with potential swallowing disorders.

Urinary Tract Infection and Functional Incontinence

Adequate and proper fluid intake is essential. For the patients using diapers or urinary catheters, appropriate perineum and catheter cleaning is important. For seniors with functional incontinence, nonpharmacologic conservative treatment should be emphasized first. Behavior therapies include attention training, bladder training, pelvic muscle exercises, scheduled and prompted voiding, and physical training in combination with ADL practicing.[35] In addition, environmental factors should be modified to improve accessibility. For example, the route from the patient to the toilet should be easily accessible and uncluttered to avoid delay or falls.

Joint Contracture

Bed positioning with posture change is essential. Stretching is an important factor for maintaining function. To realize and eliminate the factors inducing increased muscle tone or rigidity is the key for some specific groups with neurologic disorders. Orthoses can be considered in some cases.

Pressure Injury (Ulcer)

Prevention of pressure injury (ulcer) is one of the minimal requirements of nursing care especially for the subjects with consciousness change or with sensory impairment. Pressure ulcers occur at areas with bony prominence or thin skin. The areas around the sacrum, ischial tuberosity, femoral greater trochanter, fibular head, lateral malleolus, retro-calcaneus, and occiput are vulnerable sites.

Bed positioning with proper pillows and cushions, changing position every 2 h, preventing shearing force on the skin, supplying nutrition to prevent anemia or hypoalbuminemia are all important for pressure ulcer prevention.

Orthostatic Hypotension

Since bed rest is the main factor resulting in orthostatic hypotension, uprighting the trunk on the bed or tilting table should be applied once it is permitted. Patients with extensive paralysis, diabetic mellitus, cardiovascular disorders, autonomic nervous disorders, who are prone to orthostatic hypotension, should be managed for high risk of falls.

Deep Vein Thrombosis

To prevent deep vein thrombosis, lower limb pumping exercise with intermittent foot and calf muscle contraction is most important. Early and frequent walking and graduated compression stockings are also effective. For the high-risk patients, using an intermittent pneumatic compression device to improve circulation is indicated. Anticoagulation is the standard treatment if there are no contraindications.

INTENSIVE CARE UNIT REHABILITATION

Thanks to the advances in critical care medicine, more patients survive from serious illness. However, many survivors experience new or worse impairments of physical, cognitive, or psychologic functions known as post–intensive care syndrome.[36] Early rehabilitation and mobilization play important roles in preventing neuromuscular complications, reducing delirium, and shortening hospital length of stay, hence improving the quality of life.[37,38] Early rehabilitation and mobilization are safe and feasible and should be initiated immediately after stabilization of physiologic disorder, which may include the patients on mechanical ventilation.[39] The program starts with proper positioning, passive ROM exercises, breathing exercises, active arm and leg exercises, sitting on the edge of the bed, transfer to chair, mobilization out of bed, including ambulation.[38] Early intervention also decreases the negative effects of immobilization, such as pressure ulcer, deep vein thrombosis, heterotopic ossification, pulmonary complications, joint contracture, and physical deconditioning. The ICU healthcare team may include a variety of professionals, including physiatrists, primary care physicians, neurologists, surgeons, nurse practitioners, psychiatrists, pharmacists, dietitians, physical therapists, occupational therapists, speech language pathologists, and social workers. Early mobilization at ICU setting has shown to reduce morbidity and mortality, and active involvement of physiatrists in this intervention is highly recommended.

RECONDITIONING REHABILITATION AT SUBACUTE STAGE

At the subacute stage, the medical conditions become stable progressively. It is the optimal time for patients to start comprehensive rehabilitation. The aims of rehabilitation are to recondition the deteriorated general status and restore functions for independence. The tasks of reconditioning rehabilitation include integrated motor function training, cognition rehabilitation, activity of daily living training, assistive technology, and devices implementation.

Motor Function Training

For the patients with extensive paralysis, motor function training is the core strategy to prevent disability or to restore functions with adequate and appropriate exercise. Physical therapy to maintain a range of joint motion and to keep muscle strength and endurance should be applied for the trunk and upper and lower limbs. Training of trunk muscles, including respiratory muscles and core muscles surrounding the abdomen, can keep patients with a good pulmonary function and ensure good trunk supporting

mechanics. Since muscle power decays very quickly once patients become immobilized, the limb muscle training should be started as a bedside training. However, introduction of selective isotonic or isometric exercise for a variety of disease types at appropriate timing will require consultation from a rehabilitation specialist.

Cognition Rehabilitation and Psychologic Support

It is especially important for patients with stroke, traumatic brain injury, or other pathology of the central nervous system. It can be provided by rehabilitation professionals with specific training. Anxiety and depression are frequently noted in hospitalized patients, especially in cases with disease-related disability. These are known negative predictors that interfere with treatment and outcomes. Anxiety and depression can be effectively eliminated by psychologic support by the rehabilitation team and family prior to considering pharmacologic interventions. The details of cognitive impairment, depression, and delirium are described in Chapter 13, Geriatric Psychiatric and Cognitive Disorders: Depression, Dementia, and Delirium.

Family and social support have an amazing power, which can heal the body and mind. One recent study in China stated that both family and friend support are essential factors for the emotional well-being of the elderly. Family support had greater influence on reducing older people's negative affects, such as being frustrated, depressed, hostile, anxious, or impatient. Compared with family support, friend support, including colleagues or neighbors, played an important role in increasing positive effects, for example, being happy, friendly, and competent.[40]

Activity of Daily Living Training

A concept "give a chance for him or her to do activities independently as much as possible" needs to be promoted for disability prevention. ADL training is the most direct way of achieving an independent life, which requires rehabilitation professionals with special skills. Assistive technology and devices can assist the functions of patients with deconditioning for improving mobility and ADL. The details of assistive technology are described in Chapter 16, Assistive Technologies for Geriatric Population.

Nutrition and Metabolic Disorders

A chronic illness is usually accompanied with nutrition deficiency and metabolic disorders. Anemia, hypoalbuminemia, and electrolyte imbalance are the most common problems. The diseases and all of the related problems would cause a debilitated vicious cycle. Supplements of nutrition and correction of imbalanced conditions are important. Chewing and swallowing difficulty is highly prevalent among older adults, which may interfere with consuming sufficient nutrition. The details of nutritional support and dysphagia are described in Chapter 10, Nutritional Issues and Swallowing in the Geriatric Population.

CONCLUSION

Physical activity can maintain and enhance the function of various body systems of human beings. Bed rest in a supine position results in dysfunction and deterioration of multiple systems. Early mobilization is the cornerstone of prevention of deconditioning. As medical professionals, we should avoid bed rest and promote mobilization in patients in hospitals or institutions.

REFERENCES

1. Kortebein P. Functional decline: deconditioning. In: Means KM, Kortebein PM, eds. *Geriatrics*. Demos Medical Publishing; 2014.
2. WHO. http://apps.who.int/classifications/icd10/browse/ 2016/en#/R53; 2016.
3. King BD. Functional decline in hospitalized elders. *Medsurg Nurs*. 2006;15(5):265–271.
4. Inouye SK, Wagner DR, Acampora D, et al. A predictive index for functional decline in hospitalized elderly medical patients. *J Gen Intern Med*. 1993;8:645–652.
5. Gill TM, Allore HG, Holford TR, et al. Hospitalization, restricted activity, and the development of disability among older persons. *JAMA*. 2004;292:2115–2124.
6. Creditor MC. Hazards of hospitalization of the elderly. *Ann Intern Med*. 1993;118:219–223.
7. Cruz-Jentoft AJ, Baeyens JP, Bauer JM, et al. Sarcopenia: European consensus on definition and diagnosis. Report of the European Working Group on sarcopenia in older people. *Age Ageing*. 2010;39(4):412–423.
8. Han DS, Chang KV, Li CM, et al. Skeletal muscle mass adjusted by height correlated better with muscular functions than that adjusted by body weight in defining sarcopenia. *Sci Rep*. 2016;6:19457.
9. Berg HE, Larsson L, Tesch PA. Lower limb skeletal muscle function after 6wk of bed rest. *J Appl Physiol*. 1997;82(1):182–188.
10. Alkner BA, Tesch PA. Efficacy of a gravity-independent resistance exercise device as a countermeasure to muscle atrophy during 29-day bed rest. *Acta Physiol Scand*. 2004;181:345–357.
11. Kortebein P, Ferrando A, Lombeida J, et al. Effect of 10 days of bed rest on skeletal muscle in healthy older adults. *JAMA*. 2007;297(16):1772–1774.
12. Zimmers TA, Davies MV, Koniaris LG, et al. Induction of cachexia in mice by systemically administered myostatin. *Science*. 2002;296:1486–1488.
13. Han DS, Chen YM, Lin SY, et al. Serum myostatin levels and grip strength in normal subjects and patients on maintenance hemodialysis. *Clin Endocrinol*. 2011;75(6):857–863.
14. Ohira Y, Yoshinaga T, Ohara M, et al. Myonuclear domain and myosin phenotype in human soleus after bed rest with or without loading. *J Appl Physiol*. 1999;87(5):1776–1785.
15. Mack PB, Montgomery KB. Study of nitrogen balance and creatine and creatinine excretion during recumbency and ambulation of five young adult human males. *Aerosp Med*. 1973;44(7):739–746.
16. Funato K, Matsuo A, Yata Y, et al. Changes in force-velocity and power output of upper and lower extremity musculature in young subjects following 20 days bed rest. *J Gravit Physiol*. 1997;4(1):S22–S30.
17. Karpakka J, Vaananen K, Orava S, et al. The effects of preimmobilization training and immobilization on collagen synthesis in rat skeletal muscle. *Int J Sports Med*. 1990;11(6):484–488.
18. Cipriano CA, Pill SG, Keenan MA. Heterotopic ossification following traumatic brain injury and spinal cord injury. *J Am Acad Orthop Surg*. 2009;17(11):689–697.
19. Kanis JA, et al. The diagnosis of osteoporosis. *J Bone Miner Res*. 1994;9:1137–1141.
20. Chang KV, Hung CY, Chen WS, Lai MS, Chien KL, Han DS. Effectiveness of bisphosphonate analogues and functional electrical stimulation on attenuating post-injury osteoporosis in spinal cord injury patients- a systematic review and meta-analysis. *PLoS One*. 2013;8(11):e81124.
21. Taylor HL. The effects of rest in bed and of exercise on cardiovascular function. *Circulation*. 1968;38:1016–1017.
22. Van Beaumont W, Greenleaf JE, Juhos L. Disproportional changes in hematocrit, plasma volume, and proteins during exercise and bed rest. *J Appl Physiol*. 1972;33(1):55–61.
23. West JB. *Ventilation Blood Flow and Gas Exchange*. 3rd ed. Oxford, UK: Blackwell Scientific Publications; 1977.
24. Lanier JB, Mote MB, Clay EC. Evaluation and management of orthostatic hypotension. *Am Fam Physician*. 2011;84(5):527–536.
25. Greenleaf JE, Wade CE, Leftheriotis G. Orthostatic responses following 30-day bed rest deconditioning with isotonic and isokinetic exercise training. *Aviat Space Environ Med*. 1989;60(6):537–542.
26. Warlow C, Ogston D, Douglas AS. Deep venous thrombosis of the legs after strokes. Part I-incidence and predisposing factors. *Br Med J*. 1976;1(6019):1178–1181.
27. Zorbas YG, Merkov AB, Nobahar AN. Nutritional status of men under hypokinesia. *J Environ Pathol Toxicol Oncol*. 1989;9(4):333–342.
28. Dolkas CB, Greenleaf JE. Insulin and glucose responses during bed rest with isotonic and isometric exercise. *J Appl Physiol*. 1977;43:1033–1038.
29. Lerman S, Canterbury JM, Reiss JE. Parathyroid hormone and the hypercalcemia of immobilization. *J Clin Endocrinol Metab*. 1977;45(3):425–428.

30. Anderson RL, Lefever FR, Francis WR, et al. Urinary and bladder responses to immobilization in male rats. *Food Chem Toxicol.* 1990;28(8):543–545.

31. Gillick MR, Serrell NA, Gillick LS. Adverse consequences of hospitalization in the elderly. *Soc Sci Med.* 1982;16(10):1033–1038.

32. Moore JG, Datz FL, Christian PE, et al. Effect of body posture on radionuclide measurements of gastric emptying. *Dig Dis Sci.* 1988;33:1592–1595.

33. Downs FS. Bed rest and sensory disturbances. *Am J Nurs.* 1974;74(3):434–438.

34. Li CM, Chen CY, Li CY, Wang WD, Wu SC. The effectiveness of a comprehensive geriatric assessment intervention program for frailty in community-dwelling older people: a randomized, controlled trial. *Arch Gerontol Geriatr.* 2010;50(suppl 1):S39–S42.

35. Meyer P. Algorithms and urinary incontinence in the elderly. Assessment, treatment, recommendations and levels of evidence. Review. *Prog Urol.* 2017;27(3):111.

36. Needham DM, Davidson J, Cohen H, et al. Improving long-term outcomes after discharge from intensive care unit: report from a stakeholders' conference. *Crit Care Med.* 2012;40(2):502–509.

37. Tipping C, Harrold M, Holland A, Romero L, Nisbet T, Hodgson C. The effects of active mobilisation and rehabilitation in ICU on mortality and function: a systematic review. *Intensive Care Med.* 2017;43:171–183.

38. Morris PE, Goad A, Thompson C, Taylor K, et al. Early intensive care unit mobility therapy in the treatment of acute respiratory failure. *Crit Care Med.* 2008;36(8):2238–2243.

39. Parker A, Needham DM, Society of Critical Medicine. *The Importance of Early Rehabilitation and Mobility in the ICU*; 2013. Online. Available: http://www.sccm.org/Communications/Critical-Connections/Archives/Pages/Importance-Early-Rehabilitation-Mobility-ICU.aspx.

40. Li H, Ji Y, Chen T. The roles of different sources of social support on emotional well-being among Chinese elderly. *PLoS One.* 2014;9(3):e90051. https://doi.org/10.1371/journal.pone.0090051.

FURTHER READING

1. Brown CJ, Friedkin RJ, Inouye SK. Prevalence and outcomes of low mobility in hospitalized older patients. *J Am Geriatr Soc.* 2004;52:1263–1270.

2. Halar EM, Bell KR. Physical inactivity: physiological and functional impairments and their treatment. In: Frontera WR, ed. *DeLisa's Physical Medicine & Rehabilitation.* 5th ed. Lippincott Williams & Wilkins; 2010.

3. Inouye SK, Bogardus ST, Baker DI, Leo-Summers L, Cooney LM. The hospital elder life program: a model of care to prevent cognitive and functional decline in older hospitalized patients. *J Am Geriatr Soc.* 2000;48:1697–1706.

4. Bartels, Prince. Acute medical conditions. In: Cifu DX, ed. *Braddom's Physical Medicine and Rehabilitation.* 5th ed. Saunders; 2016.

CHAPTER 9

Polypharmacy and Mobility

MANISHA S. PARULEKAR, MD, FACP, CMD • CHRISTOPHER K. ROGERS, MPH

Polypharmacy is defined as the simultaneous use of multiple drugs to treat a single ailment or condition, or the simultaneous use of multiple drugs by a single patient, for one or more conditions. As the population is aging, polypharmacy has become an important risk factor for poor outcomes in the elderly.[1,2] Generally, polypharmacy in the elderly occurs because of three factors: demographic factors, health factors, and access to healthcare.[3] Important risk factors for polypharmacy are presented in Fig. 9.1. With advances in medicine, we have more medications available as prescriptions and over the counter. In addition, there is a surge in various nutritional and antiaging supplements, leading to increases in the incidence of polypharmacy and adverse events related to it. Box 9.1 provides facts on adverse drug events (ADEs) resulting from polypharmacy in the United States.

EPIDEMIOLOGY

Polypharmacy is an important health issue among the US population, especially the elderly. Currently, people aged 65 years and older make up 13% of US population, and they use 33% of prescription drugs.[2] By 2040, this will increase to 25% of population, using 50% of prescription medications[2] (Fig. 9.2). Approximately, 82% of adults living in the United States take at least one medication in a given week.[4] The prevalence of polypharmacy in the elderly across various healthcare settings has been reported in the literature (Table 9.1).[5–7] Among the elderly, 87.7% use at least one medication.[8] The prevalence of polypharmacy among the elderly in the United States is 35.8%.[8] Patients over 65 years of age take on average 2–6 prescribed medications and 1–3.4 nonprescribed medications.[9] Polypharmacy and associated adverse outcomes were recognized as a safety concern in the *Healthy People 2000 Final Review* (National Center for Health Statistics, 2001).[1]

Elderly patients are at an increased risk for ADEs and drug interactions.[10–12] ADEs account for nearly 700,000 emergency department visits and 100,000 hospitalizations each year.[13] Nearly 5% of hospitalized patients experience an ADE.[13] Table 9.2 presents the rate and percentage of ADEs for certain diseases.[14] Many factors contribute to ADEs in the elderly (Fig. 9.3), one such factor being the number of medications

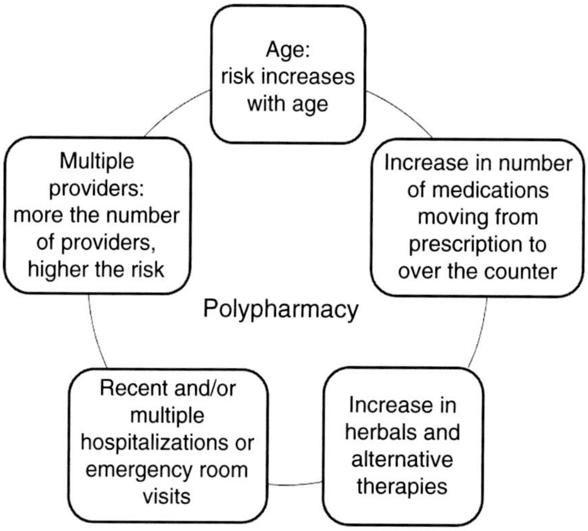

FIG. 9.1 Risk factors for polypharmacy in older adults.

> **BOX 9.1**
> **Facts on Adverse Drug Events (ADEs) Resulting From Polypharmacy in the United States**
>
> - 82% of American adults take at least one medication.
> - 25% of American adults take five or more medications.
> - ADEs cause more than 1 million emergency department visits and 280,000 hospitalizations each year.
> - $3.5 billion is spent on excess medical costs of ADEs annually.
> - 40% of costs related to ambulatory (nonhospital) ADEs can be saved.
>
> Data from Centers for Disease Control and Prevention (CDC). *Medication Safety Basics*. Available at: https://www.cdc.gov/medicationsafety/basics.html.

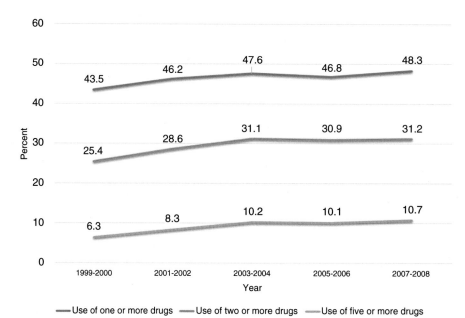

FIG. 9.2 Trends in the percentage of persons using prescription drugs in the United States, 1999–2008. (Adapted from Gu Q, Dillon CF, Burt VL. Prescription drug use continues to increase: U.S. prescription drug data for 2007-2008. *NCHS Data Brief*. 2010;(42):1.)

TABLE 9.1
Notable Studies of Polypharmacy Impacting Elderly Patients

Setting	References	Target Population	Degree of Polypharmacy	Primary Outcomes
Hospital	Flaherty et al.[5]	64 years of age and older	5 or more 7 or more 10 or more	Hospitalized patients were significantly more likely to take 7 or more medications and 10 or more medications, respectively, compared with nonhospitalized patients
Ambulatory	Kaufman et al.[3]	18 years of age and older	1 or more 5 or more 10 or more	Prescription drug use is higher in elderly women compared with men, of whom 23% took at least five in the preceding week compared with 19% in men Comorbidities were the most common reason for polypharmacy
Nursing home	Morin et al.[6]	42 years of age and older (mean age 82.5 years)	12 or more	The mean number of medications prescribed was 12.7 (range 0–30)
Nursing home	Beers et al.[7]	65 years of age and older (mean age 84 years)	7 or more	The mean number of total medications among nursing home patients was 7.2

TABLE 9.2
Causes of Drug-Related Adverse Outcomes in US Hospital Inpatient Settings, 32 States, 2011

General Causes of Drug-Related Adverse Outcomes	ADEs on Admission Number of ADEs per 10,000 Discharges	ADEs During Hospitalization Number of ADEs per 10,000 Discharges
Antibiotics and antiinfectives	90.9	28.0
Systemic agents	52.8	8.5
Hormones	46.3	20.7
Analgesics	45.5	16.2
All other general drugs and nonspecific ADE causes	215.1	64.7
Any ADE cause	**388.0**	**128.7**

ADEs, adverse drug events. Of an approximate total of 20.2 million discharges in 32 states, an estimated 782,800 ADEs were present on admission and 259,700 ADEs originated during the hospital stay.

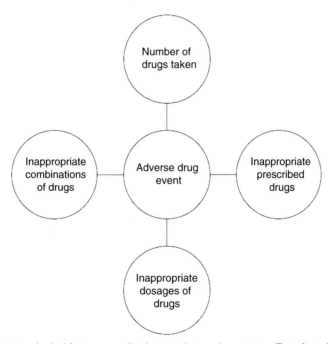

FIG. 9.3 Geropharmacological factors contributing to adverse drug events. (Data from Gallagher LP. The potential for adverse drug reactions in elderly patients. *Appl Nurs Res.* 2001;14(4):220–224.)

prescribed.[15] An estimated one-third of elderly persons will experience an adverse reaction to medication for a given year.[16] Furthermore, past research has confirmed an association between polypharmacy and ADEs and drug interactions.[17] The potential for an adverse event increases as the number of prescribed drugs increases. Elderly patients prescribed with two medications have a 6% chance of experiencing an adverse event, compared with 50% for patients prescribed with five drugs and 100% for patients prescribed with eight or more drugs.[18] One such adverse event among the elderly that results from polypharmacy is impaired mobility.[19,20]

Mobility, the ability to move around in one's environment, is the essential capacity for his or her survival. Mobility problems are most common among older adults, and the likelihood of reduced mobility and related consequences increase with polypharmacy. Consequences of reduced mobility resulting from polypharmacy are shown in Box 9.2. Elderly patients are especially vulnerable to adverse mobility events due to age-related physiologic changes resulting from the absorption, distribution, metabolism, and elimination of drugs. Montiel-Luque et al. examined polypharmacy effects on health-related quality-of-life variables in older patients and found that mobility was affected in 54.9% of the patients.[21] Herr et al. reported that having polypharmacy, in addition to frailty, markedly increases the risk of mortality. This study showed that frail people with excessive polypharmacy of 10 drugs or more were six times more likely to die.[22] This emphasizes the importance of polypharmacy among those with impaired mobility for the rehabilitation team.

AGE-RELATED PHYSIOLOGIC CHANGES AFFECTING MOBILITY

Physiologic changes of aging can impact gait and mobility adversely and make the elderly especially susceptible to adverse outcomes including falls.

- Gait changes: Shorter stride length, decreased arm swing, slower gait.
- Volume status changes: Decreased ability to maintain homeostasis, increased risk for dehydration and volume depletion, increased risk for orthostasis.
- Autonomic changes: Diminished beat-to-beat variation of heart in response to postural change, reduced vasoconstrictor response to cooling, more pronounced orthostasis.
- Central nervous system changes: Decrease in dopamine receptors, increase in α-adrenergic response and muscarinic parasympathetic response—increased tendency for Parkinsonism.
- Hearing: High-frequency hearing loss causing reduced ability to recognize speech, presbycusis—decreased sensory input for the mobility.
- Vision: Decreased lens flexibility, increased time for pupillary reflex, decreased tear production causing presbyopia, increased glare, difficulty adjusting to changes in lighting, decreased contrast sensitivity—decreased sensory input for the gait.

BOX 9.2
Consequences of Polypharmacy by System Affecting Mobility

MUSCULOSKELETAL
Muscle stiffness
Muscle soreness
Muscle apathy
Contractures
Joint pain or stiffness
Osteoporosis
Disability

RESPIRATORY
Atelectasis
Increased risk for pneumonia
Pulmonary embolism
Poor cough reflex, increased risk for aspiration

CIRCULATORY
Decreased blood pressure when standing up
Decreased sympathetic response, poor response of
    heart rate, and blood pressure changes
Cardiac arrhythmia
Hypotension
Hypertension
Deep venous thrombosis

NERVOUS
Delirium

INTEGUMENTARY
Decubitus ulcer
Decreased peripheral arterial circulation

GASTROINTESTINAL
Loss of appetite
Risk of heartburn, indigestion
Malnutrition and weight loss
Constipation
Increased aspiration due to position and inability to
    sit-up or stand after a meal

GENITOURINARY
Urinary incontinence
Urinary tract infection

MENTAL/PSYCHOSOCIAL
Confusion, irritability, or disorientation, delirium
Depression
Forgetfulness, cognitive decline
Anxiety
Decreased social interaction
Decreased self-dependence
Increased caregiver stress/burden
Increased cost of care, both health-related and custodial
    care

PHARMACOKINETIC CHANGES WITH AGING[23]

- **Absorption**: Decreased acid and pepsin secretion in stomach and decreased absorption area in small intestine may lead to impaired absorption, especially of vitamin B12, calcium, and iron.
- **Distribution**: Increased body fat percentage, decreased lean body mass and total body water.
  - Effect: Prolonged duration of action for the fat-soluble medications (e.g., opioids, benzodiazepines).
    - Recommendation: Decrease dose and frequency (longer interval between medications) when prescribing opioids and benzodiazepines.
  - Reduced albumin leading to increased availability of the active form of protein-binding medications (e.g., propranolol).
  - Reduced extracellular fluid volume allows smaller volume of distribution for the water-soluble medications (e.g., digoxin, gentamycin, cimetidine).
- **Excretion**: Impaired renal function (decreased glomerular filtration rate, tubular secretion, and blood flow).
  - Effect: Delayed excretion of the drugs requiring need for dose adjustment. A significant number of medications are excreted via kidney.
    - Recommendation: Adjustment of the dose when prescribing antibiotics.
- **Liver metabolism**: Although volume and blood supply is decreased, drug metabolism may not be affected.

PHARMACODYNAMIC CHANGES WITH AGING[23]

Impaired homeostatic capacity, which is part of physiology of aging and changes in liver and kidney metabolism, translates into increased sensitivity to various medications in the elderly. Important classes of medications include anticoagulants, antihypertensive medications, antipsychotics, and sedatives. The above changes in mobility, pharmacokinetics, and pharmacodynamics are exacerbated by chronic conditions and medications taken for the management of chronic conditions. These translate into increased risk for impaired mobility and falls. Impaired mobility and polypharmacy are independent risk factors for the disability; however, coexistence of both has much profound impact on disability.

MEDICATION CLASSES AND MOBILITY IMPAIRMENT

Medications can affect mobility by various mechanisms, and various classes of medications are commonly associated with impaired mobility. Table 9.3 presents common high-risk medications associated with impaired mobility. Benzodiazepines are commonly associated with decreased mobility.[24] They work on the central nervous system by selectively increasing the inhibitory effects of γ-aminobutyric acid.

In addition, antipsychotics have been reported as a contributing factor to drug-induced mobility problems.[25] Antipsychotics are widely used to care for elderly patients with psychiatric disorders. The use of antipsychotic drugs has been reported to be 50%–75% for elderly patients in long-term care facilities.[26] Antipsychotics work by blocking specific dopamine receptors in the brain to help normalize dopaminergic substances or actions, which in turn causes side effects such as mobility disorders, including Parkinsonism, loss of movement, akathisia, muscle spasms, and tardive dyskinesia. Elderly adults simultaneously taking one or more of the drugs outlined in Table 9.3 are at an increased risk of developing symptoms leading to mobility problems. It is important that the rehabilitation team pay attention to high-risk medications as per Beers criteria to prevent mobility impairment in patients.

Furthermore, certain classes of medications are more commonly associated with delirium and can lead to decreased mobility (Table 9.3). The rehabilitation team should become familiar with the medication classes that decrease mobility and avoid polypharmacy and functional decline.

EVALUATION OF PATIENTS FOR POLYPHARMACY AND MOBILITY IMPAIRMENT

The patient assessment begins with a comprehensive medical history review. A detailed medication history is an important part of the evaluation for polypharmacy. Any new medications, both prescription and over-the-counter ones, should be assessed and addressed. Recent hospitalization or emergency room visits are important events and can increase the risk for polypharmacy. Medication reconciliation during discharge from the hospital and at home can help minimize inappropriate medication, wrong dosage, and duplication of medications. Recent healthcare provider visits and number of healthcare providers in the care team can also increase this risk by either duplication of

TABLE 9.3
Medications May Affect Mobility in Older Adults

Category	Generic Name	Trade Name	Symptoms	Mechanisms Affecting Mobility
Benzodiazepines	Lorazepam Alprazolam Diazepam	Ativan Xanax Valium	Confusion Dizziness Lack of coordination	Disequilibrium and sedation
Antipsychotics	Haloperidol Risperidone Quetiapine	Haldol Risperdal Seroquel	Confusion/delirium	Poor insight and judgment, poor balance, unsteady gait and sedation
Opioids	Morphine sulfate Oxycodone Hydrocodone	Many trade names OxyContin, and others	Confusion/delirium	Poor insight and judgment, poor balance, unsteady gait and sedation
Vasodilators	Nitroglycerin Hydralazine Calcium channel blockers		Light-headedness Dizziness	Disequilibrium and orthostasis
First-generation antihistamines	Diphenhydramine Chlorpheniramine		Lethargy, delirium	Decreased awareness
Diuretics	Chlorothiazide Bumetanide Eplerenone	Diuril Bumex Inspra	Orthostatic hypoten- sion	Poor balance and unsteady gait

medications or drug-to-drug interaction. Special attention should also be given to the spouse or other family member medications, as medication sharing would increase the risk of adverse events. In addition, collateral history from the family and or a caregiver can help identify acute or chronic changes in mental status and mobility.

A physical assessment conducted by the rehabilitation team can identify polypharmacy and drugs that impact mobility. A gait assessment along with a special attention to mental status, heart rate, blood pressure, and checking for orthostatic blood pressure changes can provide important clues to possible medication-associated adverse events and its impact on mobility. Postural changes have been associated with syncopal episodes and can contribute to falls and impaired mobility.

INTERVENTION
Preserving Mobility Reducing Polypharmacy
Comprehensive medication review
A comprehensive medication review is the initial step that will help the rehabilitation team to promote mobility and patient safety. Box 9.3 presents details of the information needed in a comprehensive

medication review for all drugs taken. Before seeing the patient, the rehabilitation team should ask the patient to bring his/her "brown bag" to the visit for review. The "brown bag" medication review is a method of encouraging patients to bring to the visit all their medications and supplements in a bag for review.[27] For each medication contained within the bag, the clinician can determine potential adverse effects on mobility and consult with the patient's physician for possible alternative medications.

When conducting the comprehensive medication review, the clinician, if needed, should begin by briefly explaining to the patient the purpose of the medication assessment. Medical jargon should be avoided to ensure that the patient does not underreport his/her medication history. Open-ended questions should be used, such as, "What do you take for your blood clots?" and "What do you use for your heartburn?" Open-ended questions do not restrict the dimension along which the elderly answers but encourages the patient to give a full, meaningful answer using his/her knowledge, beliefs, and/or feelings concerning the medications. The clinician should encourage the patient to ask questions and when responding discuss any drug interactions and their adverse impact on mobility.

BOX 9.3
Components of Comprehensive Medication Review

- Medication names
- Strength, dosage, form, frequency, and number of tablets for all medications
- Route of administration
- Disease associated with each medication
- Contraindication for each medication
- Side effects for each medication
- Initiation of medication
- Last titration date
- Prescriber name
- Last date and time each medication was taken
- Determining if the patient is currently taking the medication
- History of allergies, interactions, and adverse reactions
- Use of over-the-counter products
- Use of vitamins, herbal, and nutritional products
- Use of topicals, liquids, injectables, and inhalants
- Name, address, website, and phone numbers of pharmacy used to fill prescriptions
- Ability to pay
- Ability to obtain medications (e.g., transportation, pharmacy delivery service)
- Missed dose of each medication
- Use of recreational drugs such as alcohol or illicit drugs

Another component of the comprehensive medication review is to determine the strength, dosage, form, frequency, and number of tablets for all medications. It is important to accurately record all medications, indications and side effects. This will help in minimizing medication use to treat side effect of another medication, an important factor in polypharmacy. The clinician should focus on any side effects, specifically those that have the potential to impact the patient's mobility, for example, muscle weakness or pain, changes in mental status, drowsiness, blurred vision, hypotension, or dizziness. In addition, the review includes obtaining information about the patient's history of allergies, interactions, and adverse reactions. If the patient reports a history of allergies, interactions, and/or adverse reactions, the clinician should document when the patient had it, how long it lasted, what medications the patient was taking,

what were the patient's signs and symptoms, and how it was treated. Prevention is the key in this situation, and information gathered should be used to reduce polypharmacy, assess the probability of future adverse events affecting the patient's mobility, and initiate interventions as needed.

Promoting safe drug use

The goal of the rehabilitation team is to educate elderly patients in the safe use of drugs to prevent mobility impairment resulting from polypharmacy. The rehabilitation team can play an important role in helping the patient to understand the effect of medications on physical functions. To the extent permitted, the rehabilitation clinician should involve the elderly patient's caretaker and family members in the education session. Together, the rehabilitation team, patient, and caretaker can collaboratively manage medication administration with careful attention to signs and symptoms of immobility resulting from polypharmacy.

Educating patients and their caretakers about their medications and the potential adverse effects on mobility requires the rehabilitation clinician to review some basic, yet important, questions about their level of understanding concerning their medication history (Box 9.4). Patients must have a basic understanding of the risks and benefits of their medications and how to communicate with their doctor when they believe they are unsure of the reasons for medications or feel they are taking too many drugs. The rehabilitation team should help the patient to identify drugs that have the potential to adversely impact his/her mobility. For example, multiple research studies have demonstrated that benzodiazepines increase the risk of self-reported mobility problems and loss of physical function.[28–30] In addition, the rehabilitation team should encourage elderly patients to use the "brown bag" technique as a way of providing their physician and pharmacist with a complete list of all drugs they take to prevent polypharmacy and assess the risk for impaired mobility. Empowering elderly patients and their caregivers to proactively monitor medications prescribed and supplements consumed and to communicate their questions and concerns to their physician or pharmacist can help prevent mobility problems and physical limitations.

SUMMARY

Once polypharmacy is identified it is essential to create an interdisciplinary plan to minimize its impact on mobility. Identifying all the members of the care

---

BOX 9.4
What Elderly Patients and Their Caretakers Should Ask and Know About Their Medications

What is the name of each drug?

What is the purpose of each drug?

How to administer each drug?

What are the risks of each drug?

What are the benefits of each drug?

Ask pharmacist for written information about the side effects of each drug.

What foods, drinks, or activities should you avoid while taking each medicine?

What should you do if a dose is missed?

How should medication be stored?

Have there been any safety problems associated with each drug reported to the US Federal and Drug Administration?

Routinely check the expiration dates for each medi and supplement.

If you have multiple prescribing physicians, bring all your medicines and supplements to your doctor visits—"brown bag."

If you have multiple pharmacist, bring all your medi and supplements to the pharmacy while filling your prescriptions—"brown bag."

Make sure your doctor knows about any medicines that have impacted your mobility in the past.

If taking more than one drug, ask your doctor to review the drugs you are taking and how your medi may impact your mobility.

If taking medicines of individual drug classes known to impact mobility such as benzodiazepines and antipsychotics, ask your doctor to review the drugs and recommend alternative drugs.

If you have a history of musculoskeletal, cardiovas respiratory, integumentary, neurologic, or metabolic illness, speak with your doctor about how your medications may alter your mobility.

Stop taking medications and report any side effects, such as muscle weakness, changes in mental sta drowsiness, blurred vision, or dizziness.

What should be done when you experience physical limitations after taking medications?

---

medication management. The following are the steps rehabilitation team may implement for patients with polypharmacy:

1. **Appointment with primary care provider**: Arranging a phone call or visit with primary care provider for medication review can be an important step in streamlining the medication list. Encouraging patients to bring the "brown bag of medications" for the visit can be extremely helpful.
2. **Pharmacy consultation** can help in monitoring drug-to-drug interactions, duplication of medications, and patient and family education.
3. **Visiting nurse visit**, when appropriate, can help with ongoing monitoring for compliance with drugs, dosage, and any new adverse events.
4. **Social worker** referral, if appropriate, can aid patients and families to comply with medical treatment regimens, including identifying financial burden and health literacy for patient and family.
5. Patient and caregiver education is a vital component in preventing polypharmacy. **Education material** for patient and family that helps them understand prescribed medications, polypharmacy, common side effects, and drug-to-drug interaction can be an immense help in preventing ADEs leading to immobility.

REFERENCES

1. National Center for Health Statistics. *Healthy People 2000 Final Review*. Hyattsville, Maryland: Public Health Service; 2001. DHHS Publication No. 01-0256. https://www.cdc.gov/nchs/data/hp2000/hp2k01.pdf.
2. Selma TP, Rochon PA. Pharmacotherapy. In: Pompei P, ed. *Geriatric Review Syllabus*. 8th ed. New York, NY: American Geriatrics Society; 2006.
3. Kaufman DW, Kelly JP, Rosenberg L, Anderson TE, Mitchell AA. Recent patterns of medication use in the ambulatory adult population of the United States. *JAMA*. 2002;287(3):337–344.
4. Slone Epidemiology Center. *Patterns of Medication Use in the United States: A Report from the Slone Survey*. Boston University; 2006. http://www.bu.edu/slone/files/2012/11/SloneSurveyReport2006.pdf.
5. Flaherty JH, Perry HM, Lynchard GS, Morley JE. Polypharmacy and hospitalization among older home care patients. *J Gerontol A Biol Sci Med Sci*. 2000;55(10):M554–M559. https://doi.org/10.1093/gerona/55.10.M554.
6. Morin L, Laroche ML, Texier G, Johnell K. Prevalence of potentially inappropriate medication use in older adults living in nursing homes: a systematic review. *J Am Med Dir Assoc*. 2016;17(9):862.e1–862.e9. https://doi.org/10.1016/j.jamda.2016.06.011.

team including family and caregiver and ongoing collaboration and communication can help minimize the adverse events associated with polypharmacy and improve patient outcomes. Primary care provider and pharmacy play a crucial role in the

7. Beers MH, Ouslander JG, Fingold SF, et al. Inappropriate medication prescribing in skilled-nursing facilities. *Ann Intern Med.* 1992;117(8):684–689. https://doi.org/10.7326/0003-4819-117-8-684.

8. Qato DM, Wilder J, Schumm LP, Gillet V, Alexander GC. Changes in prescription and over-the-counter medication and dietary supplement use among older adults in the United States, 2005 vs 2011. *JAMA Intern Med.* 2016;176(4):473–482. https://doi.org/10.1001/jamainternmed.2015.8581.

9. Stewart RB, Cooper JW. Polypharmacy in the aged. Practical solutions. *Drugs Aging.* 1994;4(6):449–461.

10. Maher RL, Hanlon JT, Hajjar ER. Clinical consequences of polypharmacy in elderly. *Expert Opin Drug Saf.* 2014;13(1):57–65. https://doi.org/10.1517/14740338.2013.827660.

11. Walsh EK, Cussen K. "Take ten minutes": a dedicated ten minute medication review reduces polypharmacy in the elderly. *Ir Med J.* 2010;103(8):236–238. http://www.lenus.ie/hse/handle/10147/122494.

12. Maeda K. Systematic review of the effects of improvement of prescription to reduce the number of medications in the elderly with polypharmacy. *Yakugaku Zasshi.* 2009;129(5):631–645. https://www.ncbi.nlm.nih.gov/pubmed/19420895.

13. AHRQ Patient Safety Network. *Medication Errors.* Agency for Healthcare Research and Quality; 2017. https://psnet.ahrq.gov/primers/primer/23/medication-errors.

14. Lucado J, Paez K, Elixhauser A. *Medication-Related Adverse Outcomes in U.S. Hospitals and Emergency Departments, 2008*HUCP Statistical Brief #109 Agency for Healthcare Research; 2011. https://www.hcup-us.ahrq.gov/reports/statbriefs/sb109.pdf.

15. Gallagher LP. The potential for adverse drug reactions in elderly patients. *Appl Nurs Res.* 2001;14(4):220–224. https://doi.org/10.1053/apnr.2001.26788.

16. The American Geriatrics Society 2012 Beers CriteriaUpdate Expert Panel. American Geriatrics Society updated Beers Criteria for potentially inappropriate medication use in older adults. *J Am Geriatr Soc.* 2012;60(4):616–631. https://doi.org/10.1111/j.1532-5415.2012.03923.x.

17. Kahl A, Blandford DH, Krueger K, Zwick DI. Geriatric education centers address medication issues affecting older adults. *Public Health Rep.* 1992;107(1):37–47. https://www.ncbi.nlm.nih.gov/pmc/articles/PMC1403599/.

18. Shaughnessy AF. Common drug interactions in the elderly. *Emerg Med.* 1992;24(21):21–32.

19. Frazier SC. Health outcomes and polypharmacy in elderly individuals: an integrated literature review. *J Gerontol Nurs.* 2005;31(9):4–11. https://www.ncbi.nlm.nih.gov/pubmed/16190007.

20. Langeard A, Pothier K, Morello R, et al. Polypharmacy cutoff for gait and cognitive impairments. *Front Pharmacol.* 2016;7(296). https://doi.org/10.3389/fphar.2016.00296.

21. Montiel-Luque A, Nuñez-Montenegro AJ, Martín-Aurioles E, et al. Medication-related factors associated with health-related quality of life in patients older than 65 years with polypharmacy. *PLoS One.* 2017;12(2):e0171320. https://doi.org/10.1371/journal.pone.0171320.

22. Herr M, Robine JM, Pinot J, Arvieu JJ, Ankri J. Polypharmacy and frailty: prevalence, relationship, and impact on mortality in a French sample of 2350 old people. *Pharmacoepidemiol Drug Saf.* 2015;24(6):637–646. https://doi.org/10.1002/pds.3772.

23. Mangoni AA, Jackson SHD. Age-related changes in pharmacokinetics and pharmacodynamics: basic principles and practical applications. *Br J Clin Pharmacol.* 2003;57(1):6–14. https://doi.org/10.1046/j.1365-2125.2003.02007.x.

24. Petrov ME, Sawyer P, Kennedy R, Bradley LA, Allman RM. Benzodiazepine use in community-dwelling older adults: longitudinal associations with mobility, functioning, and pain. *Arch Gerontol Geriatr.* 2014;59(2):331–337. https://doi.org/10.1016/j.archger.2014.04.017.

25. Saltz BL, Robinson DG, Woerner MG. Recognizing and managing antipsychotic drug treatment side effects in the elderly. *Prim Care Companion J Clin Psychiatry.* 2004;6(suppl 2):14–19. https://www.ncbi.nlm.nih.gov/pmc/articles/PMC487007/.

26. Harrington C, Tompkins C, Curtis M, Grant L. Psychotropic drug use in long-term care facilities: a review of the literature. *Gerontologist.* 1992;32(6):822–833. https://www.ncbi.nlm.nih.gov/pubmed/1478502.

27. Nathan A, Goodyer L, Lovejoy A, Rashid A. 'Brown bag' medication reviews as a means of optimizing patients' use of medication and of identifying potential clinical problems. *Fam Pract.* 1999;16(3):278–282. https://www.ncbi.nlm.nih.gov/pubmed/10439982.

28. Gray SL, LaCroix AZ, Blough D, Wagner EH, Koepsell TD, Buchner D. Is the use of benzodiazepines associated with incident disability? *J Am Geriatr Soc.* 2002;50(6):1012–1018. https://www.ncbi.nlm.nih.gov/pmc/articles/PMC4776743/.

29. Gray SL, LaCroix AZ, Hanlon JT, et al. Benzodiazepine use and physical disability in community-dwelling older adults. *J Am Geriatr Soc.* 2006;54(2):224–230. https://doi.org/10.1111/j.1532-5415.2005.00571.x.

30. Landi F, Russo A, Liperoti R, et al. Anticholinergic drugs and physical function among frail elderly population. *Clin Pharmacol Ther.* 2007;81(2):235–241. https://doi.org/10.1038/sj.clpt.6100035.

CHAPTER 10

Nutritional Issues and Swallowing in the Geriatric Population

CHRISTINA L. BELL, MD, PHD • SHARI GOO-YOSHINO, MS, CCC-SLP

INTRODUCTION

Nutritional issues in older adults can cause and compound functional decline, leading to increased morbidity and mortality. It is vital to identify and treat potentially reversible causes of weight loss and malnutrition/undernutrition as early as possible to improve outcomes. A systematic interdisciplinary approach to older adults with possible nutritional issues will ensure that important contributing factors are recognized and appropriately managed.

We will examine the issue of weight loss and malnutrition in older adults using a hypothetical patient case, Ms. Robinson.

Case Study—Initial Clinical Presentation: Ms. Robinson is 85 years old who was recently widowed and now lives alone. Last year, she was diagnosed with mild cognitive impairment and macular degeneration. She stopped driving because of her visual impairment. She also has a history of knee osteoarthritis and uses a walker intermittently "when her knees are giving her a hard time." She is independent in ADLs (activities of daily living) but relies on neighbors for rides to the market once a week, something she feels ashamed to do.

HOW COMMON IS MALNUTRITION IN OLDER ADULTS?

Malnutrition and undernutrition are synonyms and can be defined as "a state resulting from lack of intake or uptake of nutrition that leads to altered body composition (decreased fat free mass) and body cell mass leading to diminished physical and mental function and impaired clinical outcome from disease."[1] Weight loss does not always go with malnutrition, but an assessment of weight loss should consider the risk of malnutrition. The prevalence of malnutrition among ambulatory outpatient older adults has been reported to range from 5% to 30%, whereas the prevalence among hospitalized older adults has been reported to range from 23% to 60%.[2] In the long-term-care setting, the prevalence of malnutrition varied depending on how it was measured and was as high as 77% in some studies. Older adults with dementia are at particular risk of malnutrition.

The consequences of nutritional issues in older adults include higher rates of disability, morbidity, mortality, reduced quality of life, and increased healthcare costs. In the Cardiovascular Health Study, weight loss of as little as 5% over 3 years in community-dwelling geriatric patients was an independent predictor of mortality, regardless of patients' starting weight.

Case Study—Weight Loss Presentation: Ms. Robinson tells the nurse at the medical clinic that she often skips meals and lost 10 pounds in the last 4 months. She notices more fatigue and has lost her appetite. She explains to her doctor that her favorite foods just are not appetizing anymore and she feels full faster.

IS WEIGHT LOSS PART OF NORMAL AGING?

Some healthcare professionals might be tempted to think that malnutrition or weight loss is part of the normal aging process. Lean body mass normally starts to decline around the age of 30 years, whereas body fat increases until at least 65–70 years of age. However, malnutrition is not a normal part of aging. Similarly, the sense of smells declines with aging and older adults may have decreased sense of taste. However, older adults still have the ability to enjoy food that is well prepared and nicely presented. The stomach has less ability to distend and older adults may have some earlier satiety, but not to the degree that would cause malnutrition in the absence of a disease process.[3]

> **Case Study—Identification of Malnutrition:** Ms. Robinson has moderate muscle wasting, generalized weakness, and chronic arthritic changes. Her laboratory testing reveals low albumin, low cholesterol, and hypothyroidism.

WHAT IS THE BEST WAY TO IDENTIFY MALNUTRITION IN OLDER ADULTS?

Multiple measures can identify malnutrition in older adults. A body mass index (BMI; calculated as weight [kg] divided by height [m] squared or wt/[ht]^2) is a quick way to identify an older adults as undernourished (BMI < 18.5 kg/m^2), normal (18.5–24.9 kg/m^2), overweight (25–29.9 kg/m^2), or obese (30 kg/m^2 or higher).[4] In the outpatient and hospital setting, BMI is a good way to identify undernourished older adults.

Another useful and commonly used criterion for malnutrition is weight loss. In the long-term-care setting, the Medicare-mandated minimum data set defines significant weight loss as 5% body weight or more in the preceding month or 10% body weight or more in the preceding 6 months. This is considered to be one of the best measures for malnutrition in the long-term-care setting. In the outpatient setting, unintentional weight loss can also be used to raise concern for malnutrition, particularly if more than 10 pounds.[3] It is recommended that every outpatient medical visit for a community-dwelling older adult includes a screening for malnutrition and measurement of weight and BMI. In long-term-care facilities, it is recommended to check for weight loss every month. Graphing an older patient's weight over time is a very effective way to identify worrisome downward trends. The European Society of Clinical Nutrition and Metabolism recently developed diagnostic criteria for malnutrition of either BMI < 18.5 kg/m^2 or a combination of (1) unintentional weight loss (>10% of weight or >5% over 3 months) and (2) BMI under 22 kg/m^2 in adults over 70 years or low fat-free mass index. Several questionnaires also assess risk of malnutrition. The most widely used is the Mini-Nutritional Assessment or MNA. For community-dwelling elders, screening using the MNA has been shown to identify the risk of hospitalization and poor outcomes.

There are some measures that are less helpful to identify malnutrition in older adults. For example, the percentage of oral intake is often inaccurate and is not as helpful as weight loss. Trends in percentages (such as a person suddenly eating less than half or his or her food compared with usually eating all of the food) are usually more helpful than percent eaten at a single meal. Some laboratory tests, such as albumin, particularly in dementia patients, lack specificity for malnutrition, as inflammatory processes can cause the albumin to be elevated. Skinfold measurements and other anthropometric measures are also less helpful in older adults because of risk of inaccurate measurement, variation in different groups, and lack of clear-cut points for the elderly.

> **Case Study—Evaluation and Management of Malnutrition:** Ms. Robinson continues to experience slow involuntary weight loss and has now lost 16 pounds in 7 months. She discloses to the dietician that she tries to eat but does not have the energy to cook. Her current diet consists of canned soups, crackers, cereal, and coffee. Once a week she looks forward to company with her neighbor who brings fast food for their lunch. She enjoys the prepared meal but usually eats only 50% of servings.
>
> Ms. Robinson has a son who calls her weekly and drives 2 h to visit her every other week. She relies on him for decision-making in areas that her husband was responsible for such as personal finances and home maintenance problems. She prefers to be as independent as possible to avoid being a burden.

WHAT IS THE BEST APPROACH TO MALNUTRITION?

An interdisciplinary approach to malnutrition in older adults is shown in Fig. 10.1.[5]

The first step in assessing malnutrition in older adults is to determine whether caloric intake is adequate. Some medical conditions cause increased metabolism or catabolism resulting in malnutrition despite adequate oral intake, including cancer, thyroid problems, or infections, noted in Box 10.1.

If caloric intake is inadequate, the second step is to assess the older adult's access to food. Strategies for improving access to food for older adults, especially those who live alone, are summarized in Box 10.2. Bringing isolated older adults to community centers or adult day-care centers to eat with other people improves nutrition, especially when combined with activities and exercise strategies. It is essential to identify and remove dietary restrictions in older adults with malnutrition or who are at risk of malnutrition. The American Dietetic Association recommends removing restrictive, therapeutic diets in long-term-care patients as a way of improving intake, weight gain, and quality of life.[6] Supplements can sometimes be helpful, but studies have had mixed conclusions and the mortality benefit is small. Other strategies include providing favorite foods and making sure the food is served at the appropriate temperature (soups and hot meals should be hot or warm, not lukewarm,

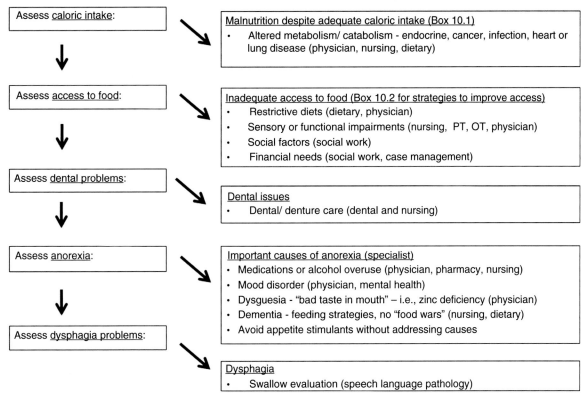

FIG. 10.1 Overview of interdisciplinary evaluation and management of nutritional issues in older adults. (Data from Omran ML, Salem P. Diagnosing undernutrition. *Clin Geriatr Med*. 2002;18(4):719–736.)

BOX 10.1
Medical Conditions Associated With Malnutrition in Older Adults

Cardiac/pulmonary diseases (i.e., congestive heart failure, cardiomyopathy, chronic emphysema)

Cancer

Infections/AIDS

Rheumatoid arthritis

Helicobacter pylori

Gallbladder disease

Malabsorption (i.e., Crohn's disease, short gut syndrome)

Hypothyroidism or hyperthyroidism

Alcoholism

Parkinson's disease

Pressure ulcers

Adapted from Omran ML, Salem P. Diagnosing undernutrition. *Clin Geriatr Med*. 2002;18(4):720; with permission.

and ice cream and frozen items should be cold). Homemade milk shakes, gravy, and sauces are other great ways to increase caloric intake. Increasing protein intake, especially with foods such as eggs, tofu, fish, or beans, can also improve nutrition. Finally, it is important to consider cultural factors, such as preferred foods, or cultural practices, that may be missing in an assisted living or nursing home setting, which can have a profound impact on an older adults' nutritional status.

Functional issues can also affect access to food by impairing an older adult's ability to feed himself or herself. Poor dexterity and arthritis can make using utensils difficult and result in reduced oral intake. Specially adapted devices and utensils can enhance the ease of self-feeding. Similarly, for patients with tremors, utensils can be modified and diet can be changed slightly to reduce frustration from spilling. Occupational therapists can provide expertise in adaptive equipment to enhance a patient's ability to eat. As much as possible, meals in bed should be avoided, as the positioning in bed tends to increase intraabdominal pressure and be uncomfortable for eating, and it is recommended to have patients sit up in a chair for meals. Completely

BOX 10.2
Strategies for Improving Access to Food for Older Adults

Meal programs/Meals on Wheels

Senior centers or adult day care if home-dwelling

Serve food attractively and at the correct temperature

Companionship and congregate dining

Comfortable seating, warm lighting, ambient music, and use of china plates

Family-style or cafeteria-style meals better than fixed-portion trays

Special utensils if arthritis impairs the use of utensils

Assist or enable self-feeding if tremors impair feeding

Cues for hearing and visual impairment

Positioning if bed-bound (upright, alert, comfortable, able to see the plate)

Make diet as liberal as possible (remove restrictive therapeutic diets)

Smaller more frequent meals and snacks

Provide favorite foods, milk shakes, gravy, and sauces to increase calories

bed-bound patients need to be carefully positioned to be able to see what they are eating, control foods and liquids in their mouths, and remain comfortable throughout a meal.

The third step in evaluating and managing malnutrition in older adults is to assess for dental problems. The dental team is an integral part of the management of malnutrition, as carefully assessing and treating broken or rotten teeth, poorly fitting dentures, dry mouth, oral lesions, and candidiasis can improve oral intake and quality of life. Ongoing oral care improves dysgeusia (bad taste in the mouth) and dry mouth, and family and/or caregivers may need to help older adults with monitoring, cleaning, and rinsing out the teeth, mouth, and dentures. Edentulousness is an independent risk factor for weight loss; therefore evaluating community-dwelling and more functional nursing home patients for dentures may help improve nutrition. In addition, oral care is one of the best methods for preventing pneumonia among nursing home patients.

The fourth step is to assess for anorexia. Anorexia is not a normal part of aging. It is common for health professionals to wonder if appetite stimulants may be an option for older malnourished adults with anorexia. Before considering an appetite stimulant, it is important to first work closely with the pharmacist and

medical team to reduce or stop any medications that may be affecting appetite. Depression, substance abuse, and other psychologic disorders need to be identified and treated if present. Mirtazapine for depression can stimulate appetite and improve the mood and can be a good choice if an older adult has depression, malnutrition, and trouble sleeping. Appetite stimulants such as megestrol have potentially dangerous side effects in older adults, including risk of thromboembolism, and are generally not recommended as an initial treatment for malnutrition or weight loss for most older adults. Artificial nutrition and hydration can be considered in appropriate clinical situations, such as reversible postoperative malnourished states where clinical improvement is expected. Use of long-term artificial nutrition and hydration in end-stage dementia or terminal cancer is generally not recommended in the geriatric population. Discussions about artificial nutrition and hydration in frail older adults should be approached by the team using sensitivity, high-level communication skills, and a careful appraisal of risks versus benefits. A detailed discussion of artificial nutrition and hydration in the geriatric population is beyond the scope of this chapter, but training programs to enhance communication skills in this area can be very helpful.

Older adults with dementia have additional factors that need to be considered in addressing malnutrition. Mood disorders, adjustment to new care settings, understimulation or overstimulation, misperceptions, paranoia, and other behavioral issues can contribute to feeding difficulties in older adults with dementia. The Edinburgh Feeding Evaluation in Dementia can help identify challenging behaviors related to feeding in older adults with dementia. There are some feeding strategies that can be particularly helpful in older adults with dementia (Box 10.3).[7]

Case study—New Concern: Ms. Robinson calls her neighbor after awakening and feeling "too weak" to get out of bed. Her neighbor calls 911 for emergency care. She is taken to a hospital and admitted for a stroke. During the review of her history, involuntary weight loss, reduced appetite, and fatigue over the past 7 months were noted. Her admitting team wonders if the stroke may have affected her swallowing as well.

Swallowing problems (dysphagia) are particularly important to recognize and address in older adults, especially when evaluating and managing malnutrition. Oropharyngeal dysphagia is defined as a swallowing difficulty that affects the transport of foods and liquids from the mouth to the esophagus. According to a position document developed by the Dysphagia Working Group, oropharyngeal dysphagia is included in the World Health Organization's classification of diseases and meets the criteria of a geriatric syndrome including high frequency of occurrence in older adults, multiple causal factors, poor outcomes, and multidisciplinary treatment.[8] The processes and methods for management of oropharyngeal dysphagia in the geriatric population are discussed in this section and are aimed to support interprofessional practice in prevention, early identification and diagnosis, and intervention of dysphagia to reduce consequences that are both costly and compromise health and quality of life.

HOW COMMON IS DYSPHAGIA IN OLDER ADULTS?

Oropharyngeal dysphagia is a clinical symptom of an underlying disease process that affects 1 in 25 adults.[9] In a systemic review by Takizawa et al.,[10] the prevalence of oropharyngeal dysphagia was high in patients with a history of stroke (8%–80%), Parkinson's disease (11%–81%), traumatic brain injury (27%–30%), and community-acquired pneumonia (92%). A systematic review by Alagiakrishnan, Bhanji, and Kurian indicated 13%–57% of persons with dementia also have dysphagia.[11] Although aging is not a disease, age-related diseases such as these exacerbate, predispose, and increase the risk of dysphagia in the elderly population.

As a result, the prevalence of swallowing impairment increases with age. As older adults are the fastest-growing segment of the overall population, oropharyngeal dysphagia is becoming a critical healthcare issue.

Complications resulting from dysphagia include aspiration pneumonia, chronic lung disease, malnutrition and dehydration, and compromised general health prompting treatment with possible hospitalization. Choking and death are also morbid outcomes. Furthermore, dysphagia can disrupt quality of life for affected individuals with diminished satisfaction of eating and drinking and in activities surrounding meals such as grocery shopping, cooking, and social engagements. Collectively, these complications extend beyond the patient by adding to caregiver burden.

HOW DOES AGING AFFECT SWALLOWING?

The swallowing process has four phases that occur in a controlled, timed, and overlapping sequence of events requiring central and peripheral sensory-motor activity. Any compromise in this dynamic process can result in oropharyngeal or esophageal dysphagia:

- First phase: Oral preparation phase consists of chewing and mixing food with saliva. Foods and liquids (i.e., bolus) are then gathered and controlled on the tongue (Fig. 10.2A).[12]
- Second phase: Oral phase is the transfer of bolus from anterior to posterior of the tongue (Fig. 10.2B and C).
- Third phase: Pharyngeal phase starts when the bolus enters and then passes through the pharynx (Fig. 10.2C–E).
- Fourth phase: Esophageal phase refers to passage of the bolus through the esophagus and lower esophageal sphincter (Fig. 10.2F).

Presbyphagia refers to changes in the swallowing process of healthy adults related to a natural course of aging that includes alteration in the central nervous system, head and neck anatomy, physiology, and sensory-motor function.[13,14] Swallowing in older adults may be slower in all phases and result in pooling in the pharynx but is not considered a disorder.[13-16] However, these differences reduce functional reserve and can compromise safe and efficient swallowing when a vulnerable system is challenged with "physical exertion, injury, infection, starvation, and dehydration."[17]

WHAT ARE CAUSES OF DYSPHAGIA IN OLDER ADULTS?

Although aging is not a disorder, adults are at risk for comorbid conditions related to aging that increase

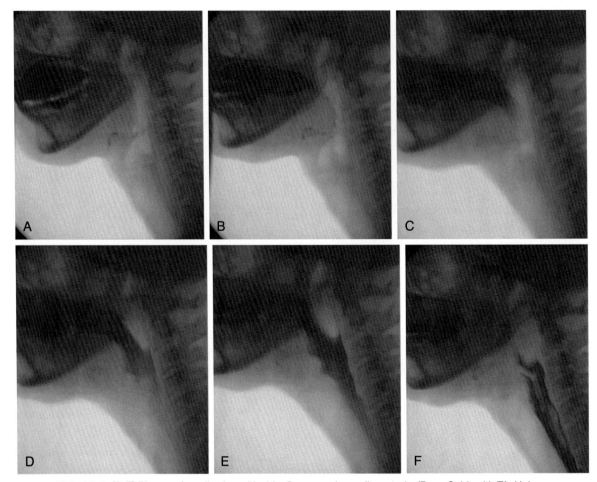

FIG. 10.2 **(A–F)** Phases of swallowing with videofluoroscopic swallow study. (From Goldsmith TA, Holman AS, Nunn D. Videofluoroscopic evaluation of oropharyngeal swallowing. In: Som PM, Curtin HD, eds. *Head and Neck Imaging*. 5th ed. St. Louis: Mosby, Inc.; 2011; with permission.)

their risk for dysphagia and aspiration pneumonia. The most common causes of dysphagia in adults include neurologic, medical, and surgical conditions and head and neck cancer treatment.[18] Although it may be difficult to identify the main cause of dysphagia in an older adult with a complex history, it is critical to the evaluation and management of oropharyngeal dysphagia. Box 10.4 lists medical conditions that may contribute to dysphagia.

Case Study—Identification of Swallowing Difficulties: Ms. Robinson is alert for a swallow screening by the nurse. After the final swallow of water, she coughs. This is considered a failed screening test at this hospital, triggering a referral for a clinical swallow evaluation.

HOW IS DYSPHAGIA IDENTIFIED?

A swallow screen is a pass/fail procedure that identifies individuals who require a comprehensive swallow assessment or a referral for other professional and/or medical services. Although systematic reviews did not result in agreement on the best screening tool for oropharyngeal dysphagia, instruments developed for diverse age groups were identified. Because the absence of consensus does not mean screening should not be performed, it is imperative that professionals select a process that is appropriate for their patient population and reliable in identifying or ruling out dysphagia.[19] If a screening is positive, a follow-up comprehensive swallow assessment is warranted. Fig. 10.3 shows a workup process from identification to treatment of dysphagia.

BOX 10.4
Medical Conditions That May Contribute to Dysphagia in Older Adults

Alzheimer's disease

Cardiothoracic surgery

Cognitive decline—other dementias

Deconditioning

Delirium

Dentition absent or in poor condition

Developmental disabilities (e.g., cerebral palsy)

Frailty

Gastroesophageal reflux

Head and neck cancer or cancer treatment

Lung disease—respiratory compromise

Medication related

Multiple sclerosis

Parkinson's disease

Post–polio syndrome

Pulmonary diseases

Sarcopenia

Stroke

Traumatic brain injury

WHAT ARE SYMPTOMS AND SIGNS OF DYSPHAGIA?

Although symptoms and signs of dysphagia can be present, problems may still go undetected. Elders may be unaware of or unable to report difficulties. For these reasons, a caregiver report of changes in food preparation or preferences (e.g., soft, moist over dense, chewy foods), eating habits (e.g., chewing foods well and frequent sips of liquid), and extended mealtime and effort level can be revealing. It is essential to consider symptoms and signs of dysphagia in the context of other clinical indicators, rather than relying on a single symptom or sign. Refer to Table 10.1 for a list of common symptoms and signs of dysphagia in the elderly.

Case study—Evaluation: A speech-language pathologist conducts a clinical swallow evaluation. Although Ms. Robinson attributed coughing to "just old age," she acknowledged some fear when swallowing. Her son noted problems about a year ago that gradually

worsened. He was mostly concerned about his mother's weakened state and ability to continue independent living.

Ms. Robinson is alert to participate in the intake and examination. Her speech is understood although mildly imprecise in articulation. Her son indicates no communication changes with the exception of slurred speech that significantly improved over the past 24 h.

An oral motor examination reveals reduced tongue strength and control. Dentition is compromised for chewing with no opposing molars. Ms. Robinson acknowledges having dentures but prefers not to wear them.

To evaluate swallow function, Ms. Robinson is offered various liquids and foods. Using a systematic approach, texture and bolus size are increased to safely challenge her swallow. She exhibits both oral preparation and oral phase dysphagia with prolonged chewing and food residue on her tongue. After successive liquid swallows, her voice changes to a wet quality. She also coughs when swallowing liquids with preexisting food in her mouth and reports sensation of food sticking in her throat.

Therapeutic intervention trials and training are introduced in the session. Wet vocal quality and cough decreases with compensatory strategies (individual sips of liquid to improve bolus control, two swallows per teaspoon of food to eliminate oral and sensation of pharyngeal residue), postural adjustments (chin tuck), and texture modification (nectar-thick liquid).

Ms. Robinson and her son, speech-language pathologist, physician, nurse, and dietician collaborate in developing a plan of care that includes the following:
1. Modify the diet order to cohesive, moist, minced foods, requiring minimal chewing. Meals will include personal preferences of coffee, soup, oatmeal, mashed potato, and cottage cheese.
2. Initiate dysphagia intervention to establish compensatory strategies (individual sips and two swallows per teaspoon of food).
3. Assess barriers to oral care and wearing dentures.
4. Continue nutrition therapy to optimize oral intake to meet nutrition and hydration needs with an addition of healthy and calorie-dense snacks.
5. Perform an instrumental swallow examination to evaluate oral and pharyngeal phases of swallow and assess effectiveness of therapeutic interventions to improve swallow efficiency and safety.

HOW IS DYSPHAGIA DIAGNOSED?

Evaluation and management of dysphagia is a complex and multidimensional process that is best accomplished with an interprofessional approach. The team includes the patient, their support network, speech-language pathologist, physician, nurse, dietician, radiologist, gastroenterologist, otolaryngologist, neurologist, and others depending on the patient's needs.

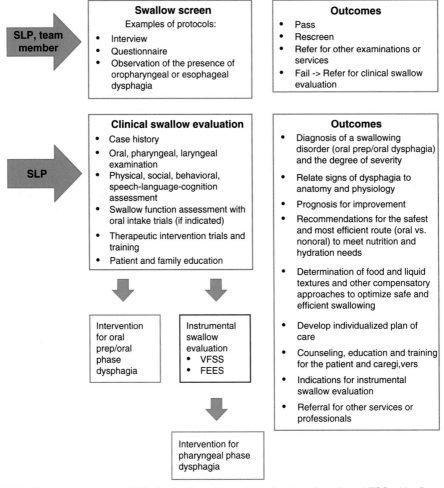

FIG. 10.3 Dysphagia workup. *FEES*, fiberoptic endoscopic evaluation of swallow; *VFSS*, videofluoroscopic swallow study.

Based on the primary symptoms, the initial step may be a referral to the speech-language pathologist for an evaluation of oral and pharyngeal phases of swallowing or gastroenterologist for gastrointestinal concerns. This section focuses on the evaluation of oropharyngeal dysphagia.

Clinical (or Bedside) Swallow Evaluation

If signs and symptoms are more consistent with an oropharyngeal dysphagia (vs. esophageal dysphagia), the first step in diagnosis is a clinical swallow evaluation conducted by a speech-language pathologist specializing in swallowing. Critical elements involve:
- a review of medical records and interview with patient, family, and caregivers;

- an assessment of alertness, speech, language, and cognitive abilities;
- an examination of oral structures and function involved in swallowing;
- a systematic evaluation of swallow during intake of various food and liquid textures based on swallow safety and patient's acceptance; and
- a trial of compensatory strategies to reduce or eliminate symptoms or clinical signs of swallowing difficulty.

To gather accurate and relevant information from older adults, it is important for healthcare providers to be mindful of their patients' communication needs without ageist assumptions. The following can enhance engagement and evaluation results[20]:

TABLE 10.1
Symptoms and Signs of Dysphagia

GENERAL SYMPTOMS AND SIGNS OF DYSPHAGIA
Coughing
Choking
Hoarse voice
Globus sensation
Complaints of pain with swallowing
Repeated swallows per sip of liquid or teaspoon of food
Involuntary weight loss and difficulty gaining weight
Recurring pneumonia, respiratory infection or fever

Symptoms and Signs of Oropharyngeal Dysphagia	Symptoms and Signs of Esophageal Dysphagia
• Coughing during or shortly after eating and drinking • Complaints of food "sticking" in the pharynx • Reduced mouth opening or labial seal around spoon or cup • Holding food or liquid in mouth • Prolonged chewing • Spill of food or liquid from the lips or nasal cavity • Food or liquid residue in the mouth • Fear of eating or swallowing • Drooling or extra secretions • Dysarthria • Wet voice during or after swallow • Difficulty coordinating breathing and swallowing	• Chronic coughing • Complaints of food "sticking" in the throat or chest • Pressure or burning in chest • Progressive difficulty in swallowing solids to liquids • Vomiting • Hiccups • Bone pain • Black stool • Anemia • Fatigue

- optimize sensory information (e.g., placement of glasses or hearing aids as needed);
- focus attention (e.g., greet the older adult using his/her name, establish eye contact, reduce distractions);
- encourage autonomy (e.g., include the older adult in conversation, share decision-making); and
- support participation (e.g., provide simple directions; allow additional time for processing, comprehension, and expression; ask open-ended questions; model or use visual aids; and verify exchanges).

Reports and observations are integrated to determine the presence of oral preparation and oral phase dysphagia, symptoms or clinical signs of pharyngeal phase dysphagia, nature of impairment, and etiology of the disorder. Outcomes also include recommendations for an oral diet (if indicated), support and intervention to improve swallow safety and efficiency, patient and family education, and direction of next steps such as an instrumental swallow examination. In addition, a referral and consultation with other specialists and follow-up for dysphagia may be indicated based on presentation. For example, if a patient complains of

sensation of slow clearance through the esophagus, a referral to a gastroenterologist should be considered.

> **Case Study—Instrumental Swallow Examination:** A videofluoroscopic swallow study (VFSS) is selected based on clinical questions (e.g., Is cough related to aspiration? If yes, is it resulting from oral impairment, pharyngeal impairment, or both? What impact do strategies have on bolus flow through oropharynx?) and Ms. Robinson's preference. Before the study, Ms. Robinson's son and a nursing assistant helped with the placement of her dentures with adhesive. She was encouraged to wear them as tolerated during meals. A speech-language pathologist provided education and training to establish individual sips of liquid, two swallows per teaspoon of food, and coordinate chin tuck with swallows.
>
> The speech-language pathologist and radiologist conducted the VFSS. Radiographic visualization of the oral, pharyngeal, and laryngeal structures and function confirmed oral phase dysphagia with residual of food on her tongue. Visualization also showed entrance of liquids into the airway and trace aspiration before the swallow. These signs are related to reduced tongue movement and strength. Pharyngeal phase dysphagia is

characterized by liquid and food residue in the vallecula related to reduced tongue base retraction. Ms. Robinson is aware of this residue to swallow again. Swallows evaluated with compensatory strategies improved safety and efficiency of swallow. The chin tuck in particular reduced the spill of liquids deep into the pharynx and eliminated aspiration and residue in the vallecula.

Results of the study are discussed with the medical team. Based on her history, it is determined that dysphagia is likely resulting from a combination of preexisting sarcopenia exacerbated by malnutrition before this admission and further impaired by the stroke.

Additional recommendations included:
1. resumption of thin liquids with chin tuck;
2. continuation of therapy for dysphagia with exploration of restorative treatment;
3. occupational therapy for assessment and assistance with ADL training including increasing independence in oral care and denture placement;
4. physical therapy to support safe and independent mobility within her home and community settings.

Instrumental Swallow Examination

An instrumental swallow examination is used to evaluate all phases of swallowing. The aim is to clarify the nature of the disorder with related anatomic and physiologic impairment. Unlike a clinical swallow evaluation, an instrumental swallow examination provides direct visualization of the pharyngeal and laryngeal structures to determine the presence, severity, and characteristics of pharyngeal phase dysphagia. It is also sensitive to identifying aspiration, which is critical because approximately 40% of patients who aspirate do so without cough response.[21] This is called silent aspiration.

Guidelines for the appropriate use of instrumental procedures have been developed with consensus.[22] Refer to Table 10.2 for indications and contraindications for an instrumental swallow evaluation.

Instrumental swallow evaluations consist of two primary procedures that allow the provider to view the anatomy and physiology of swallowing structures to determine the nature and severity of oropharyngeal dysphagia and aspiration. In hospital and clinical settings, common options include VFSS also known as modified barium swallow study (MBSS) and fiberoptic endoscopic evaluation of swallow (FEES):
- VFSS or MBSS (Fig. 10.2)
  - A radiographic procedure conducted by a speech-language pathologist, frequently in collaboration with a radiologist performed in a radiology suite. Images of the oral, laryngeal, pharyngeal, and upper esophageal structures and movement are

TABLE 10.2
Indications and Contraindications for an Instrumental Swallow Evaluation

Indications	Contraindications
History of medical conditions associated with high risk for dysphagia and aspiration	Medical instability
Uncertainty in safety and efficiency of swallowing	Unable to participate or cooperate
Differential diagnosis of dysphagia to guide management and treatment	Outcome would not change management or treatment
Symptoms or signs are inconsistent with clinical presentation	

viewed in the lateral and anterior-posterior planes as foods and liquids (mixed with barium or water-soluble contrast medium) are swallowed.
- FEES (Fig. 10.4)
  - A procedure conducted by a speech-language pathologist, frequently in collaboration with an otolaryngologist. It is an examination that can be performed at bedside with portable equipment. The examiner passes a flexible endoscope through the nasal pharynx for direct visualization of the anatomy of the larynx and pharynx at rest and with swallowing tasks.

Both procedures result in diagnosis, understanding of the nature and severity of the problem, and assessment of the effect of strategies on swallow safety and efficiency. Given the availability of both evaluations within a facility, refer to Table 10.3 for the benefits of VFSS versus FEES.

Case Study—Intervention: Ms. Robinson is now consuming about 75%–90% of minced foods and nectar-thick liquid meals, more than her intake at home. After being cleared to drink thin liquids with chin tuck, she often accepts sips of water throughout the day with snacks.

Although Ms. Robinson does not mind modified diet textures, she expressed a desire to eat "regular" foods such as grilled ham and cheese sandwich and stew. Meals are liberalized with inclusion of soft filled sandwiches and other soft, moist foods as her risk of choking has decreased with two swallows to clear residual of food from her tongue.

She agrees to start a restoration program with exercises intended to improve and maintain muscle function for swallowing. Oral and pharyngeal motor exercises are selected based on impairments noted on the swallow evaluation. Ms. Robinson responds well to models and brief written instructions to optimize her accuracy and independence in demonstrating exercises. The speech-language pathologist's role of coaching Ms. Robinson through exercises is gradually transferred to her son to optimize follow-through at home.

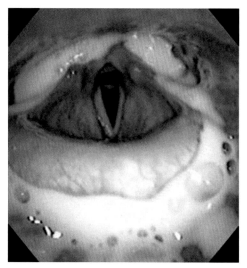

FIG. 10.4 Fiberoptic endoscopic evaluation of swallowing. Liquid residue in the vallecula and pyriform sinuses. (From Leder SB, Murray JT. Fiberoptic endoscopic evaluation of swallowing. *Phys Med Rehabil Clin North Am*. 2008;19(4):792; with permission.)

TABLE 10.3

Comparison of Videofluoroscopic Swallow Study (VFSS) Versus Fiberoptic Endoscopic Evaluation of Swallow (FEES)

Clinical Indications	VFSS	FEES
Can be performed in patients with • Movement disorder • Bleeding disorder or recent epistaxis • Recent craniofacial trauma • Bilateral nasal obstruction	+	
Poor tolerance for nasal endoscopy	+	
Global complaints	+	
Evaluate oral preparation and oral phases	+	
Screen esophageal phase	+	
Evaluate pharyngeal phase	+	+
Identify aspiration	+	+
Evaluate swallow of secretions (high risk of aspiration)		+
Real-time patient and family education, strategy training, and biofeedback without radiation exposure		+
Barium allergy or intolerance		+
Claustrophobia		+
Imaging equipment cannot accommodate patient's size or posture limitations		+

HOW IS DYSPHAGIA TREATED?

Effective treatment of dysphagia is guided by comprehensive evaluation results and ongoing assessment of the individual's interest and response to intervention. In older adults, developing and executing an individualized patient-centered plan of care must consider primary condition(s) related to the dysphagia and their goals, priorities, and resources.

Key treatment goals of intervention are to minimize related consequences of oropharyngeal dysphagia. This includes a safe and efficient oral intake of a least restrictive diet (textures) to meet nutrition and hydration needs. Treatment includes education and compensatory and rehabilitative approaches.

Education and Counseling

Within an interdisciplinary process, information about conditions and diseases likely affecting nutrition and swallowing, the nature and the consequences of dysphagia, and intervention options are shared with patients (and their families and caregivers). Discussions also include feeding and swallowing guidelines, instructions for thickening liquids (if recommended), and suggestions to incorporate palate preferences to optimize adherence.

Compensatory Approaches

Strategies used to offset impairment improve swallow safety without altering physiology. Simple and quick strategies include smaller bites of foods or sips of liquid to improve bolus control or follow-up dry or liquid swallows to clear oral and pharyngeal residue. In a review of these types of compensatory strategies, Lazarus reported positive outcomes with reduction in medical consequences of oropharyngeal dysphagia such as aspiration pneumonia and enhanced nutritional

> **BOX 10.5**
> **General Strategies to Optimize Safe Oral Intake**
>
> Offer meals when individual is alert and ready
>
> Place dentures (that fit comfortably)
>
> Sit upright during and after eating and drinking
>
> Mouth should be clear of food before next bite or sip
>
> Swallow food and liquid before talking or next bite of food or sip of liquid
>
> Allow more time to swallow and complete meals
>
> After meal, clear mouth of residual food
>
> Maintain healthy oral care and hygiene

> **Case Study—Ongoing Assessment and Support:** Ms. Robinson reports feeling "good" and "ready to go home." Her laboratory testing reveals improvement in prealbumin level along with an increase in her appetite, weight, and energy level. Her son agrees with plans for her discharge to home with home care rehabilitation (OT, PT, and speech-language pathology). Social work will continue to assist her in identification and utilization of community resources such as transportation for medical appointments and meal deliveries while she contemplates a move to an assisted living center.
>
> Nutrition recommendations include more frequent smaller meals (i.e., 4–6 meals a day), making sure to get sources of protein and fluids in her diet, and keeping meals social by eating with others and limiting isolation.
>
> Speech-language pathology recommendations include follow-up for (1) swallow reassessment including a repeat VFSS and (2) initiating cognitive-communication assessment and intervention for mild cognitive impairment to optimize cognitive function.

status.[23] Refer to Box 10.5 for general strategies to optimize safe oral intake.

Diet modification, such as thickening liquids and downgrading food textures, is frequently used during the acute phase of an illness and adjusted as swallow function improves or other compensatory strategies are established.[24] In the context of progressive disease with a decline in cognitive and swallow function, diet modifications may be used long term. Systematic reviews of oropharyngeal dysphagia management concluded that the use of thickened liquids may be advantageous in addressing dysphagia and reducing aspiration.[11,24] Although supported in research, texture changes may not be well accepted by individuals, particularly in elders who may already have appetite changes from reduced sense of smell and taste. Older adults often have poor compliance with thickened liquids because of dissatisfaction and inaccessibility. With this in mind, it is important to determine if the benefits outweigh the risks such as refusal to eat and drink, anxiety, and social isolation that can add to further functional decline.

Other compensatory strategies include postures and maneuvers that can also be helpful in the management of dysphagia. Although chin-tuck and airway-protection maneuvers (e.g., supraglottic swallow) may improve swallow function, effects in preventing aspiration are variable. In addition, these intentional modifications may be difficult to execute consistently in individuals with memory and endurance challenges. For individuals who demonstrate the ability to promptly and consistently follow instructions and retain new information, it may be reasonable to provide them with training opportunities to support their independence in using behavioral strategies as a first option rather than thickened fluids.

Rehabilitative Approaches

The principles of neuroplasticity—use it or lose it; use it and improve it; and repetition, intensity, and saliency matter—are applied to improve swallow physiology.[15] Swallow function exercises are selected based on the underlying impairment. For example, resistance and range-of-motion exercises for labial and lingual weakness or swallowing with "effort" to increase posterior tongue base movement may be prescribed. Exercises can take weeks to months to take effect.

In approaching swallowing issues in older adults, it is important to broaden the focus beyond the act of swallowing. Physical therapy and occupational therapy are crucial in enhancing a patient's ability to sit upright, use utensils, and feed oneself. Nursing, dental, pharmacy and medical professionals need to review and manage oral care, medications and reversible medical conditions affecting the mouth, swallowing, or mental alertness, which may contribute to eating or swallowing problems. Dietary specialists should continue to monitor the nutritional quality of the older adult's diet. In addition, as the older adult's condition stabilizes and swallowing improves, ongoing monitoring for malnutrition and weight loss remains essential.

The most common reversible causes of malnutrition in older adults are summarized with the mnemonic "Meals on Wheels" in Fig. 10.5.[25] Healthcare professionals need to work as a team to identify and treat factors contributing to malnutrition, weight loss, and dysphagia in older adults. A continued team approach toward the older adult, with attention to the medical,

Medication (digoxin, theophylline, psychotropics)	**W**andering (dementia/ behavior)
	Hyperthyroidism/ hyperparathyroidism
Emotional (depression)	**E**nteric problems (malabsorption)
Anorexia/ alcoholism	**E**ating problems
Late-life paranoia	**L**ow-salt or restricted diets
Swallowing disorders	**S**ocial/ shopping/ food prep problems
Oral and dental disease	
No money	

FIG. 10.5 Reversible causes of malnutrition: "Meals on Wheels." (Adapted from Morley JE, Silver AJ. Nutritional issues in nursing home care. *Ann Intern Med.* 1995;123(11):850–859; with permission.)

functional, and social aspects of eating and nutrition, is necessary to maintain gains made in nutrition and weight. A clear, stepwise approach, such as the one outlined in this chapter, will help to ensure that important factors are not missed and that the team is able to work together to improve quality of life for our older adults.

REFERENCES

1. Cederholm T, Barazzoni R, Austin P, et al. ESPEN guidelines on definitions and terminology of clinical nutrition. *Clin Nutr.* 2017;36(1):49–64. https://doi.org/10.1016/j.clnu.2016.09.004.
2. Agarwal E, Miller M, Yaxley A, Isenring E. Malnutrition in the elderly: a narrative review. *Maturitas.* 2013;76(4):296–302. https://doi.org/10.1016/j.maturitas.2013.07.013. PMID: 23958435.
3. Medina-Walpole A, Pacala JT, Potter JF, eds. *Geriatrics Review Syllabus: A Core Curriculum in Geriatric Medicine.* 9th ed. New York: American Geriatrics Society; 2016.
4. https://www.cdc.gov/healthyweight/assessing/bmi/adult_bmi/index.html.
5. Omran ML, Salem P. Diagnosing undernutrition. *Clin Geriatr Med.* 2002;18(4):719–736.
6. Alzheimer's Association Website. http://www.alz.org/national/documents/brochure_DCPRphases1n2.pdf.
7. Niedert KC. Position of the American Dietetic Association: liberalization of the diet prescription improves quality of life for older adults in long-term care. *J Am Diet Assoc.* 2005;105(12):1955–1965.
8. Baijens LW, Clavé P, Cras P, et al. European Society for Swallowing Disorders – European Union Geriatric Medicine Society white paper: oropharyngeal dysphagia as a geriatric syndrome. *Clin Interv Aging.* 2016;11:1403–1428.
9. Bhattacharyya N. The prevalence of dysphagia among adults in the United States. *Otolaryngol Head Neck Surg.* 2014;151:765–769.
10. Takizawa C, Gemmell E, Kenworthy J, et al. A systematic review of the prevalence of oropharyngeal dysphagia in stroke, Parkinson's disease, alzheimer's disease, head injury, and pneumonia. *Dysphagia.* 2016;31:434–441.
11. Alagiakrishnan K, Bhanji RA, Kurian M. Evaluation and management of oropharyngeal dysphagia in different types of dementia: a systematic review. *Arch Gerontol Geriatr.* 2013;56:1–9.
12. Goldsmith TA, Holman AS, Nunn D. Videofluoroscopic evaluation of oropharyngeal swallowing. In: Som PM, Curtin HD, eds. *Head and Neck Imaging.* 5th ed. St. Louis: Mosby, Inc.; 2011.
13. Humbert IA, Robbins J. Dysphagia in the elderly. *Phys Med Rehabil Clin North Am.* 2008;19:853.
14. McCullough GH. Normal swallowing in the geriatric population. *Perspect Swal Swal Dis (Dysph).* 2001;10(1):14–18. https://doi.org/10.1044/sasd10.1.14.
15. Robbins J, Butler SG, Daniels SK, et al. Swallowing and dysphagia rehabilitation: translating principles of neural plasticity into clinically oriented evidence. *J Speech Lang Hear Res.* 2008;51(1):S276–S300. https://doi.org/10.1044/1092-4388(2008/021).
16. Ortega O, Martín A, Clavé P. Diagnosis and management of oropharyngeal dysphagia among older persons, state of the art. *J Am Med Dir Assoc.* 2017;18:576–582.
17. Murray J. Frailty, functional reserve, and sarcopenia in the geriatric dysphagic patient. *Perspect Swal Swal Dis (Dysph).* 2008;17(1):3–11.
18. American Speech-Language-Hearing Association. *Roles of Speech-Language Pathologists in Swallowing and Feeding Disorders* [Technical Report]; 2001. Available from: www.asha.org/policy.
19. Etges CL, Scheeren B, Gomes E, Barbosa LDR. Screening tools for dysphagia: a systematic review. *CoDAS.* 2014;26(5):343–349.
20. Harwood, et al. https://changeagents365.org/resources/ways-to-stay-engaged/the-gerontological-society-of-america/Communicating%20with%20Older%20Adults%20Low_GSA.pdf; 2017.
21. Splaingard M, Hutchins B, Sulton L, Chaudhuri G. Aspiration in rehabilitation patients: videofluoroscopy vs bedside clinical assessment. *Arch Phys Med Rehabil.* 1988;69(8):637–640.
22. American Speech-Language-Hearing Association. *Guidelines Clinical Indicators for Instrumental Assessment of Dysphagia.* Rockville, MD: American Speech-Language-Hearing Association; 2000.
23. Lazarus CL. History of the use and impact of compensatory strategies in management of swallowing disorders. *Dysphagia.* 2017;32:3–10.
24. Anderson UT, Beck AM, et al. Systematic review and evidence based recommendations on texture modified foods and thickened fluids for adults (≥18 years) with oropharyngeal dysphagia. *e-SPEN J.* 2013;8(4):e127–e134.
25. Morley JE, Silver AJ. Nutritional issues in nursing home care. *Ann Intern Med.* 1995;123(11):850–859.

CHAPTER 11

Diagnosis and Rehabilitation of Hearing Disorders in the Elderly

CHIEMI TANAKA, PHD • LISA D. TANIGUCHI, AUD • HENRY L. LEW, MD, PHD

INTRODUCTION

According to the National Institute on Deafness and Other Communication Disorders,[1] disabled hearing loss was reported by about 8.5% of adults aged 55–64 years, increasing to about 25% of the population in the 65- to 74-year-old range and 50% of those who are 75 years and older. With increasing longevity, the number of older adults who suffer from hearing impairment is expected to increase tremendously. In this chapter, the authors will briefly describe the diagnosis and rehabilitation of age-related hearing loss (ARHL). Accumulation of research studies indicated that audiologic management of ARHL is more crucial than what we used to think because untreated ARHL could result in negative consequences, such as depression, anxiety, lethargy, social dissatisfaction, poor social interaction,[2-7] and, more importantly, dementia.[8,9] Besides ARHL, this chapter will briefly cover information about other ear disorders that may be commonly observed in the elderly population (e.g., cerumen impaction and ear infection). For those who need basic audiologic knowledge, please refer to the book chapter by Lew et al.[10]

AGE-RELATED HEARING LOSS

Definition of Age-Related Hearing Loss

ARHL, also known as presbycusis, is an age-related degeneration of the auditory function without any effects of other ear diseases. Therefore, ARHL is a diagnosis of exclusion and "an umbrella term for multiple forms of auditory pathology manifest in aging individuals."[11]

Symptoms and Impact of Age-Related Hearing Loss

ARHL exhibits a slow onset and is normally bilateral, symmetrical, progressive, and permanent because aging of the auditory system affects both ears simultaneously and at a similar rate. Typically, the type of hearing loss is sensorineural. High frequencies are usually affected most, and then the hearing loss gradually progresses to the low frequencies. Despite the high-frequency hearing loss being a prevalent form, some individuals with ARHL can exhibit other hearing configurations, such as flat hearing loss (all frequencies are affected by the similar degree).[12-14] Typical complaints of the patient with hearing impairment are summarized in Box 11.1. Patients with ARHL report the same complaints as younger ones with hearing loss. However, more difficulty understanding with speech, especially in noisy environment, is observed in older adults with ARHL.

The fact that some patients with ARHL may be unaware of the presence of hearing loss is noteworthy. This may be, in part, due to an asymptomatic condition and/or self-denial/indifference of hearing loss. Some patients, especially Asian older adults with ARHL, may not seek a medical attention because they accept hearing loss as part of natural aging. In addition, others may view hearing aids as a stigma of old age, leading to delay in treating their hearing loss. Basically, the lack of understanding of the impact of hearing loss in general could increase the population of untreated hearing loss and consequently impair one's quality of life (QOL).

The impact of hearing loss in older adults has been described well in literature: depression, anxiety, lethargy, social dissatisfaction/isolation, poor social interaction, loss of independence, reduced emotional and social well-being, and cognitive dysfunction. [2-7] Negative effects, such as social deprivation, on the spouse and caregivers of individuals with ARHL were also reported.[15-17] Moreover, various studies revealed a link between hearing impairment in older adults and dementia,[6] and recent studies found that hearing loss is associated with incident all-cause dementia and an increased risk of developing dementia in the elderly.[8,9] Even more, longitudinal studies reported an association between hearing loss and cognitive decline.[18,19]

Pathology, Etiology, and Contributing Factors of Age-Related Hearing Loss

ARHL is known to show the variability in its pathology. Human temporal bone examination revealed degeneration and/or damage to different structural elements in the auditory pathway, such as hair cells, especially in the basal end of the cochlea, neurons, and cochlear lateral wall tissues including stria vascularis.[12,13] What makes ARHL complex is that these pathologies can occur in different elements simultaneously. Genetic susceptibility modified by environmental effects (e.g., noise exposure, diseases, and lifestyle) was considered to be contributing to the observed variability.[11] Recently, the free radical, mitochondrial dysfunction, and oxidative stress were reported to be in association with ARHL.[20]

Exact etiology of ARHL is still under investigation. However, Van Eyken[21] proposed that ARHL is a complex sensory disorder caused by the interaction of a variety of factors, including genetic and nongenetic factors (environmental and medical) such as noise exposure, exposure to ototoxic agents, smoking, alcohol use, renal failure, diabetes, cardiovascular diseases, bone mineral density, head trauma, immune system, diet, hormones, and socioeconomic status. Fig. 11.1 shows the complexity of ARHL.

Evaluation of Age-Related Hearing Loss

Clinical evaluation for an elderly patient with hearing impairment is performed with case history intake, otoscopic examination, and audiologic testing. Physicians or audiologists take case history and examine the ears, depending on types of practice, and audiologic testing is almost always performed by audiologists. Diagnosis of ARHL is given by the physicians such as an otolaryngologist and otologist who also perform a head and neck examination.

Case history

Questioning about hearing loss (onset, ear, severity, progression, previous hearing test results) and other related symptoms, such as otalgia (ear pain), otorrhea (ear drainage), tinnitus, vertigo, dizziness, and facial nerve dysfunction, is necessary to rule out other otologic disorders. Inquiring about past and present otologic disorders, such as ear infections (acute/chronic), impacted cerumen (accumulation of excessive ear wax), Eustachian tube dysfunction, and ear trauma, is helpful. Information about medical and occupational history, history of noise exposure, prior ear surgery, ototoxic medication/chemical intake, and a family history of hearing loss can be used to determine the contributing factors to ARHL and aid in differential diagnosis. Questions about previous experience in amplification and psychosocial impact of hearing loss, such as activity limitation due to hearing loss, are also important to understand the patient's psychologic status, feeling about hearing aid use, and any effects that hearing loss might have caused on individuals. Information on the patient's cognitive status is also important because hearing loss and cognitive dysfunction have similar manifestation sometimes. Warning signs that physicians should note regarding possible hearing impairments during hearing evaluation are shown in Box 11.2.

Otoscopic examination

During the otoscopic examination, external and internal ear structures are inspected to detect the presence of any anomalies with pinna, ear canal, tympanic membrane, ossicular landmarks, and middle ear space. The otoscopic examination is useful to note the evidence of impacted cerumen, ear infection, and structural anomaly. For external ear structures, such as pinna, any

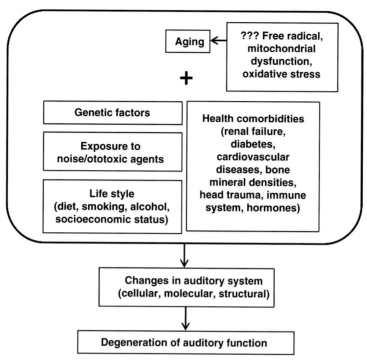

FIG. 11.1 Complexity of age-related hearing loss.

abnormalities (atresia, anotia, microtia), set (position) of the ears, skin tags, nodule (possible carcinoma) or sinuses, tenderness, redness, signs of drainage, or cerumen buildup are detected. For internal ear structures, the presence of an obstruction, drainage or blood, stenosis, damage, and signs of inflammation in the ear canal are examined. Normal landmarks (cone of light, translucent/pearly gray tympanic membrane, handle of malleus), signs of inflammation (red/bulging), retraction, perforation, and bubbles behind the tympanic membrane are noted during the examination of the tympanic membrane.

Normal ear examination or age-appropriate changes in the ear structures is expected in the older adults with ARHL. Normal age-related changes in the outer ear and tympanic membrane include enlargement of the pinna, loss of elasticity and strength in the ear canal, loss of secretory ability in the sebaceous and cerumen glands in the ear canal, and excessive hair growth along the edge of the helix and at the tragus (mostly seen in elderly males).

Beyond ARHL, owing to the changes in the glands in the ear canal, hardening or impaction of cerumen is commonly observed in the older adults.[22] Before audiometric evaluation, a blockage of the ear canal (e.g.,

excessive cerumen) should be checked with an otoscope because severe blockage can elevate air-conduction thresholds, causing a conductive or mixed hearing loss. Excessive cerumen needs to be removed before the audiometric testing to ensure accurate results. Healthcare providers routinely use different techniques such as irrigation, suction, cerumen-removal ear drops, and curettage to remove cerumen. In case of severe cerumen impaction, the patient needs to be referred to an otolaryngologist to avoid serious side effects of cerumen removal (e.g., bleeding of the ear canal, damaging the tympanic membrane).

Besides cerumen impaction, collapsed ear canal is another popular functional condition in the elderly population. This is due to the decreased elasticity in the cartilaginous portion of the ear canal. It is common practice to use insert earphones in the older adults for an audiometric testing to avoid pressure from the headphones that may cause the ear canal to collapse resulting in an inaccurate audiogram. Moreover, owing to less effective immune system in the elderly population,[23] indicative of ear infections, such as red tympanic membranes and/or ear canal, bubbles behind the tympanic membrane, may be found commonly in the elderly population. The

---

BOX 11.2
Signs That Physicians Should Note Regarding Possible Hearing Impairments

- Cannot hear or understand you when you ask them to enter your office for the appointment
- Not very talkative
- Does not reply when spoken to
- Does not respond appropriately to the questions you are asking
- Does not understand you when you speak with them on the telephone
- Looks closely at your face or lips when you speak
- May appear confused when giving an inappropriate response
- May have a hearing aid but does not use it
- May strain to understand or place the hand behind the ear in an attempt to amplify your voice
- Needs occasional repetition or a louder speaking voice to understand
- Needs frequent prompting multiple repetitions or restatement of what was said
- Not able to understand what is being said; asks you to write the message down to facilitate understanding
- Appears to have difficulty understanding fast speech and accented speech

From Weinstein BE. Primary care physicians and audiologists: partners in care. In: Weinstein BE, ed. *Geriatric Audiology*. 2nd ed. New York: Thieme Medical Publishers, Inc.; 2013; with permission.

BOX 11.3
Red Flags: Warnings of Ear Disease

1. Hearing loss with a positive history of ear infections, noise exposure, familial hearing loss, TB, syphilis, HIV, Meniere's disease, autoimmune disorder, ototoxic medication use, otosclerosis, von Recklinghausen's neurofibromatosis, Paget's disease of bone, ear or head trauma related to onset.
2. A history of pain, active drainage, or bleeding from an ear.
3. Sudden onset or rapidly progressive hearing loss.
4. Acute, chronic, or recurrent episodes of dizziness.
5. Evidence of congenital or traumatic deformity of the ear.
6. Visualization of blood, pus, cerumen plug, a foreign body, or other materials in the ear canal.
7. An unexplained conductive hearing loss or abnormal tympanogram.
8. Unilateral or asymmetric hearing loss (a difference of greater than 15 dB pure-tone average between ears) or bilateral hearing loss >30 dB.
9. Unilateral or pulsatile tinnitus.
10. Unilateral or asymmetrically poor speech discrimination scores (a difference of greater than 15% between ears) or bilateral speech discrimination scores <80%.

The red flags do not include all indications for a medical referral and are not intended to replace clinical judgment in determining the need for consultation with an ENT physician (otolaryngologist).

Reprinted with permission. Copyright © 2017 American Academy of Otolaryngology–Head and Neck Surgery. Reproduction or republication strictly prohibited without prior written permission.

American Academy of Otolaryngology–Head and Neck Surgery or Foundation (AAO-HNS/F) provides the position statement regarding the medical referral recommendation to a specialist for possible ear diseases (Box 11.3). It is recommended that patients who show these warning signs be referred to an otolaryngologist.

Standard audiologic evaluation

The standard audiologic evaluation is composed of pure-tone (air and bone conduction) and speech audiometry.

Pure-tone audiometry. The pure-tone audiometry, including air- and bone-conduction testing, is conducted to characterize type, degree (severity), and sidedness (unilateral or bilateral) of hearing loss. Clinically, pure-tone hearing thresholds (lowest decibel hearing level [dB HL] at which the patient detects the pure tone at least 50% of the time) at frequencies from 250 to 8000 Hz, important frequency range to understand speech, are determined in air- and bone-conduction pathways, using headphones/insert earphones and bone conductor, respectively. Occasionally, pure-tone average (PTA) is calculated by simply averaging air-conduction hearing thresholds at 500, 1000, and 2000 Hz. The AAO-HNS/F listed unilateral or asymmetrical hearing loss as a red flag of ear diseases, if a difference of greater than 15 dB PTA between ears or bilateral hearing loss >30 dB is detected (Box 11.3).

Three types of hearing loss are conductive, sensorineural, and mixed. Conductive hearing loss results because of obstruction, damage, or infection of the outer ear (ear canal) and/or middle ear (tympanic membrane, ossicular chain, middle ear space), which can be seen as 15 dB or more of air-bone gap in an audiogram (elevated air-conduction thresholds with

TABLE 11.1
Examples of Drugs Known to Be Associated With Ototoxicity

Type/Group	Subclass of Drug	Examples
Chemotherapeutics	Platinum complex	Cisplatin, carboplatin
	Vinca alkaloids	Vinblastine, vincristine, vinorelbine
	Difluoromethylornithine	Eflornithine
Antibiotics	Aminoglycosides	Gentamicin, kanamycin, neomycin, streptomycin, tobramycin, amikacin, netilmicin
	Macrolides	Erythromycin, azithromycin, clarithromycin
	Others	Vancomycin
Diuretics	Loop diuretics	Ethacrynic acid, furosemide, bumetanide
Nonnarcotic analgesics	NSAIDs	Salicylates (aspirin), ibuprofen
Antimalarials		Quinine, chloroquine

NSAIDs, nonsteroidal antiinflammatory drugs.
This list is not all-inclusive, and ototoxicity depends on various factors, such as dose (daily/life time), duration of intake, kidney function, age, drug interactions, preexisting hearing loss, and genetic susceptibility.
From Campbell KCM, ed. *Pharmacology and Ototoxicity for Audiologists*. 1st ed. New York: Cengage Learning.

TABLE 11.2
Examples of Industrial Chemicals and Solvents Known to Be Associated With Ototoxicity

Type/Group	Examples
Chemical asphyxiants	Carbon monoxide, cyanide
Metals	Lead, mercury, manganese
Organic solvents	Styrene, toluene, ethyl benzene, xylene, trichloroethylene, n-hexane
Acrylonitrile	

This list is not all-inclusive, and ototoxicity depends on various factors, such as dose (daily/life time), duration of intake, kidney function, age, drug interactions, preexisting hearing loss, and genetic susceptibility.
From Campbell KCM, ed. *Pharmacology and Ototoxicity for Audiologists*. 1st ed. New York: Cengage Learning; 2007.

normal bone-conduction thresholds). On the other hand, sensorineural hearing loss (SNHL) is characterized by elevated air- and bone-conduction thresholds with 10 dB or less of air-bone gap. This type of hearing loss results because of damage/deterioration of the cochlea and/or in the retrocochlear pathway. Almost all patients with ARHL, drug-induced hearing loss, and noise-induced hearing loss exhibit high-frequency SNHL. Therefore, it is important to find out about a history of ototoxic medication intake (Tables 11.1 and 11.2) and traumatic noise exposure for differential diagnosis. Lastly, mixed hearing loss is a mixture of conductive hearing loss and SNHL, characterized by elevated air- and bone-conduction

thresholds with an air-bone gap of 15 dB or greater. Examples of otologic disorders that can cause a conductive or mixed hearing loss in the older adults are cerumen impaction, perforation of the tympanic membrane, Eustachian tube dysfunction, ear infections, and otosclerosis. The patient with unexplained conductive hearing loss may need a medical referral to an otolaryngologist based on the AAO-HNS/F recommendation (Box 11.3).

Severity of hearing impairment is described by a degree of hearing loss (mild, moderate, moderately severe, severe, profound), and there is no uniform classification system. However, hearing threshold of 25 dB HL or better is commonly considered normal hearing in adults, followed by mild (26–40 dB HL), moderate (41–55 dB HL), moderately severe (56–70 dB HL), severe (71–90 dB HL), and profound (>90 dB HL) hearing losses.[24] Fig. 11.2 shows age-related changes in hearing thresholds in different age-groups. Note that elderly males exhibit greater hearing loss than females, and high-frequency hearing is mostly affected, continuing to progress following aging. Auditory rehabilitation is considered for a patient with any degree of hearing impairment based on healthcare professional's clinical judgment and the patient's needs.

Speech audiometry. Speech audiometry is performed to obtain the speech recognition (reception) threshold (SRT) or speech detection (awareness) thresholds (SDTs) using spondee (bisyllabic) words and suprathreshold speech recognition. The SRT measures the lowest dB HL at which a patient can correctly repeat or identify spondee 50% of the time, while the

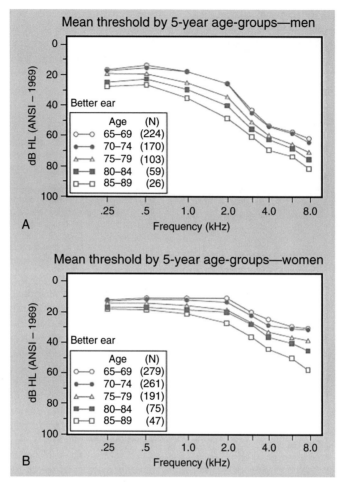

FIG. 11.2 Age-related changes in hearing thresholds in different age-groups. **(A)** Men; and **(B)** women. (From Gates et al. Hearing in the elderly: the Framingham cohort, 1983-1985 Part I. Basic audiometric test results. Ear Hear 11:247-56, 1990; Lew HL et al. Auditory, vestibular, and visual impairments. In: Cifu DX, Kaelin DL, Kowalske KJ, et al., eds. *Braddom's Physical Medicine and Rehabilitation*. 5th ed. Philadelphia: Elsevier; 2016; with permission.)

SDT assesses the lowest dB HL at which a patient can correctly detect the presence of speech. The SDT is used when the SRT cannot be obtained owing to the patient's inability to repeat or identify words. The SRT or SDT is used to cross-check the accuracy of the pure-tone thresholds and determine the presentation level of the speech recognition (discrimination) scores that are typically obtained at suprathreshold level (40 dB above the SRT). For speech discrimination, an audiologist scores the percentage of words that are correctly repeated or identified from phonetically balanced word lists (25 or 50 words), such as Northwestern University Auditory Test No. 6 (NU-6) and the Central Institute for the Deaf Auditory Test W-22. Although

there is no consensus about the categorization of the speech recognition scores, 90%–100% is typically considered as excellent or within normal limits. According to the AAO-HNS/F, a medical referral to an otolaryngologist is recommended to rule out ear diseases if unilateral or asymmetrically poor speech discrimination scores (a difference of greater than 15% between ears) are observed or bilateral speech discrimination scores are < 80% (Box 11.3).

Immittance audiometry

Immittance audiometry includes tympanometry and acoustic reflexes. Tympanometry assesses the volume of the ear canal, integrity of the tympanic membrane, and the middle ear pressure, while the acoustic reflexes examines the presence of retrocochlear and facial nerve pathology by using the reflexive contraction of the stapedius muscle in the middle ear in response to loud sound. Compared with the acoustic reflexes, tympanometry, in most cases, is ordered more often when clinically indicated a condition that cannot be explained solely by age-related changes (e.g., presence of a conductive or mixed hearing loss and any signs of ear infection mostly detected by the otoscopic examination, or higher risks indicated by the case history). It is important for clinicians to keep in mind that the elderly population is susceptible to ear infection owing to less efficient immune system.

Other auditory testing and questionnaires

Other auditory testing such as otoacoustic emissions and auditory brain stem response test may be performed for the purpose of differential diagnosis. For testing details, please refer to Lew et al.[10]

Management of Age-Related Hearing Loss
Auditory rehabilitation

Informative counseling is an important part of auditory rehabilitation. The patient should be informed the process of ARHL and the absence of any more serious ear pathology. Because ARHL is progressive and irreversible, it is crucial to explain to the patient the appropriate care of residual hearing and encourage him/her to audiologically manage hearing loss to maintain a high QOL. For example, avoiding excessive noise exposure (e.g., usage of ear plugs or protective ear muffs) and maintaining a healthy lifestyle may increase the chance of conserving residual hearing. Some patients with ARHL may be reluctant to try a hearing aid or hearing assistance (assistive) technology (HAT) owing to the negative stigma of the usage of a hearing aid or acceptance of ARHL as a natural course of aging. Surprisingly, fewer than 30% have ever used hearing aids among adults aged 70 years and older with hearing impairment who could benefit from hearing aids.[25] To prevent the patient from experiencing serious consequences of untreated ARHL, such as depression and social isolation, a clinician can play a significant role in encouraging him/her to actively seek a way to manage his/her hearing loss by amplification or other means.

Furthermore, compensatory communication strategies that refer to behavioral and listening modifications need to be discussed with the patient. These strategies work with or without hearing aid use. Box 11.4 shows common communication strategies that can be used by both the patient and conversation partner to enhance the understanding of conversation. More importantly,

---

BOX 11.4
Compensatory Communication Strategies

1. Address the person with hearing loss.
   - Get the person's attention before starting to communicate. His/her brain must be alerted to be ready to focus and listen.
2. Have face-to-face communication.
   - The more important high-pitched sounds of speech are very directional (only propagate well in the direction the speaker is facing) and the production of the high-pitched sounds is visible on the mouth.
   - Do not obscure the lips with hands or other objects.
   - Make certain that light shines directly on the speaker's face, not from behind the speaker.
3. Start with the topic.
   - It is easier for the listener to fill in missed information if he/she knows the context.
4. Use a slightly slower rate of speaking.
   - It gives more time for the listener's brain to process and keep up with the flow of information.
   - Avoid shouting because it will not help.
5. Use appropriate distance.
   - The more important high-pitched sounds are very weak and are not able to travel far from the speaker.
6. Control noise (unwanted sounds).
   - Noise will always interfere with communication and many of these unwanted sounds will also be picked up by a hearing aid.
7. Spell words out, use gestures, or write down.
8. Repeat back or change phrasing if the listener does not understand at first.
9. Speak toward the better ear, if applicable.

From Lew HL et al. Auditory, vestibular, and visual impairments. In: Cifu DX, Kaelin DL, Kowalske KJ, et al., eds. *Braddom's Physical Medicine and Rehabilitation*. 5th ed. Philadelphia: Elsevier; 2016; with permission.

---

it is beneficial for healthcare providers and staff members to use these communication strategies to accommodate an elderly patient's communication need.

On top of the informational counseling, there are two major aspects in the auditory rehabilitation:
1. technical, including hearing aids, HAT, and cochlear implants (CI);
2. perceptual, such as speech and language therapy and auditory training.

This chapter will mainly describe the technical aspects of auditory rehabilitation.

Hearing aid. Hearing aids are personally worn electrical devices that process and amplify the incoming sound based on an individual's hearing configuration. Before hearing aid consultation, ear diseases should be treated medically and surgically if treatments are available. Hearing aids are designed to improve speech understanding of the patient with hearing impairment and the most commonly used noninvasive devices. The majority of hearing aids dispensed in the United States are digital hearing aids that use a computer chip to process incoming sounds. Generally, the incoming sound is picked up by a microphone(s) and converted to a digitized signal by an analog-to-digital converter for further processing in the computer chip. Sophisticated sound processing algorisms are available, such as feedback management, noise reduction/suppression, and speech enhancement. Then, the processed sound is converted to an analog signal by a digital-to-analog converter and sent to a final-stage amplifier and receiver (speaker). Batteries provide power for amplification, and a single battery typically lasts approximately 7–10 days, depending on duration of the hearing aid use.

For patients who suffer from tinnitus, it is well known that the hearing aid can help managing tinnitus because amplified background noise delivered by the hearing aid provides a masking effect for the tinnitus. However, for patients with severe tinnitus, a combination device (a hearing aid equipped with a sound generator) is used for either sound therapy or traditional tinnitus masking. In the sound therapy, various sounds, such as oceanlike noise, fractal tones, and soothing sounds, are used to promote the distraction of attention to tinnitus, habituation to tinnitus, and relaxation. On the other hand, in the traditional tinnitus masking, a band of noise, such as steady white/speech noise that surrounds the pitch of the tinnitus, is used to mask (cover up) tinnitus. The volume of the sounds for tinnitus management can be adjusted by the patient directly on the hearing aid or via remotes/applications (iOS, android).

Fig. 11.3 shows the different styles of hearing aids. The behind-the-ear (BTE) hearing aid has a microphone located behind the pinna, and a custom earmold with a tube conducts sound to the ear. A thinner tube and small dome are used for an open-fit mini BTE hearing aid that works especially for high-frequency hearing loss with relatively good low-frequency hearing. In-the-ear (ITE), in-the-canal, completely-in-the-canal, and invisible-in-the-canal hearing aids are customized to a patient's ear and house all parts inside. The receiver-in-the-ear (RITE) hearing aid, also known as receiver-in-the-canal (RIC)

hearing aid, has the BTE component, but the tubing of the BTE hearing aid is replaced with a wire attached to the receiver that is inserted in the ear canal. The RITE/RIC hearing aids are becoming more popular owing to various advantages (e.g., more features available over the custom hearing aids, less occluded feeling in the ear).

Some hearing aids are cosmetically appealing than others in terms of visibility because many people still consider a hearing aid as a sign of aging. However, the size and cosmetics may not be the first thing to consider during the hearing aid selection for elderly patients with dexterity and vision problems that may affect device manipulation, such as inserting/removing a hearing aid, changing a battery, and cleaning the hearing aid. In addition, smaller hearing aids use smaller batteries, leading to less power and amplification. Therefore, bigger hearing aids with more power may be suitable for individuals with severe to profound hearing loss.

Because most of the patients with ARHL have symmetrical bilateral hearing loss, binaural fitting of hearing aids is recommended to benefit from spatial hearing unless contraindicated. To maximize the benefit of binaural hearing, some digital hearing aids have features to exchange data between the right and left hearing aid worn by the patient. Besides improvement of audibility, recent studies found that listening effort can be reduced by the hearing aids.[26,27] Other studies reported that hearing aids worn by the older adults can reduce the negative effects of hearing loss on both their spouses/significant others and themselves.[28,29] Interestingly, a 25-year longitudinal study was published recently to indicate that the hearing aid use attenuates accelerated cognitive decline seen in the older adults.[30]

Despite the variety of advantages in hearing aid usage, not everyone benefits from hearing aids because of various factors. Consultation with an audiologist for careful selection of the hearing aid is a crucial step for success in hearing aid use. First and foremost, the hearing aids need to be programmed appropriately by an audiologist or a hearing specialist, according to a prescriptive formula or a manufacturer's algorithm to set proper amplification for the individual's needs and preference. Without this process, benefits of the hearing aids cannot be maximized to the point of successful hearing aid use.

Hearing assistance/assistive technology. HAT refers to personal devices that assist an individual to communicate more effectively regardless of hearing loss. These devices can be used alone or to supplement hearing aids. One of these useful devices that can be coupled

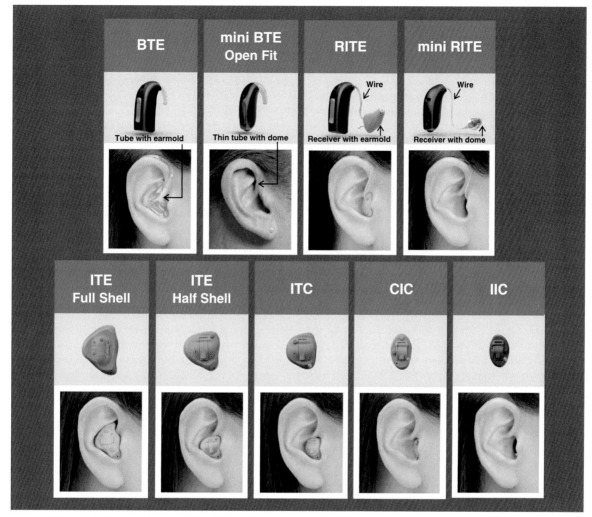

FIG. 11.3 Types of hearing aids. *BTE*, behind-the-ear style; *CIC*, completely-in-the-canal style; *IIC*, invisible-in-the-canal style; *ITC*, in-the-canal style; *ITE*, in-the-ear style; *RITE*, receiver-in-the-ear style (also known as *RIC*, receiver-in-the-canal). (With permission by Oticon, Inc., Somerset, NJ.)

with a hearing aid is a personal FM system that transmits a speaker's voice directly to an individual's ear. A listener wears an FM receiver that can be coupled directly to the listener's ear via hearing aids and other means (e.g., earphones, ear buds, induction loop, or CI) and the speaker wears a microphone and FM transmitter.[31] Wireless FM signal carries speech information between the speaker and listener to avoid significant interference from environmental sounds.

Besides the FM system, a portable personal amplifier may be a simple HAT to be used for non–hearing aid users. The device is composed of a wireless or hard-wired amplifier device, a microphone, and a headset.

The speaker talks to the microphone directly and the speech is directly delivered to the listener's ear through the headset. The portable personal amplifier can be a great help in a physician's office to assist communication with a patient with ARHL.

Because the hearing aid technology is advancing in full speed, it is noteworthy to discuss Bluetooth technology here. To help a patient with hearing loss hear more clearly on his/her iOS devices, such iPhone, iPad, or iPod touch, "Made for iPhone hearing aids" (see https://support.apple.com/en-us/HT201466 for compatible hearing aid devices) can be paired with the patient's iOS devices via Bluetooth technology. The advantage of this pairing is that the patient can hear the speaker's voice or sound through his/her hearing aid that is already adjusted and customized to his/her hearing loss. Moreover, the volume of the paired hearing aids can be controlled by the iPhone. Patients with non-iOS device, such as Android phones, can still have access to Bluetooth technology by wearing a discrete Bluetooth transmitter around their neck. Such devices can also be clipped to a patient's shirt or even hidden under a thin article of clothing. The Bluetooth transmitter is paired to a patient's cell phone that supports Bluetooth and also paired to the patient's hearing aids. As the patient receives the call, he/she can answer the call by pushing a button on the transmitter and the conversation is streamed to his/her hearing aid/s directly, allowing for hands-free conversations.

The manufacturer-specific Bluetooth transmitter can also connect a patient's hearing aid and other devices, such as a television and remote microphone, to accommodate patients' communication needs. The television device can be paired to the transmitter and stream sound from the patient's television directly to his/her hearing aid. This will allow for the patient to listen TV sounds at an increased volume level through the hearing aids, while family members can listen to the television at a regular volume that is not disruptive. A remote microphone accessory could also be useful in noisy environments, such as inside a car, classrooms, meetings, places of worship, or any place where noise or distance can interfere with communication, because it reduces the speaker-to-listener distance. The microphone is paired to the transmitter and clipped on or placed in front of the speaker. The speaker's voice would then stream directly to the patient's hearing aid to enhance communications.

Lastly, in patients with a severe or profound ARHL, nonauditory alerting devices may be useful to promote their safety and independence. These devices convert auditory signals to nonauditory ones, such as light or vibration. For example, sounds from alarm clock, microwave oven, doorbell, or even smoke detector can be converted to either vibration or flash/strobe light that are noticeable by these patients.

Surgical and medical treatment
Cochlear implant. Basically, the CI is a choice for a patient with severe to profound SNHL who received limited benefits from hearing aid use, as well as with sufficient anatomical structures to support CI function. To receive the CI, the patient needs to pass the CI candidacy criteria that are set by each CI manufacturer (Cochlear Ltd., MED-EL, and Advanced Bionics in the

US market). The CI is a FDA-regulated surgically implanted device that is designed to electrically stimulate the auditory nerve via electrodes inserted into the scala tympani of the cochlea. A patient with ARHL is thought to be a good CI candidate because direct stimulation of the auditory nerve by the CI bypasses the cochlear hair cells that are found to be pathologic in those patients. Benefits of the CI range from full communication function to only the detection of environmental sounds, depending on individuals. The patient with ARHL can benefit from the CI, but extra caution needs to be taken for those with chronic health conditions owing to surgical risks.

The CI is consisted of external portions (ear-level/body-worn speech processor with a microphone and transmitting coil) and internal ones (receiver/simulator and electrode array). The external speech processor processes acoustic sound that was picked up by the microphone. The transmitter and receiver/simulator receive processed signals from the speech processor and convert them into electric pulses that are sent to electrode array in the cochlea for electrical stimulation of different regions of the auditory nerve. After the surgery, the CI speech processor is programmed by an audiologist based on objective and subjective measurements. New CI users are required to learn speech through auditory training because electric hearing by the CI is different from the natural sound perceived by the ears.

In addition to the traditional CIs mentioned earlier, the FDA approved a new type of the CI, called Cochlear Nucleus Hybrid Implant System (Cochlear Ltd.) and EAS (electric acoustic stimulation) Hearing Implant System (MED-EL Corp.). This new type of the CI is suitable for an individual with residual hearing in low frequencies, sloping to severe to profound SNHL in high frequencies. Amazingly, this new technology combines the CI with the hearing aid to provide amplification in low frequencies through the hearing aid component and electrically stimulate high-frequency regions of the cochlea via the shorter CI electrode arrays in the same ear. For more information, visit manufacturer's websites.

Middle ear implantable hearing aids. The middle ear implantable hearing aids are mainly used for individuals with SNHL who received limited benefits from conventional hearing aid use but do not have enough hearing loss to warrant the CI. Basically, the implanted portion is attached to one of the ossicles in the middle ear and drives the ossicles directly to deliver sound to the cochlea. Currently, Vibrant Soundbridge (MED-EL Corp.), Esteem middle ear implants (Envoy Medical), Maxum hearing implant (Ototronix LLC), and Carina middle-ear implant (Cochlear Ltd.) are in the US market. For further details, please refer to manufacturers' websites or a review article.[32]

Regeneration of the cochlear hair cell and auditory nerve. The cochlear hair cells (mechanoreceptors in the auditory system) play an important role in sound perception. The human temporal bone studies in a patient with ARHL revealed missing and damaged hair cells, especially in the basal turn of the cochlea, contributing to high-frequency hearing loss.[12,13] It is known that mammalian cells in many organs are constantly replenished or regenerated following injury, but no mammalian hair cell replacement or cell proliferation was observed. Researchers found that hair cells in other vertebrates, such as avian, regenerate,[33] and ongoing human hair cell regeneration research is taking place in animal studies, facing progress and challenges.[34] On the contrary, the auditory nerve is known to degenerate after hair cell death. Research studies in preservation and regeneration of auditory nerve, as well as hair cell regeneration, are advancing forward. Following translational and large-scale clinical trials, regeneration of the cochlear hair cell and auditory nerve may become a medical treatment option in the future.[35]

Prevention of Age-Related Hearing Loss

The prevention of ARHL is not possible at this point because the exact etiology of ARHL is unknown. However, minimizing the contributing factors of ARHL that were discussed previously in this chapter is thought to reduce a risk of developing ARHL. New prevention strategy is on the way, using pharmacologic agents such as antioxidants. Although pharmacologic protection of ARHL seems promising, large-scale clinical trials are still needed for these agents to be used clinically.[20]

CASE STUDY

The following two case studies illustrate successful management of ARHL.

Case Study: Age-Related Hearing Loss
Background

Mr. S.P. is a 70-year-old recently retired male who reported a history of gradual hearing loss over several years. He and his wife moved to a new state after retirement, and he started to notice communication difficulties in new social situations. In particular, he was mishearing names and street names, which caused frustration and embarrassment. He admitted to withdrawing

from social events, especially with elevated background noise, to avoid people he could not understand.

Mr. S.P. reported bilateral hearing loss in the high frequencies and indicated that both parents had gradual hearing loss. No history of tinnitus, dizziness, noise exposure, or other significant medical history was reported.

Evaluation

A head and neck examination was unremarkable. Otoscopic examination was also unremarkable in both ears. Fig. 11.4 illustrates Mr. S.P.'s audiologic testing results. Pure-tone audiometry revealed a mild to severe SNHL in both ears (see Pure-tone audiometry section for the definition of SNHL). His SRTs were in good agreement with his PTAs, bilaterally. His word recognition scores using NU-6 were 88% in the right ear and 84% in the left ear. Tympanograms indicated normal tympanic membrane mobility and middle ear function in both ears. Acoustic reflex thresholds were elevated or absent in the higher frequencies, consistent with audiologic results.

Management

His physician diagnosed Mr. S.P. with ARHL owing to no indication of serious otologic disorders based on the evaluation. Informative counseling was provided to explain his hearing status and management of his hearing loss. Based on the audiologic evaluation, hearing aids were recommended for Mr. S.P. After hearing aid consultation with his audiologist, Mr. S.P. decided on binaural amplification with smartphone compatibility to satisfy his communication needs. The RIC-style hearing aids were selected owing to hearing configuration (relatively good hearing in low frequencies with high-frequency hearing loss), comfort, and cosmetics.

Hearing aids were fit to target and confirmed with real-ear measurement. Devices were paired to his Android phone and iPod. Hearing aid use and care were reviewed with him. At initial fitting appointment, Mr. S.P. was counseled on communication strategies, need for consistent use, and realistic expectations with hearing aid use. During his follow-up appointment, Mr. S.P. reported that overall he is doing well with music and one-on-one communication; however, he still noted slight difficulty understanding speech in background noise. Directional microphone program was added, and he was reminded of the phone application use where he could control the directionality beam. During the second follow-up, Mr. S.P. reported satisfaction with the last adjustments and noted improvement in social situations. Mr. S.P.'s wife also reported that she is

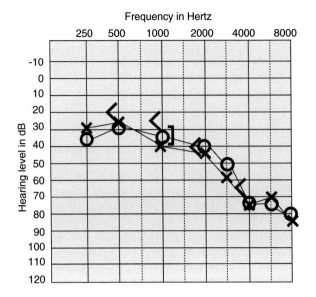

	PTA	SRT	WRS % correct	Level	Test material
Right	36	35	88%	75 dB HL	NU-6
Left	35	35	84%	75 dB HL	NU-6

FIG. 11.4 Audiologic testing results for case study: age-related hearing loss. *PTA*, pure-tone average; *SRT*, speech recognition (reception) threshold; *WRS*, word recognition (speech discrimination) score.

not repeating herself as frequently and is less frustrated with Mr. S.P. during communication. He is no longer embarrassed but proud to show his technology to his new friends. It was recommended that Mr. S.P. return to the clinic for audiologic evaluation, if any changes in his hearing are noted.

Case Study: Age-Related Hearing Loss With Severe Tinnitus

Background

Ms. R.M. is an 82-year-old female with long-standing history of hearing loss and tinnitus. She had tried amplification several years ago with no success. She admitted that she was wearing the devices inconsistently. Ms. R.M. visited the clinic to seek amplification and management of her tinnitus (constant bilateral high-pitched ringing, louder in the right ear). She explained that her hearing loss and tinnitus are seriously affecting her daily activities and causing frustration and stress.

Ms. R.M. reported a history of asymmetrical hearing loss with negative MRI results. No history of dizziness, noise exposure, or other significant medical history was reported.

Evaluation

A head and neck examination was unremarkable. Otoscopic examination was also unremarkable in both ears. Fig. 11.5 illustrates Ms. R.M.'s audiologic testing results. The pure-tone audiometry revealed a mild to moderately severe SNHL in the left ear and moderate to severe SNHL in the right ear. Her SRTs were in good agreement with her PTAs, bilaterally. Word recognition scores were 76% in the right ear, 84% in the left ear, and 88% binaurally. Tympanograms indicated normal tympanic membrane mobility and middle ear function, bilaterally. Acoustic reflex thresholds were elevated or absent, bilaterally, consistent with her audiometric results.

Management

Her physician diagnosed Ms. R.M. with ARHL owing to no indication of other serious otologic disorders based on the evaluation. Informative counseling was provided to explain her hearing status and management of her hearing loss and tinnitus. Based on the audiologic evaluation, hearing aids were recommended for Ms. R.M. After hearing aid consultation with her audiologist, she decided on binaural amplification with Bluetooth transmitter to

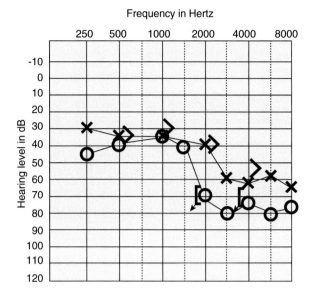

	PTA	SRT	WRS % correct	Level	Test material
Right	48	45	76%	85 dB HL	NU-6
Left	36	35	84%	75 dB HL	NU-6
Binaural			88%	80/70 dB HL	NU-6

FIG. 11.5 Audiologic testing results for case study: age-related hearing loss with severe tinnitus. *PTA*, pure-tone average; *SRT*, speech recognition (reception) threshold; *WRS*, word recognition (speech discrimination) score.

stream sounds from her television and cell phones. ITE half shell style with larger battery size was chosen to compensate her hearing loss and dexterity concerns.

Hearing aids were fit to target and confirmed with real-ear measurement. Hearing aids were paired to TV accessory and cell phone via Bluetooth transmitter. Hearing aid use and care were reviewed with her. At her initial fitting appointment, Ms. R.M. was counseled on communication strategies, need for consistent use, and realistic expectations with hearing aid use. During her follow-up appointment, Ms. R.M. reported improvement in communication and better management of tinnitus in background noise. However, tinnitus was still bothersome when she was in quiet situations, such as at home by herself. Because her hearing aids were combination devices with amplification and sound generator, sound therapy was added to control her tinnitus. The audiologist helped Ms. R.M. to select the most effective sound to manage her tinnitus. She was shown how to change the volume of the sound and asked to adjust the level as needed. Ms. R.M. was extensively counseled on tinnitus management and when to

use sound generator. At the second follow-up, Ms. R.M. reported great control of tinnitus as well as her hearing loss and satisfaction with her combination devices.

CONCLUDING STATEMENT

This chapter described diagnosis and rehabilitation of ARHL. With increasing longevity, the number of older adults who suffer from hearing impairment is growing. To maintain a high QOL, audiologic management of ARHL is crucial for the prevention of negative consequences on individuals with ARHL and their spouse/caregivers. Although specialists, such as otolaryngologists and audiologists, are working on detecting and rehabilitating patients with ARHL, it is very important for other healthcare providers to detect hearing impairment earlier by conducting hearing screening. Performing simple audiometric screening by using a portable audiometer and screening questionnaires, such as the Hearing Handicap Inventory for the Elderly—Screening version,[36] at the physician's office is beneficial for the older adults to promote earlier audiologic management of hearing loss.

REFERENCES

1. NIDCD. *Quick Statistics about Hearing*; 2016. https://www. nidcd.nih.gov/health/statistics/quick-statistics-hearing.
2. Heine C, Browning CJ. Communication and psychosocial consequences of sensory loss in older adults: overview and rehabilitation directions. *Disabil Rehabil.* 2002;24(15):763–773.
3. Kiely KM, Anstey KJ, Luszcz MA. Dual sensory loss and depressive symptoms: the importance of hearing, daily functioning, and activity engagement. *Front Hum Neurosci.* 2013;7:837.
4. Li CM, Zhang X, Hoffman HJ, Cotch MF, Themann CL, Wilson MR. Hearing impairment associated with depression in US adults, National Health and Nutrition Examination Survey 2005-2010. *JAMA Otolaryngol Head Neck Surg.* 2014;140(4):293–302.
5. Strawbridge WJ, Wallhagen MI, Shema SJ, Kaplan GA. Negative consequences of hearing impairment in old age: a longitudinal analysis. *Gerontologist.* 2000;40(3): 320–326.
6. Weinstein BE. *Audiological rehabilitation/communication management: an integrated approach. Geriatric Audiology.* 2nd ed. New York: Thieme Medical Publishers; 2013:153–204.
7. Weinstein BE, Ventry IM. Hearing impairment and social isolation in the elderly. *J Speech Hear Res.* 1982;25(4): 593–599.
8. Deal JA, Betz J, Yaffe K, et al. Hearing impairment and incident dementia and cognitive decline in older adults: the health ABC study. *J Gerontol A Biol Sci Med Sci.* 2017;72(5):703–709.
9. Lin FR, Metter EJ, O'Brien RJ, Resnick SM, Zonderman AB, Ferrucci L. Hearing loss and incident dementia. *Arch Neurol.* 2011;68(2):214–220.
10. Lew HL, Tanaka C, Hirohata E, Goodrich GL. Auditory, vestibular, and visual impairments. In: Cifu DX, ed. *Braddom's Physical Medicine and Rehabilitation.* 5th ed. Philadelphia: Elsevier; 2016:1137–1161.
11. Yang CH, Schrepfer T, Schacht J. Age-related hearing impairment and the triad of acquired hearing loss. *Front Cell Neurosci.* 2015;9:276.
12. Nelson EG, Hinojosa R. Presbycusis: a human temporal bone study of individuals with downward sloping audiometric patterns of hearing loss and review of the literature. *Laryngoscope.* 2006;116(9 Pt 3 suppl 112):1–12.
13. Schuknecht HF, Gacek MR. Cochlear pathology in presbycusis. *Ann Otol Rhinol Laryngol.* 1993;102(1 Pt 2):1–16.
14. Suga F, Lindsay JR. Histopathological observations of presbycusis. *Ann Otol Rhinol Laryngol.* 1976;85(2 Pt 1): 169–184.
15. Lazzarotto S, Baumstarck K, Loundou A, et al. Age-related hearing loss in individuals and their caregivers: effects of coping on the quality of life among the dyads. *Patient Prefer Adherence.* 2016;10:2279–2287.
16. Scarinci N, Worrall L, Hickson L. The effect of hearing impairment in older people on the spouse. *Int J Audiol.* 2008;47(3):141–151.

17. Scarinci N, Worrall L, Hickson L. Factors associated with third-party disability in spouses of older people with hearing impairment. *Ear Hear.* 2012;33(6):698–708.
18. Lin FR, Thorpe R, Gordon-Salant S, Ferrucci L. Hearing loss prevalence and risk factors among older adults in the United States. *J Gerontol A Biol Sci Med Sci.* 2011;66(5):582–590.
19. Valentijn SA, van Boxtel MP, van Hooren SA, et al. Change in sensory functioning predicts change in cognitive functioning: results from a 6-year follow-up in the maastricht aging study. *J Am Geriatr Soc.* 2005;53(3):374–380.
20. Tavanai E, Mohammadkhani G. Role of antioxidants in prevention of age-related hearing loss: a review of literature. *Eur Arch Otorhinolaryngol.* 2017;274(4): 1821–1834.
21. Van Eyken E, Van Camp G, Van Laer L. The complexity of age-related hearing impairment: contributing environmental and genetic factors. *Audiol Neurootol.* 2007;12(6): 345–358.
22. Ballachanda B. Cerumen and the ear canal secretory system. In: Ballachanda B, ed. *Introduction to the Human Ear Canal.* San Diego: Singular; 1995.
23. White J, Regan M. Otological considerations. In: Mueller G, Geoffrey V, eds. *Communication Disorders in Aging: Assessment and Management.* Washington, DC: Gallaudet University Press; 1987.
24. Goodman A. Reference zero levels for pure-tone audiometer. *Am Speech Lang Hear Assoc.* 1965;7:262–263.
25. NIDCD. *Use of Hearing Aids by Adults with Hearing Loss*; 2014. https://www.nidcd.nih.gov/health/statistics/use-hearing-adults-hearing-loss.
26. Ng EH, Rudner M, Lunner T, Ronnberg J. Noise reduction improves memory for target language speech in competing native but not foreign language speech. *Ear Hear.* 2015;36(1):82–91.
27. Lunner T, Rudner M, Rosenbom T, Agren J, Ng EH. Using speech recall in hearing aid fitting and outcome evaluation under ecological test conditions. *Ear Hear.* 2016;37(suppl 1):145S–154S.
28. Brooks DN, Hallam RS, Mellor PA. The effects on significant others of providing a hearing aid to the hearing-impaired partner. *Br J Audiol.* 2001;35(3):165–171.
29. Stark P, Hickson L. Outcomes of hearing aid fitting for older people with hearing impairment and their significant others. *Int J Audiol.* 2004;43(7):390–398.
30. Amieva H, Ouvrard C, Giulioli C, Meillon C, Rullier L, Dartigues JF. Self-reported hearing loss, hearing aids, and cognitive decline in elderly adults: a 25-year study. *J Am Geriatr Soc.* 2015;63(10):2099–2104.
31. Johnson CE. Introduction to hearing assistive technology. In: Johnson CE, ed. *Introduction to Auditory Rehabilitation: A Contemporary Issues Approach.* Upper Saddle River: Pearson; 2012:229–263.
32. Bittencourt AG, Burke PR, Jardim Ide S, et al. Implantable and semi-implantable hearing AIDS: a review of history, indications, and surgery. *Int Arch Otorhinolaryngol.* 2014;18(3):303–310.

33. Stone JS, Cotanche DA. Hair cell regeneration in the avian auditory epithelium. *Int J Dev Biol.* 2007;51(6–7):633–647.

34. Groves AK. The challenge of hair cell regeneration. *Exp Biol Med (Maywood)*. 2010;235(4):434–446.

35. Geleoc GS, Holt JR. Sound strategies for hearing restoration. *Science.* 2014;344(6184):1241062.

36. Ventry IM, Weinstein BE. Identification of elderly people with hearing problems. *ASHA.* 1983;25(7):37–42.

CHAPTER 12

Rehabilitation in Musculoskeletal and Sports Injuries in Older Adults

WILLIAM MICHEO, MD • LUIS A. SÁNCHEZ, MD

INTRODUCTION

Individuals aged 65 years and older make up 13% of the US population according to the US Census in 2010. This trend is expected to continue, and this population will double to 72 million over the next 25 years, with 20% of the total population by the year 2030 being considered old.[1,2]

Advancing age leads to physiologic changes that result in loss of functional capacity, change in body composition, decrease in physical activity volume, intensity, and risk of chronic disease.[3] Sedentary behavior also increases with age, making older adults the most sedentary population, with 65%–80% of their waking time spent sitting.[4] Sedentary behavior has negative effects on cardiometabolic health, muscle-tendon health, functional fitness, physical independence, body composition, and all-cause mortality. Conversely, physical activity and exercise have been well established as strategies to reduce the risk of chronic disease, increase life expectancy, and improve functional capacity and cognitive function as well as a medical intervention to counteract the detrimental effects of aging.[2,5]

Organized sports participation plays an important role in promoting exercise activity in older adults. Common sports practiced by masters athletes such as swimming and racquet sports have proven beneficial for improving all-cause mortality and cardiovascular risks, whereas swimming has shown reduction in all-cause mortality.[6] In addition, higher quality of life, reduced smoking, and getting regular medical evaluations have been reported for masters athletes.[7] Playing team sports contributes more to the person's motivation compared with individual exercise activity in older adults. These benefits may be associated to the social interactions during team sports activity.[8]

The masters athlete is commonly defined as an individual older than 35 years, who either trains or participates in sports competitions specifically designed for older athletes.[9] The American College of Sports Medicine defines the masters athlete as those aged 50 years or older who desire to exercise and expect high levels of performance in sports practice and competition. They also expect good quality sports medical care once they are injured, which will allow them to return to the competition.[10] Many sports, including tennis, golf, swimming, long-distance running, and track and field, have age-based individual and team competitions for athletes starting by age 25 years in swimming, above age 50 years in golf, and extending to categories for individuals in their 80s in tennis.[11–13] Participation in masters sports competition carries risk of injury, with 50%–60% or more of athletes suffering an injury, which requires stopping training and competition for at least 1 week.[7,14]

The goal of management of sports injury in the older athlete is to safely return the individual to normal form and function. The injured athlete should have no symptoms at rest and with activity, achieve normal flexibility, strength, muscle balance, and neuromuscular coordination and exhibit psychologic readiness before returning to participation in sports.

The process of rehabilitation should start as early as possible after the injury to minimize functional losses associated with acute or chronic recurrent injury. Evaluation, management, and rehabilitation of sports injury require an accurate diagnosis and specific treatment addressing not only the area of injury but also the complete kinetic chain.

The purpose of this chapter is to review basic concepts of sports injury in the older athlete and how they relate to planning and implementation of a rehabilitation program, describe the phases of rehabilitation, present return to play criteria, and the components of an injury prevention program.

BASIC CONCEPTS OF SPORTS INJURY IN THE OLDER ADULT

Epidemiology of Sports Injury

Understanding the incidence and prevalence of injuries based on variables, such as type and nature of the injury, age group, type of sports, sex, and time since the onset of symptoms, among others, has contributed to the development of programs aimed at prevention, treatment, and rehabilitation of sports injuries.[15] Athletic injuries occur from acute or chronic overload on the muscles, nerves, tendons, bones, or joints. The shoulder, knee, back, and ankle are common sites of injury in older athletes, and frequent diagnoses include rotator cuff injuries, Achilles tendinopathies, meniscal tears, and osteoarthritis.[9]

The location and type of injuries seen in athletes is influenced by the particular sport involved. Adult recreational tennis players have been reported to suffer three injuries per 1000h of play, overuse injuries, which affect the upper extremities, and acute injuries, which affect the lower extremities. Increasing skill level may increase injury risk, specifically of acute injuries. Common anatomic sites of injury included the elbow, shoulder, knee, and back.[16,17]

Amateur golfers most frequently report injuries to the lower back and elbow. Lateral epicondyle injuries are more common than medial epicondyle injuries in amateur athletes, whereas professional players exhibit similar frequency of both injuries. The nondominant shoulder is commonly injured in the golf swing, as the shoulder is positioned in internal rotation, flexion, and horizontal adduction.[18]

Masters runners have a reported injury rate of 46%, are injured more frequently than younger runners, and suffer multiple injuries. The knee and foot are the most common location of injury in these athletes, with a high prevalence of soft tissue injuries to the calf, Achilles tendon, and hamstring muscles.[19] The incidence of osteoarthritis in runners is not clear, but it has been reported to be associated with high volume of activity and elite level of competition.[20]

Identification of Risk Factors

The incidence of athletic injury can be affected by physiologic, biomechanical, anatomic, or genetic intrinsic factors, which may include muscle weakness and imbalance, inflexibility, age, gender, prior injury, and kinetic chain abnormalities. Extrinsic risk factors for injury include the inherent demands of the sport, intensity of training and competition, environmental conditions, and equipment.[21] Psychologic factors have also been found to influence injury risk through attentional and somatic changes, muscle fatigue, and reduced coordination. These include psychologic stressors such as negative life events, sports-related stress, personality variables such as trait anxiety, and maladaptive coping strategies.[22]

TABLE 12.1 Risk Factors for Injury in Older Adults	
Intrinsic Factors	**Extrinsic Factors**
• Age[a] • Gender[a] • BMI • Previous injury[a] • Anatomic misalignment[a] • Muscle fatigue and weakness • Inadequate flexibility	• Sport-specific demands • Volume of activity • Playing surface • Training and competition equipment

[a]Nonmodifiable.

Intrinsic factors can be modifiable (poor flexibility, muscle weakness, body mass index) or nonmodifiable (sex, height, ligamentous laxity, previous injury, and anatomic malalignment). Extrinsic factors that are modifiable include training and competition load, playing surface, and sports equipment (Table 12.1).

In tennis players, intrinsic risk factors, such as scapular dyskinesis, glenohumeral internal rotation deficits (GIRDs), and weakness of the external rotators of the shoulder are associated to rotator cuff impingement in the subacromial space.[17] Golfers with abnormal swing mechanics and poor conditioning present with low back and upper extremity injuries.[18] Training errors have been reported to account for 60% of running injuries. Excessive running distance, high training intensity, and rapid increases in running distance or intensity significantly increase the rate of injury.[23] Masters athletes that participate in sports with high torsional loads, such as tennis and basketball, those that have suffered a prior joint injury, and those that have high body mass index are at a higher risk of osteoarthritis of the knee and hip.[24]

Classification of Injury

A sports injury can be defined as a pathologic process that interrupts training or competition and may lead the athlete to seek medical treatment. Sports injuries are usually divided into two basic types: those resulting from macrotrauma and those associated with overuse and repetitive microtrauma. In traumatic injuries, there is a clear inciting event that results in damage to previous normal tissue. Microtraumatic overuse injury occurs when repetitive exposure to sports activity results in a failure of normal homeostasis and an inability of tissue to recover from sports-related trauma. Acute injury can be defined as one that occurred within 2 weeks of evaluation, subacute injury is associated with symptoms of 2–6 weeks duration, and chronic injury has symptoms that persist after 6 weeks.[25,26]

Injury definitions for use in epidemiologic studies have been standardized in different sports. A definition of a recordable injury in athletics is a physical complaint or observable damage to body tissue produced by the transfer of energy experienced or sustained by the athlete during participation in training or competition, regardless of whether it received medical attention or its consequences with respect to impairments in connection with competition or training. Severity of injury can be related to the time lost from full participation in sports. It can be classified into slight (1 day), minimal (2–3 days), mild (4–7 days), moderate (8–28 days), serious (>28 days–6 months), and long-term (>6 months) injury severity.[27]

Using the International Classification of Functioning, Disability and Health, Timpka defined athletic injury as a sports impairment associated with pain and functional limitations and participation restriction with inability to compete as a result of acute trauma or chronic overuse injury. If not managed appropriately within the health system, the athlete may present with chronic recurrent symptoms, residual sports impairment, participation restriction, and finally sports-related disability.[28]

Patient Evaluation

The history and physical examination are very important in evaluating an injured athlete. Pertinent information that should be obtained in the history includes the type of sport, the mechanism of injury, the severity of the injury, and prior treatment. In addition, information regarding previous history of similar or related injury, associated medical problems, and use of medications should be obtained.[10] Psychologic issues that should be investigated include history of anxiety, depression, and feeling vulnerable to injury.[21]

The physical examination should identify postural asymmetry, anatomic malalignment, lack of flexibility, muscle weakness and imbalance, neurologic as well as proprioceptive deficits, and ligamentous laxity. It is also important to evaluate core trunk and pelvic muscle strength, neuromuscular control, and sports-specific techniques.

The treating physician also has the responsibility of ordering and interpreting the appropriate diagnostic studies to complement the history and physical examination and aid in treatment planning. These include laboratory tests, X-rays, musculoskeletal ultrasound, bone scan, computerized tomography, and magnetic resonance imaging. In the older athlete, it is important to understand that abnormalities in diagnostic studies may be present, associated to the aging process, and not necessarily the cause of the patient's symptoms.

TABLE 12.2 Musculoskeletal Injuries Complex	
Clinical symptoms	Pain Instability Swelling
Anatomic alterations	Tissue injury Tissue overload
Functional alterations	Biomechanical deficits Subclinical adaptations

From Kibler WB. A framework for sports medicine. *Phys Med Rehabil Clin North Am*. 1994;5(1):1–8; with permission.

Complete diagnosis of athletic injury can be established using a modification of the musculoskeletal injury complex model described by Kibler.[26] This model identifies the anatomic site of injuries, the clinical symptoms, and the functional deficits (Table 12.2).

The clinical symptoms complex addresses the main complaints of the injured athlete. Symptoms such as pain, swelling, feeling unstable, numbness, weakness, or change in performance should be identified to be appropriately treated. The anatomic alterations complex identifies the site of the primary injury causing the patient's symptoms and the associated areas of tissue overload. The functional alterations complex addresses the biomechanical deficits that result from an athletic injury, the adaptations used by the athletes to try to continue to participate in sports, and the changes in sports and exercise performance.

Phases of Sports Rehabilitation

Rehabilitation of sports injury can be divided into acute, recovery, and functional phases. Each phase has specific goals and criteria for progression and can be correlated with the inflammatory, repair, and remodeling stages of tissue injury[29] (Table 12.3). Rehabilitation combines physical modalities, therapeutic exercise, assistive devices, and functional sports-specific training. Its principal goal is to restore optimal function and should begin immediately after the injury or surgery to minimize the deleterious effects of inactivity and facilitate the return to training and competition.[30]

During the acute phase of treatment, the primary focus is to decrease pain and swelling, protect the injured structures, and allow the tissue to heal. In this phase, treatment strategies include the use of analgesics, nonsteroidal antiinflammatory drugs (NSAIDs) for a short period of time, and physical modalities, such as cryotherapy and electrical stimulation, which limit secondary tissue damage, reduce muscle inhibition,

TABLE 12.3
Rehabilitation of Sports Injury

Phases	Goals
Acute	Treat symptom complex Protect anatomic injury site
Recovery	Correct biomechanical deficits Improve muscle control and balance Retrain proprioception Start sports-specific activity
Functional	Increase power and endurance Improve neuromuscular control Work on entire kinematic chain Return to competition

and allow the initiation of therapeutic exercise. Isometric strengthening exercises can be started during this phase. This static muscular training helps preserve muscle mass and strength, usually is well tolerated, and should be performed at multiple joint angles. Additionally, pain-free range of motions exercises can be implemented actively or with assistance, with no load or minimal external load. Aerobic exercise, flexibility, strengthening, and balance training of uninjured components of the kinetic chain can be started in this stage of rehabilitation. In addition, the use of orthotic equipment may be required to protect the injured part.[30,31] Control of pain, swelling, and tolerance of therapeutic exercise are required prior to progressing to the next stage of treatment.

The recovery phase aims to achieve full range of pain-free motion, improve flexibility, and regain normal muscle strength and balance. If pain persists with activity, analgesic medications and physical modalities, such as superficial heat (i.e., hydrocollator packs, paraffin), deep heat (i.e., ultrasound), and electrical stimulation can be utilized. These interventions help to reduce edema, increase circulation to the healing tissues, and improve collagen flexibility. Biomechanical and functional deficits are addressed during this phase. Static flexibility exercises with emphasis on muscles that cross two joints and dynamic flexibility training that works on sagittal, frontal, and transverse planes of motion should be integrated into the treatment program. Dynamic strengthening using open chain exercises that isolate weak muscles and train both eccentric and concentric muscle activities and closed kinetic chain exercises that involve multiple joints and muscle co-contraction in functional range of motion are key components in this phase. Neuromuscular training that addresses proprioceptive and muscle firing deficits

that result from injury to the ankle, knee, shoulder, and spine is also a component of rehabilitation.[32,33] Progression of functional training without recurrence of symptoms is required prior to advancing to the next phase of rehabilitation.

Finally, the functional phase aims to increase power and endurance, improve neuromuscular control in functional activities, and prepare the athlete to return to sports-specific training and competition. This phase emphasizes work on the entire kinetic chain and addresses residual biomechanical deficits and abnormal adaptations in sports technique. Most of the training during this phase takes place in the gym or sports venues and may include sports-specific drills, such as kicking, jumping, running, or throwing. The resolution of functional deficits or breaks in the kinetic chain is required prior to allowing the athlete to return to unrestricted participation in sports.[34]

REHABILITATION OF INJURIES COMMON IN THE OLDER ATHLETE
Rotator Cuff Injury

Rotator cuff injury is one of the most common pathologies seen in older athletes, particularly in those who perform overhead activities such as tennis. This lesion can range from tendinopathy to tears that could be partial or full-thickness. It is described that aging has been associated with an increase in rotator cuff tears, but not all are symptomatic.[35] Symptomatic rotator cuff disease can be secondary to biomechanical deficits that include tight posterior shoulder structures and pectoral muscles, GIRD, weak rotator cuff and scapular stabilizers, and weak and tight pelvic girdle muscles.[36,37] A tennis player who suffers a rotator cuff injury will also show a performance decline, such as difficulty with serve, overhead, and backswing.[16]

The rehabilitation program should focus on combining stretching and strengthening exercises, with the aim of restoring shoulder range of motion, reduce pain, maintain stability, improve function, and prevent further injury. In the acute phase, treatment strategies include physical modalities (i.e., cryotherapy, electrical stimulation) to decrease pain and inflammation, with subsequent addition of isometric and closed chain exercises to the rotator cuff and scapular stabilizers muscles. These should be performed within a nonpainful range of motion, with the goal of preventing muscle atrophy. Additionally, strengthening of the trunk and lower extremities should be started. Biomechanical abnormalities, such as scapular dysfunction, can be addressed during this phase.[38–40]

During the recovery phase, biomechanical and functional deficits, such as GIRD and throwing motion abnormalities can be addressed. Treatment strategies during this phase consist of heat modalities, shoulder joint mobilization, posterior capsule stretching, and strengthening exercises. Goals are directed to achieve a normal passive and active glenohumeral range of motion, scapular muscle control, and recover normal muscle strength and balance. The range of motion and stretching program should include internal/external rotation with a stick, cross-arm, and sleeper stretches to address flexibility deficits of the pectoralis, rotator cuff, and scapular stabilizer muscles.[38-40] An adequate strengthening program includes closed kinetic chain exercises for the rotator cuff and scapular stabilizers, such as pushups against a wall. Additionally, strengthening of the rotator cuff muscles and scapular stabilizers can be performed in an open kinetic manner using light weights or surgical tubing progressing to functional ranges of motion.

In the functional phase, the entire kinetic chain must be worked and sports-specific training should be started, including squats, lunges, and rotational exercises to improve core, pelvic girdle, and lower extremity muscles' neuromuscular control and strength. Normal motion, flexibility, strength, and symptom-free participation in sports practice should be achieved prior to returning to play.[38-40]

Knee Osteoarthritis

Osteoarthritis is a multifactorial disease, affected by activity, exercise, sports, and previous injury. OA in the lower extremities is associated to activities that increase joint loading, such as high-impact sports, particularly in older athletes. Knee osteoarthritis is commonly reported and is the result of biomechanical changes, muscle weakness, increased joint loading, alteration in the gait pattern, and an increase in knee adduction moment.[9] Development of OA is associated to previous injuries and recurring microtrauma, and not necessarily to an increase in physical activity.[9]

A comprehensive approach needs to be implemented during rehabilitation, and exercise is an essential component of knee OA management.

In the acute phase, the treatment should focus on decreasing pain and swelling with NSAIDs, cryotherapy, electrical stimulation, and relative rest. In some instances, athletes present with knee effusions and a knee joint aspiration could be considered to improve joint mobility and pain. Isometric exercises are started during this phase to promote quadriceps activation, thus preventing arthrogenic inhibition.

The recovery phase program consists of pain-free range of motion exercises and stretching of hip flexors, iliotibial band, quadriceps, and hamstrings. Strengthening is emphasized on quadriceps, hamstrings, and pelvic girdle muscles, using open and closed chain exercises.[41-44] It has been described that a reduction in cartilage damage is seen in those who have greater quadriceps strength. In addition, patients who perform strengthening exercises show improvement in balance, proprioception, reduced pain intensity, and improved patient functionality.[9,41-44] Athletes can combine stretching and strengthening exercises with cross-training strategies. Aerobic and neuromuscular training is recommended for the older athletes for relieving joint loading and improving function.[41-44]

There are other alternatives for the management of patients with Knee OA. Among them are cycling, aquatherapy, and Tai Chi. Aquatherapy provides benefits in the functional status and patient's quality of life, although the results regarding improvement of pain symptoms are controversial.[24]

Furthermore, weight loss and mechanical interventions, such as knee bracing and insoles (i.e., lateral wedge) may be considered with the goal of decreasing knee joint loading. There is some evidence that an unloader brace provides stability to the knee, decreases medial compartment loading, and improves functional levels in the runner.[24]

Older athletes who present with severe degenerative joint disease could be candidates for knee joint arthroplasty. Joint replacement is a cost-effective treatment option, which has been shown to improve pain, mobility, function, psychologic well-being, and most importantly, quality of life. Undergoing a joint replacement does not necessary means having to stop masters athletic participation, but activity modification is required to prevent hardware loosening, fracture, and reduced prosthetic survival. These athletes should avoid high-impact activity such as running, but swimming, golf, and cycling are recommended.[9,45] Return to activity should be performed after restoration of the muscle strength of the quadriceps, hamstring, and pelvic girdle. There should be a balance between too little activity (due to a predisposition to decreased bone mineral density) and too much activity (due to increase wear and loosening). Usually, learning a new sport is associated with high joint loads, thus it is not recommended that athletes start participation in new high-impact sports after the surgical procedure. In addition, it is unclear if tennis players can return to singles play after knee joint replacement; however, return to doubles is allowed.[9,45]

Lumbar Spine Injury

Lumbar spine injuries are associated to damage to multiple structures and a complexity of clinical symptoms. This results in a broad differential diagnosis in the older athlete that includes facet joint syndrome, lumbosacral radiculopathy, and spinal stenosis. Biomechanical deficits, such as tight hip flexors and hamstrings, weak pelvic girdle and core muscles, predispose older athletes to develop lumbar spine symptoms, resulting in performance decline.[46] For example, a tennis player could demonstrate loss of serve velocity, ability to volley, and difficulty reaching low balls.[16]

Initial management consists of limited bed rest, ice, analgesics, NSAIDs, muscle relaxants, physical modalities, and a decrease in activities that involve repetitive movements, such as back extension, rotation, and flexion. Isometric and static exercises should be initiated to retrain proper muscle firing patterns in patients with muscle inhibition and abnormal firing patterns. Painless light aerobic exercise can also be included in the treatment program. In addition, spine-positioning abnormalities are identified, and proper spine biomechanics education is provided.[47,48]

Typically, as part of the aging process, older athletes tend to lose the ability to compensate for the instability generated by a perturbation process, particularly if there is a chronic low back pain history. Therefore strengthening of core muscles is highly recommended, as they provide lumbar stability.[49] For example, adequate core stability is vital for the golfer, particularly to improve trunk flexion velocity during the downswing.[50] Low back stability is achieved by the combination of static and dynamic components, static stability provided by structures such as bones and ligaments, and dynamic stability associated with neuromuscular control. Particularly, dynamic stabilizers work on maintaining joint position or proper alignment through an equalization of forces.[32]

The muscles that are targeted for strengthening include the multifidi, quadratus lumborum, abdominals, and hip girdle muscles. Dynamic flexibility training in sagittal, frontal, and transverse planes of motion are started gradually as the pain subsides. Then, tightness of the hip flexors, rotators, and hamstrings, and gastro-soleus complex are addressed. Exercise training with gym balls, rotational patterns, and eccentric loading of the spine are implemented. Normal spine mechanics for sports activities should be restored, and progression of sports-specific training fulfilled prior to completion of rehabilitation.[46,49,50]

Return to Play Considerations

Once the athlete completes a rehabilitation program, the decision to return to safe sports participation must be made. This includes returning patients to the practice of their sport, and finally the clearance to participate in competition. This important decision should be based on clinical evaluation, results of objective tests, and psychologic factors, and not rely solely on the absence of symptoms, and the time elapsed from injury or surgery.

Factors to consider include the type of sport and position played, the treatment or surgery offered to the patient, absence of symptoms at rest and with sports activity, normal flexibility, strength and neuromuscular control based on clinical evaluation, isokinetic dynamometry and functional tests that may include jumping, running, and changing direction. Patient satisfaction with the treatment offered, sense of confidence with sports activity, and psychologic readiness to participate in sports need to be addressed prior to returning to play, and may require the use of validated questionnaires.[51,52]

Prevention of Sports Injury

For the athlete that returns to practice and competition, prevention of recurrent injury is very important. Prevention programs have been developed for athletes that have not been injured (primary prevention) and for those that have been injured (secondary prevention). Prehabilitation is defined as conditioning strategies for athletes susceptible to injury because of sports-specific demands, and in formerly injured athletes, to prepare them for the stresses and demands of their sport. Prevention programs focus on modifiable risk factors, neuromuscular deficits, and sports-specific techniques focusing in areas at risk or already injured in a specific sport.[53]

Components of a prehabilitation program include stretching, strengthening, proprioception, and plyometric exercises. Static stretching as a clinical intervention has been found to improve flexibility, but it has not been conclusively shown to reduce the risk of injury, and should be combined with dynamic stretching, which works in sport-specific ranges of motion.[32]

Strengthening exercises are known to reduce the risk of injury. Eccentric exercise, in particular, has been found to reduce the risk of hamstring strains in elite athletes.[54] Balance training, learning how to fall from a jump, modifying cutting techniques, and plyometric exercises that activate the hamstrings have been found to reduce the risk of anterior cruciate ligament injuries, and should be integrated into injury prevention programs.[53]

Finally, education about modifiable risk factors, such as frequency and intensity of activity, sports technique, type of playing surface, and equipment should be integrated into the prevention program.

SUMMARY

- The aging population continues to increase.
- Older age is associated to chronic illness, functional loss, and sedentary lifestyle.
- Exercise and sports participation lead to improved health, increased life expectancy, reduction in disability, improved mental health and cognition.
- Risk of injury to the older athlete is associated with sports participation.
- Identification of injury patterns and modifiable risk factors associated to sports participation is key in management.
- Rehabilitation of sports injury in the older athlete is a criteria-based progression associated to meeting specific goals.
- Return to play decisions are based on objective criteria, and prevention of injury programs should be instituted combining education, correction of risk factors, and an exercise program.

REFERENCES

1. US Census Bureau. *The Older Population 2010. 2010 Census Brief*; 2011.
2. Centers for Disease Control and Prevention. *The State of Aging and Health in America 2013*. Atlanta, GA: Centers for Disease Control and Prevention, US Dept. of Health and Human Services; 2013.
3. Chodzko-Zajko W, Proctor DN, Fiatarone Singh MA, et al. Exercise and physical activity for older adults. *Med Sci Sports Exerc*. 2009;41(7):1510–1530.
4. Wullems JA, Verschueren SMP, Degens H, et al. A review of the assessment and prevalence of sedentarism in older adults, its physiology/health impact and non-exercise mobility countermeasures. *Biogerontology*. 2016;17:547–565.
5. Nelson ME, Rejeski WJ, Blair SN, et al. Physical activity and public health in older adults: recommendations from the American College of Sports Medicine and the American Heart Association. *Med Sci Sports Exerc*. 2007;39(8):1435–1445.
6. Oja P, Kelly P, Pedisic Z, et al. Association of specific types of sports and exercise with all-cause and cardiovascular disease mortality: a cohort study of 80, 306 British adults. *Br J Sports Med*. 2016;0:1–7.
7. Shephard RJ, Kavanagh T, Mertens DJ, et al. Personal health benefits of masters athletics competition. *Br J Sports Med*. 1995;29(1):35–40.
8. Pedersen MT, Vorup J, Nistrup A, et al. Effects of team sports and resistance training on physical function, quality of life and motivation in older athletes. *Scand J Med Sci Sports [Internet]*. 2017:1–13. Available in: http//11doi.wiley.com/10.111/sms.12832.
9. Tayrose GA, Beutel BG, Cardone DA, Sherman OH. The masters athlete: a review of current exercise and treatment recommendations. *Sports Health*. 2014;7(3):270–276.
10. Herring SA, Kibler WB, Putukian M, et al. Selected issues for the master athlete and team physician: a consensus statement. *Med Sci Sports Exerc*. 2010;42(4):820–833.
11. https://www.fina.org.
12. https://www.usga.org.
13. https://www.usta.com.
14. Galloway MT, Jokl P. Aging successfully: the importance of physical activity in maintaining health and function. *J Am Acad Orthop Surg*. 2000;8:37–44.
15. Frontera WR. Epidemiology of sports injuries: implications for rehabilitation. In: Frontera WR, ed. *Rehabilitation of Sports Injuries: Scientific Basis*. Blackwell: Massachussets; 2003:3–9.
16. Jayanthi N, Esser S. Racket sports. *Curr Sports Med Rep*. 2013;12(5):329–336.
17. Changstrom B, Jayanthi N. Clinical evaluation of the adult recreational tennis player. *Curr Sports Med Rep*. 2016;15(6):437–445.
18. Wadsworth LT. When golf hurts: musculoskeletal problems common to golfers. *Curr Sports Med Rep*. 2007;6:362–365.
19. McKean K, Manson NA, Stanish WD. Musculoskeletal injury in masters runners. *Clin J Sports Med*. 2006;16(2):149–154.
20. Ni GX. Development and prevention of running related osteoarthritis. *Curr Sports Med Rep*. 2016;15(5):342–349.
21. Herring SA, Kibler WB, Putukian M, et al. Selected issues in injury and illness prevention: a consensus statement. *Med Sci Sports Exerc*. 2016;48(1):159–171.
22. Soligard T, Schwellmus M, Alonso JM. How much is too much? (Part 1) International Olympic Committee consensus statement on load in sport and risk of injury. *Br J Sports Med*. 2016;50:1030–1041.
23. Hreljac A. Etiology, prevention, and early intervention of overuse injuries in runners: a biomechanical perspective. *PMR Clin NA*. 2005;16:651–667.
24. Straker JS, Vannatta CN, Waldron K. Treatment strategies for the master athlete with known arthritis of the hip and knee. *Top Geriatr Rehabil*. 2016;32(1):39–54.
25. Frontera WR, Micheo WF, Amy E, et al. Patterns of injury evaluated in an interdisciplinary clinic. *PR Health Sci J*. 1994;3:65–70.
26. Kibler WB. A framework for sports medicine. *PMR Clin NA*. 1994;5:1–8.
27. Timpka T, Alonso JM, Jacobsson J, et al. Injury and illness definitions and data collection procedures for use in epidemiologic studies in athletics (track and field): consensus statement. *Br J Sports Med*. 2014;48:483–490.
28. Timpka T, Jacobson J, Bickenbach J, et al. What is a sports injury? *Sports Med*. 2014;44(4):423–428.
29. Dugan SA, Frontera WR. Rehabilitation in sports medicine. In: Micheli L, Smith A, Bachl N, et al., eds. *Team Physician Manual*. Hong Kong: Lippincott Williams & Wilkins, Asia; 2001:162–186.
30. Frontera WR. Exercise and musculoskeletal rehabilitation: restoring optimal form and function. *Phys Sports Med*. 2003;31(12):39–45.

31. Micheo W, Esquenazi A. Orthosis in the prevention and rehabilitation of injuries. In: Frontera WR, ed. *Rehabilitation of Sports Injuries: Scientific Basis*. Blackwell: Massachussetts; 2003:301–305.

32. Micheo W, Baerga L, Miranda G. Basic principles regarding strength, flexibility, and stability exercises. *PMR*. 2012;4(11):805–811.

33. Kibler WB. Closed kinetic chain rehabilitation for sports injuries. *PMR Clin North Am*. 2000;11:369–384.

34. Kibler WB, Chandler TJ. Functional rehabilitation and return to training and competition. In: Frontera WR, ed. *Rehabilitation of Sports Injuries: Scientific Basis*. Blackwell: Massachussetts; 2003:288–300.

35. Tokish JM. The mature athlete's shoulder. *Sports Health*. 2014;6:31–35.

36. Wilk KE, Macrina LC, Fleisig GS, et al. Correlation of glenohumeral internal rotation deficit and total rotational motion to shoulder injuries in professional baseball pitchers. *Am J Sports Med*. 2011;39(2):329–335.

37. Kibler B, Wilkes T, Sciascia A. Mechanics and pathomechanics of the overhead athlete. *Clin Sports Med*. 2013;32:637–651.

38. Wilk KE, Meister K, Andrews JR. Current concepts in the rehabilitation of the overhead throwing athlete. *Am J Sports Med*. 2002;30:136–151.

39. Krabak BJ, Sugar R, McFarland EG. Practical nonoperative management of rotator cuff injuries. *Clin J Sports Med*. 2003;13(2):102–105.

40. Sciascia A, Thigpen C, Namdari S, et al. Kinetic chain abnormalities in the athletic shoulder. *Sports Med Arthrosc Rev*. 2012;20:16–21.

41. Fransen M, McConnell S, Harmer AR, et al. Exercise for osteoarthritis of the knee. *Br J Sports Med*. 2015;49(24):1554–1557.

42. Vincent KR, Vincent HK. Resistance exercise for knee osteoarthritis. *PMR*. 2012;4:S45–S52.

43. Semanik PA, Chang RW, Dunlop DD. Aerobic activity in prevention and symptom control of osteoarthritis. *PMR*. 2012;4:S37–S44.

44. Ageberg E, Roos EM. Neuromuscular exercise as treatment of degenerative knee disease. *Exerc Sport Sci Rev*. 2015;43(1):14–22.

45. Jassim SS, Douglas SL, Haddad FS. Athletic activity after lower limb arthroplasty: a systematic review of current evidence. *Bone Joint J*. 2014;96-B:923–927.

46. Nadler SF, Malanga GA, Bartoli LA, et al. Hip muscle imbalance and low back pain in athletes: influence core strengthening. *Med Sci Sports Exerc*. 2002;34(1):9–16.

47. McGill S. *Low Back Disorder: Evidence-Based Prevention and Rehabilitation*. Champaign, IL: Human Kinetics; 2002.

48. Donelson R. The McKenzie approach to evaluating and treating low back pain. *Orthop Rev*. 1990;19(8):681–686.

49. Akuthota V, Ferreiro A, Moore T. Core stability exercise principles. *Curr Sports Med Rep*. 2008;7:39–44.

50. Finn C. Rehabilitation of low back pain in golfers: from diagnosis to return to sport. *Sports Health*. 2013;5(4):313–319.

51. Creighton DW, Shrier I, Shultz R, et al. Return-to-play in sport: a decision-based model. *Clin J Sport Med*. 2015:379–385.

52. Sepúlveda F, Sánchez L, Amy E, et al. Anterior cruciate ligament injury: return to play, function and long-term considerations. *Curr Rep Sport Med*. 2017;16(3):172–178.

53. Acevedo R, Rivera-Vega A, Miranda G, et al. Anterior cruciate ligament injury: identification of risk factors and prevention strategies. *Curr Rep Sport Med*. 2014;13(3):186–191.

54. Chu SK, Rho ME. Hamstring injuries in the athlete: diagnosis, treatment, and return to play. *Curr Sports Med Rep*. 2016;15:184–190.

CHAPTER 13

Geriatric Psychiatric and Cognitive Disorders: Depression, Dementia, and Delirium

YEONSIL MOON, MD, PHD • MOOYEON OH-PARK, MD • JONGMIN LEE, MD, PHD

DEPRESSION

Definition of Depression

Depression can refer to both a symptom and a disease. As a symptom, depression is recognized as a mood that stands on a continuum from sadness to pathologically severe depression,[1] whereas as a syndrome, requisite condition is needed. According to the fifth edition of the Diagnostic and Statistical Manual of Mental Disorders (DSM-5), depression is diagnosed when the depressive symptoms persist over at least a two-week period and other related symptoms, such as weight loss or gain without changes in diet, insomnia or hypersomnia, psychomotor agitation or retardation, fatigue, feeling of worthlessness or excessive or inappropriate guilt, diminished ability to think or concentrate, or recurrent thoughts of death or suicidal ideation, should be added.

Depression is far more common and easily ignored than dementia, although dementia is regarded as a characteristic disease of the elderly. The prevalence of depression is estimated to be 1% of older adults aged 65 years and over living in the community. Depression also adds to the morbidity of the patient's comorbid disease, and vice versa. In addition, depression is associated with a decline in mobility and cognition, and it needs to be taken into consideration for the preservation of physical and cognitive function.

Clinical Features of Depression

In elderly patients, clinical features of depression are different from those in young patients. Elderly patients tend to minimize depressive moods and additional symptoms related with somatic concerns such as hypochondriasis. Psychomotor retardation is also common. Several physical illnesses accompany aging, and these comorbid diseases overlap with depression or could be the cause of depression. Hence, depression is usually complained as or with pain (such as headaches and/or musculoskeletal pain on joints) or dyspepsia rather than depressive mood.[2]

Another typical feature of elderly depression is combined cognitive decline. Depression causes the patients to lose the power to think appropriately; hence, elderly with depression usually present slowed mental processing speed and diffuse cognitive dysfunction. Indifferent attitude to cognitive decline, dominant retrieval type of memory loss, and self-report of cognitive decline without objective report by caregivers could be clues to differentiate "pseudodementia: dementia due to depression." However, it is not easy to distinguish, as Alzheimer's disease (AD) also accompanies depressive mood in the early stages of the disease.

Suicide is another issue to be evaluated carefully in elderly patients with depression. In the elderly, even one suicide gesture to attract concern is enough to cause fatality although the rate of suicide is much different based on the age, gender, and country. Moreover, the suicide rate in the elderly who are not treated with antidepressants is relatively higher than in young patients.[3]

Causes of Depression

Increasing age is the most robust risk factor for depression in the elderly, and this may be explained by disability, poor health conditions, medical comorbidities, poor social support, and loneliness by bereavement.[4] A physically disabled state causes depression in the elderly; furthermore, depression can worsen the outcome of a health condition. This includes not only physical disability such as gait disturbances and hearing and visual loss, but also medical comorbidities such as ischemic heart disease, cerebrovascular disease (CVD), or obstructive pulmonary disease, which are very common in the elderly. Among these diseases, CVD particularly contributes to elderly depression. This, called "vascular depression," is supported by considerable evidence of relationship between depression and a cerebrovascular imaging marker, and the interaction is also bidirectional.[5]

The vicious cycle between physical disability, medical comorbidities, and depression is mediated by a synergistic interaction between health handicap and social activity. Decreased social support due to the disability and medical comorbidities causes depressive mood in elderly patients, which exacerbates the prognosis of the disease. Economic problems might not be the immediate cause that affects elderly depression; however, the elderly who are not well supported by caregivers because of socioeconomic problems are very vulnerable to depression.[6] Loneliness and bereavement, which many elderly undergo, are common triggers for depression. Likewise, loss of significant beings such as pets or friends could be a stressful life event, resulting in depression. Healthy elderly also become depressive after bereavement or separation; however, a normal depressive response does not persist beyond 2–6 months after an event. At all ages, depression is more frequent in women than in men.

Diagnosis of Depression

Recording substantial history is important to examine patients with depression. Clinicians should note the onset, progression, attitude, accompanied mood, and personal characteristics. Validated tools, such as the Patient Health Questionnaire 9, which reflect the diagnostic criteria of DSM-5, are used to evaluate depression comprehensively.[7] The Geriatric Depression Scale (GDS) is one of the most commonly used tools, and it has been developed specifically for elderly depression. The 15 questions containing a "short version of GDS" as well as the original version of 30 questions are widely used and have been translated into the various languages of the world. In the case of the original version of GDS (30 questions), the cutoff score of normal are 0–9; mild depressives, 10–19; severe depressives, 20–30. In the case of the short version of GDS (15 questions), scores over 5 points is suggestive of depression and should warrant a follow-up interview for clinical purpose. Scores over 10 are almost always depression.

There is even a version of 4-questions, which includes the most sensitive items from the original GDS: "Are you basically satisfied with your life?" "Do you feel that your life is empty?" "Are you afraid that something bad is going to happen to you?" and "Do you feel happy most of the time?"[8] The interpretation of GDS-4 questions is as follows: Score 0 is not indicative of a depressive status; however the patient should be monitored further for any more signs displayed and also for their evolution. Score 1

is not consistent with a depressive status; however, there should be some concerns raised in regard to the mental health of the patient and further assessment is required. Score over 2 is indicative of the presence of a depressive status. The patient needs to be referred to further specialist consultation. Besides, the Hospital Anxiety and Depression Scale, the World Health Organization Well-Being Index, and the Cornell Scale for Depression in Dementia are also widely used to evaluate depression.

Laboratory tests such as those for anemia, glucose level, vitamin B12, and thyroid-stimulating hormone levels are necessary to rule out systemic disease that can contribute or worsen depressive symptoms. As mentioned earlier, cognitive decline is a typical feature of elderly depression; neuropsychological testing is useful to define comorbid dementia. However, it is recommended that comprehensive neuropsychological testing be avoided during an acute or severe phase of depression.

Treatment of Depression

Pharmacotherapy is a very effective treatment for patients with depressive disorder. Age should not be a barrier for pharmacotherapy; however, clinicians should be familiar with precautions in prescribing medications to older adults. The number and affinity of most receptors decrease with age; changes in pharmacodynamics should be observed. Moreover, polypharmacy is a characteristic of geriatric medicine. Hence, clinicians should be always aware of drug-drug interactions, reduced renal clearance rate, and decreased metabolism. Selective serotonin-reuptake inhibitors (SSRIs) are the first-line treatment of depressive disorder. Sertraline, fluoxetine, and paroxetine are effective in treating depression. Escitalopram tends to be more effective in treating severe depression.[9] Side effects of SSRIs include nausea, headache, or diarrhea, and these symptoms are common in the elderly. The second-line medicines are serotonin-norepinephrine reuptake inhibitors (SNRIs): duloxetine and venlafaxine. Although there are no significant differences between the effects of SSRIs and SNRIs, SNRIs show more frequent adverse effects than SSRIs.[10] Tricyclic antidepressants (TCAs), an older generation of antidepressants, also have beneficial effects on depression. However, the side effects of TCAs including dry mouth and orthostatic intolerance are much greater than SSRIs or SNRIs. Atypical antipsychotics are also used to treat patients nonresponsive to antidepressants. Treatment typically lasts between 6 and 12 months, or over 12 months in some cases. The clinical pharmacology of these drugs is described in Table 13.1.

TABLE 13.1
Clinical Pharmacology of Medications for Depressive Disorder

Drug		Starting Dose (mg/day)	Maximal Dose (mg/day)	Adverse Effects
TCA	Desipramine	10–25	300	Hypotension, urinary retention
	Nortriptyline	10–25	200	
RIMA	Moclobemide	150	600	
SSRI	Escitalopram	5	20	Sexual dysfunction, insomnia
	Sertraline	25	200	
SNRI	Venlafaxine	37.5	375	Nausea, constipation, anorexia, dizziness
	Duloxetine	20–30	60	
NaSSA	Mirtazapine	15	45	
DNRI	Bupropion	100	300	Seizure, anorexia, constipation
SARI	Trazodone	150	400	Hypersomnia, sedation, weight gain

DNRI, dopamine and norepinephrine reuptake inhibitor; *NaSSA*, norepinephrine and specific serotonergic antagonist; *RIMA*, reversible inhibitor of monoamine oxidase-A; *SARI*, serotonin blockade and serotonin-reuptake inhibitor; *SNRI*, serotonin and norepinephrine reuptake inhibitor; *SSRI*, selective serotonin-reuptake inhibitor; *TCA*, tricyclic antidepressant.

Psychotherapy is as effective as medication. Cognitive behavioral therapy focusing on identifying and reframing negative, dysfunctional thoughts and encouraging participation in pleasurable and social activities is a successful strategy to reduce depressive symptoms in the elderly. Interpersonal therapy, problem solving treatment, dynamic psychotherapy, and family therapy have shown efficacy for the treatment of depressive disorder.

Prevention of Depression

As mentioned earlier, the risk factors of depression are multiple, mixed, and interlaced. Among these factors, some factors including socioeconomic support or loneliness are somewhat controlled by public health for the primary prevention of depression. In patients with depressive disorder, there is considerable evidence that maintaining medication is effective in preventing the recurrence of depressive symptoms.

DEMENTIA
Definition of Dementia

Dementia is a syndrome defined as a decline in mental ability severe enough to interfere with a person's ability to perform daily activities. Dementia is not a specific disease; rather, it is a general term that describes various symptoms of epistemic or neuropsychiatric decline. Although patients with dementia have decreased higher cortical functions, they have an alert mental status unlike patients with delirium who have clouded consciousness. Dementia usually occurs because of disease of the brain, usually of a chronic or progressive nature, in which there is disturbance in multiple higher cortical functions, including memory, thinking, orientation, comprehension, calculation, learning capacity, language, and judgment. Memory loss is the most common and representative symptom; however, the impairment in cognitive function is accompanied, and occasionally preceded, by deterioration in emotional control, social behavior, or motivation.[1]

According to the International Statistical Classification of Diseases and Related Health Problems 10th Revision (ICD-10), dementia is classified as organic, including symptomatic, mental disorders and coded by each cause of dementia.[11] However, DSM-5, which was recently released by the American Psychiatric Association, replaced the term "dementia" with "major neurocognitive disorder and mild neurocognitive disorder." The new terms focus on a decline, rather than a deficit, in function. The new criteria focus less on memory impairment, allowing for variables associated with conditions that sometimes begin with a decline in speech or language usage ability.[12]

Nevertheless, the use of term "dementia" is still retained; the Alzheimer's Association, which is one of the leading voluntary health organizations in Alzheimer's care, support, and research, and the National

Institute on Aging, an agency of the US National Institutes of Health, continue to use the term when they issued the new research criteria and guidelines for the diagnosis of AD.[13]

Mild Cognitive Impairment

Mild cognitive impairment (MCI) is one of the syndromes that describe the decline in cognitive function based on the age and education of the individual but are not significant enough to interfere with their daily activities. This concept was proposed by Peterson in 1999 and has been in use until now.[14]

MCI is four times more prevalent than dementia[15] and is a very heterogenous group. MCI is mostly on the neurodegenerative spectrum from subjective cognitive decline to dementia and shares the causes of dementia. However, the contribution of nonneurodegenerative or nonvascular causes, such as depression or anxiety, is much higher in MCI than dementia.

MCI is important, as it progresses to dementia preferentially than normal cognition in the elderly. Because MCI is a transitional stage evolving into dementia and usually convert to dementia with a conversion rate of 10%–16% per year, it has important implications for patients and their families.[16,17] The medical intervention for MCI is still not available. No drug, including cholinesterase inhibitors, ginkgo biloba, or testosterone, has proven effective in the treatment of MCI. Only controlling vascular risk factors, including stroke prevention strategy such as blood pressure control, glucose control, smoking cessation, and antiplatelet medication, may reduce risk of progression from MCI to dementia.[18]

Causes of Dementia
Neurodegenerative disease
Alzheimer's disease. AD is the most common cause of dementia, accounting for 50%–56% of cases at autopsy and in clinical series. Another 13%–17% of the cases are also accounted for when combined with intracerebral vascular disease.[19] The most powerful and crucial risk factor for AD is age. The incidence of the disease doubles every 5 years after 65 years of age.[20]

The most representative molecular mechanism of AD is the β-amyloid (Aβ) theory. Aβ peptides originate from proteolysis of the amyloid precursor protein (APP) and are divided into two types of proteins by the sequential enzymatic actions. If APP is cleaved by α-secretase and γ-secretase, the sequence initiates nonamyloidogenic processing; however when sliced by beta-site APP–cleaving enzyme 1 (BACE-1), a β-secretase, and γ-secretase, the aggregation-prone

and toxic Aβ is produced. Because the cleavage by γ-secretase is somewhat imprecise, it results in a heterogenous peptide population.[19] Among many different Aβ species, those ending at position 40 (Aβ40) are much more abundant than 42 (Aβ42), which are more hydrophobic and fibrillogenic and the principal species deposited in the brain.[21] Oligomer are more readily formed from Aβ42 than Aβ40. These soluble and diffusible oligomers are cytotoxic, especially when these form fibrils through assemblage. Because these Aβ oligomers and fibrils are unlikely to occur in a healthy brain, the microglia and astrocytes would recognize these peptides as a foreign material and start forming neuritic plaques, which are the representative biomarkers of AD. However, it is important to note that certain level of neuritic plaques are also common in asymptomatic patients older than 75 years and in those with other neurodegenerative disorders such as cerebral amyloid angiopathy (predominantly diffuse plaques), dementia with Lewy bodies (DLB), and Parkinson's disease (PD).[22]

Another protein abnormality observed in AD is neurofibrillary tangles. It occurs in various neurodegenerative disorders including AD. The hyperphosphorylated tau causes microtubules to destabilize and disrupt. The aggregates of abnormal tau protein form helical filaments, which then become neurofibrillary tangles.[23] Unlike the total Aβ burden not being correlated with cognitive impairment, these neurofibrillary tangles are a pathologic marker of the severity of AD.[19]

Besides protein abnormalities, mitochondrial dysfunctions including oxidative stress, an insulin-signaling pathway, vascular factors, inflammation, calcium, axonal-transport deficits, aberrant cell-cycle reentry, and cholesterol metabolism are also detected as molecular mechanisms of AD.[19] Genetic factors are also one of the important factors of AD; however, the dementia symptoms due to genetic mutation–based AD tend to occur before the age of 60–65 years.

Although memory decline is a predominant symptom of AD, executive and visuospatial dysfunction along with neuropsychiatric symptoms such as apathy, depression, anxiety, and agitation is common in AD. Although the general neurologic examination is normal at the early stage of AD, motor symptoms including dysarthria, dysphagia, and gait disturbance are noted in patients with advance AD.

Dementia with Lewy bodies. Dementia with Lewy bodies (DLB) accounts for 20% of dementia. As suggested by the name, the pathologic hallmark of DLB is Lewy bodies. PD has Lewy bodies primarily affecting

TABLE 13.2

Comparison Between Neurodegenerative Disease (Alzheimer's Disease and Dementia With Lewy Bodies) and Vascular Dementia

Causes of Dementia	Alzheimer's Dementia	Dementia with Lewy Bodies	Vascular Dementia
Essential features	Dementia with cognitive decline that disrupts activities of daily living		
Patterns of cognitive deficit	Prominent and early involvement of memory decline	More deficits in attention, executive function, and visuospatial ability	Various patterns depending on the lesion of CVA
Accompanying features	Depression or apathy at early stage	RBD, loss of atonia during REM sleep-neuroleptic sensitivity	Early involvement of gait disturbance, urinary frequency, neurologic deficit
Main pathophysiology	Cholinergic deficit due to neuronal loss within the cholinergic nucleus basalis of Meynert	Low dopamine transporter uptake in the basal ganglia with neocortical cholinergic deficit	Decreased cerebrovascular perfusion and neuronal degeneration
Characteristics of brain MRI	Medial temporal atrophy on coronal T2	Marked deficits in the occipital regions with relative sparing of the medial temporal lobe when compared with AD	Evidence of ischemic damage including small vessel disease, cerebral infarction, lacunar infarction, intracerebral hemorrhage

CVA, cerebrovascular attack; *MRI*, magnetic resonance imaging; *RBD*, REM sleep behavior disorder; *REM*, rapid eye movement.

the substantia nigra, locus ceruleus, and raphe nuclei, whereas DLB is characterized by limbic, paralimbic, and neocortical Lewy bodies. Symptoms in patients with DLB are somewhat overlapping with AD and PD. According to the consensus diagnostic criteria for DLB, the core features include fluctuating cognition or level of consciousness, visual hallucinations, and parkinsonian motor signs.[24] Patients with DLB show more severe impairment in visuospatial and executive function than those with AD (which show more prominent memory decline) and earlier involvement of progressive cognitive decline appearing before or within one year of parkinsonian symptoms compared with PD dementia.

As patients with DLB show severe reduction in acetylcholine levels in the brain network, the response to acetylcholinesterase inhibitors (AChEIs) is quite acceptable to cognition and neuropsychiatric symptoms.

Vascular dementia

Vascular cognitive impairment (VCI) is defined as a syndrome with evidence of clinical stroke or subclinical vascular brain injury and cognitive impairment affecting at least one cognitive domain. VCI encompasses all stages of cognitive decline, and vascular dementia (VD) refers to the "dementia" stage of cognitive impairment.[25] VD is the second most common cause of dementia after AD and tends to be more prevalent

in Asia than Europe or North America.[26] Because AD shares the risk factors with stroke and patients with AD often show concurrent stroke, especially in the elderly, numerous patients with dementia show mixed pathology (CVD with other neurodegenerative pathology, such as AD). It is not easy to clarify this overlapped pathologies and symptoms; however, the most decisive point to diagnose VD is the association between CVD and cognitive impairment. Hence, the clinical neurocognitive deficit of patients with VD is much linked with the location of their stroke lesions. However, the most common form of VCI is the subcortical type, which is revealed as white matter changes, lacunar infarcts, and cerebral microbleeds on brain magnetic resonance imaging (MRI).[27]

Decreased speed of mentation, executive dysfunction, and retrieval memory impairment rather than input dysfunction are the features of cognitive dysfunctions of VD; however, it is not easy to identify, as elderly patients usually have multiple brain pathologies including CVD, subcortical cerebrovascular injury, and asymptomatic neurodegenerative disease. Relatively early involvement of gait disturbance, urinary difficulties, and poststroke psychiatric disturbances such as depression could be clues to diagnosis of VD in the elderly.

A brief comparison of the three types of diseases that cause dementia is presented in Table 13.2.

TABLE 13.3
Medications That May Trigger Cognitive Impairment

Categories of Medication	Examples of Medication
Anticholinergics	Benztropine, tolterodine
Benzodiazepines	Lorazepam, diazepam,
Anticonvulsants	clonazepam
Antidepressants	Carbamazepine,
Antihistamines	phenobarbital, phenytoin
Chemotherapeutic agents	Fluoxetine, sertraline, citalopram
Narcotics	Diphenhydramine,
Nonbenzodiazepine sedatives	chlorpheniramine
	Busulfan, cytarabine
	Oxycodone, morphine, codeine
	Pentobarbital, mephobarbital

Other causes of dementia

The causes of dementia are numerous, from the irreversible causes to reversible causes such as medication, hypothyroidism, or vitamin deficiencies. Almost all cases of dementia are due to irreversible causes such as neurodegenerative disease and CVD. Among neurodegenerative diseases, AD and VD are the most common types; however, many other diseases could cause cognitive decline in patients. Besides DLB, **frontotemporal dementia** that is characterized by the early atrophy of frontotemporal lobes and noticeable personality changes or language dysfunction, **Huntington's disease** that shows executive dysfunction, or **Creutzfeldt-Jakob disease** that progresses very rapidly, could be causes of dementia. However, these diseases manifest dementia symptoms relatively early, before the age of 65 years, in patients.

Some causes of dementia could be reversed or improved with appropriate treatment. **Metabolic and endocrine-related diseases** such as hyponatremia, hypoglycemia, or hypothyroidism; **infectious and inflammatory diseases** such as meningitis, encephalitis, or autoimmune disease; **nutritional disturbances** including vitamin deficiencies, or dehydration; or **medication reaction** (Table 13.3) could be a cause or concomitant factors affecting symptoms of dementia.

Diagnosis of Dementia

The first goal of patient evaluation is to establish whether dementia is present or not. To diagnose a patient with dementia, the comprehensive history obtained from patient and family members or caregivers is necessary. As many patients with dementia deny their cognitive decline, and many clinicians tend to interpret and ignore the elderly's cognitive complaints because of aging, the key tip to obtain accurate information is to interview credible caregivers who could provide much more information about the patients. During their review, the clinicians should focus on three categories: **activities of daily living, behavioral changes, and cognitive decline**, which are called as the "ABC of dementia." (Table 13.4) Based on the patient's daily life, the clinician assesses the daily activities that patient can and cannot execute any more only because of cognitive decline. Changes in patient's character, mood, or behavior different from before should be apprehended. Cognitive decline is usually categorized into five domains: executive, memory, language, attention, and visuospatial function. It could be divided and clustered in various ways; however, the important consideration is to evaluate the diverse cognitive domains as much as possible.

After a diagnosis of dementia, the next step is to enumerate the possible causes of dementia. A **neurologic examination** is important to evaluate the causes of dementia, especially detecting focal neurologic signs for cerebrovascular contribution to dementia. If the patient has no lateralizing signs, the clinician could suspect the causes of dementia as more diffuse pathology, such as AD or DLB. Laboratory tests include vitamin B12 and thyroid-stimulating hormone levels, and structural brain imaging. MRI is more preferred than computed tomography (CT); however, both are recommended to diagnose dementia and classify the cause by the American Academy of Neurology.[30] The widely used cognitive tests are the Mini-Mental State Examination[28] and Montreal Cognitive Assessment.[29] Comprehensive neuropsychological testing, usually applied as a battery of tests, is not mandatory but valuable for cognitive assessment. Laboratory tests include vitamin B12 and thyroid-stimulating hormone levels, and structural brain imaging are also needed to clarify the causes of dementia. MRI is more preferred than computed tomography (CT); however, both are recommended to diagnose dementia and classify the cause by the American Academy of Neurology.[30]

Treatment of Dementia

Current medications approved by the US Food and Drug Administration (FDA) are of only two types: the **cholinesterase inhibitors**—donepezil,

TABLE 13.4
ABC of Assessing the Impact of Dementia on Lives of Older Adults

Category	Description Examples	Tools
A, ADL	• What changes have occurred in his/her abilities to perform household chores? • Do you have any problems managing your home finances? • Did you have trouble driving because of poor judgment?	• IADL • Barthel Index • BADLS
B, Behavior	• Do you feel sad or depressive? • Are you less interested in your usual activities or in the activities and plans of others? • Is the patient resistive to help from others or hard to handle?	• NPI • BEHAVE-AD • CMAI
C, Cognition	• Do you have a problem with your memory or thinking? • Can you recall recent events? • Do you often lose your way? • Is it difficult to buy things and get change exactly? • Is it difficult to get clothes that suit the situation? • Is it difficult to concentrate for a short time?	**Screening** MMSE MoCA Mini-Cog **Overall dementia severity** CDR GDS

ADL, Activities of Daily Living; *BADLS*, Bristol Activities of Daily Living Scale; *CDR*, Clinical Dementia Rating; *CMAI*, Cohen-Mansfield Agitation Inventory; *GDS*, Global Deterioration Scale; *IADL*, Instrumental Activities Of Daily Living; *MMSE*, Mini-Mental State Examination; *MoCA*, Montreal Cognitive Assessment; *NPI*, Neuropsychiatric Inventory (Questionnaire).

rivastigmine, and galantamine—and moderate affinity, uncompetitive N-**methyl-D-aspartate (NMDA) receptor antagonist**—memantine. Moreover, these drugs are not for all causes of dementia, but only for AD dementia, based on the cholinergic hypothesis of memory decline[31] and neuroprotective mechanism against glutamate and calcium-mediated neurotoxicity via NMDA receptors.[32] Donepezil, the most frequently prescribed medication, has been tested in other disorders such as DLB and VD; however, there is no current approval yet. The clinical pharmacology of these drugs is described in Table 13.5. In case of cholinesterase inhibitors, cholinergically mediated gastrointestinal adverse effects such as nausea, vomiting, and anorexia are relatively common, and precautions in patients with bradycardia, obstructive pulmonary disease, or high risk for gastrointestinal bleeding are needed.

Nonpharmacologic interventions, such as physical exercise, cognitive training, music therapy, or aromatherapy, seem to be efficient methods to improve cognitive function and control the abnormal behavior and moods in patients with dementia. More evidence regarding the long-term effects are needed using a refined, objective, and comprehensive manual. As dementia is a multifactorial disease, the combination of two or more nonpharmacologic interventions is important along with pharmacologic treatments.

Prevention of Dementia

The most efficient modifiable strategies to prevent dementia are controlling lifestyle risk factors (especially education and physical activity) and cardiovascular factors. Smoking cessation and a balanced diet with adequate supplement of antioxidants and vitamins can prevent cognitive decline in the elderly. These are not only effective primary preventions that protect neurodegeneration but also valuable secondary preventions that prevent dementia in the elderly showing cognitive decline, as well as tertiary preventions that retard further progressive deficits in patients with dementia.[7]

DELIRIUM
Definition of Delirium

Delirium is a clinical syndrome, which is a transient, usually reversible mental disturbance that results in a confused mental state and/or a wide range of neuropsychiatric abnormalities. It is a commonly encountered serious problem; about 20% of hospitalized patients develop delirium.[33] Elderly in the intensive care unit (ICU) have especially high risk with increasing incidence to 80%. It is not only a marker of severe sickness but also associated with poor outcomes: increased mortality, prolonged hospitalization, frequent discharge to the nursing home, and a high risk of developing dementia.[34]

The pathophysiology of delirium is quite complex and not well understood, yet. Changes to the

TABLE 13.5
Clinical Pharmacology of Medications for Alzheimer's Disease (AD) Dementia

	Drug	DOSAGE AND ADMINISTRATION		Adverse Effects	Contraindications
Cholin-esterase inhibitors (all stages of AD dementia)	Donepezil	Route	Oral	Diarrhea, loss of appetite, muscle cramps, nausea, trouble in sleeping, unusual tiredness or weakness, vomiting	Neuroleptic malignant syndrome, epileptic seizure, atrioventricular heart block, torsades de pointes, sick sinus syndrome, sinus bradycardia, asthma
		Starting dose	5 mg/day		
		Maximal dose	10 mg/day, 23 mg/day (only in moderate to severe cases)		
		Half-life (h)	70–80		
	Rivastigmine	Route	Oral, transdermal	Diarrhea, indigestion, loss of appetite, loss of strength, nausea and vomiting, weight loss, fainting	Symptoms of Parkinson's disease, extrapyramidal reaction, sick sinus syndrome, slow heartbeat, abnormal heart rhythm, asthma, stomach or intestinal ulcer
		Starting dose	1.5 mg bid, 4.6 mg patch/24 h		
		Maximal dose	6 mg bid, 9.5 mg patch/24 h, 13.3 mg patch/24 h (only in moderate to severe cases)		
		Half-life (h)	2–8, 3–4 (patch)		
	Galantamine	Route	Oral	Chest pain or discomfort; light-headedness; dizziness; fainting; shakiness in the legs, arms, hands, or feet; shortness of breath; slow or irregular heartbeat; unusual tiredness	Epileptic seizure, atrioventricular heart block, slow heartbeat, asthma, obstructive pulmonary disease
		Starting dose	4 mg bid		
		Maximal dose	12 mg bid		
		Half-life (h)	5–7		
N-methyl-D-aspartate receptor antagonist (moderate to severe AD dementia)	Memantine	Route	Oral	Tiredness, body aches, joint pain, dizziness, nausea, vomiting, diarrhea, constipation, loss of appetite	Epileptic seizure, liver problems, severe renal impairment
		Starting dose	5 mg/day		
		Maximal dose	10 mg bid		
		Half-life (h)	60–80		

neurotransmitter system—reduced cholinergic function, excess release of dopamine or norepinephrine, and both decreased and increased serotonergic and gamma-aminobutyric acid activity—caused by hypoxia or metabolic disturbance are taking an axis. Thereon, increased cerebral secretion of cytokines due to a wide range of physically stressful events can influence the activity of various neurotransmitter systems; these mechanisms may interact. Neuroinflammation induced by cytokines secretes systemic inflammatory factors and activates the action of microglial cells in the brain, which results in blood-brain barrier breakdown and neuronal death. Furthermore, additional medications to treat a medical disease also cause neurotransmitter imbalance and disruption of synaptic communication.

Clinical Features of Delirium

The clinical hallmarks of delirium are changes in the level of consciousness and a change in baseline cognition, which usually rapidly starts within a few days. The fluctuating confusion ranges from a hypoactive type with lethargy, stupor, or coma to a hyperactive type characterized by agitation, aggression, and belligerent with existence of mixed type. Delirium is reported to be undiagnosed in a clinical setting, because hypoactive delirium is typically unrecognized or misattributed as dementia. Acute impairment in cognition includes various domains with primary involvement of inattention, and executive, memory, language, and visuospatial function are also often impaired. Psychotic symptoms are relatively common; visual hallucinations and changes in sleep patterns are the most frequently observed. All these confusion and restless symptoms tend to worsen at night; therefore it is called as the sundown phenomenon.

Causes of Delirium

The most important risk factors for delirium are aging and preexisting cognitive dysfunction. Visual and hearing impairment, disability, depression, malnutrition, and alcohol abuse are also risk factors of delirium.[34] Individuals with baseline risk factors might have delirium after aggravated by various precipitating factors. Medications are the most common cause of delirium, accounting for 12%–39% of all cases of delirium. The most common precipitating drugs include high-dose narcotics, benzodiazepines, and anticholinergic medications, and these drugs triple the risk of delirium in the elderly.[34] Numerous other drugs including antihistamines, antiepileptic drugs, muscle relaxants, dopamine agonists, and steroids could be a precipitating candidate.[36] Among these drugs, anticholinergic drugs are frequently mentioned and are associated with the occurrence and severity of delirium.[37] Both hyperactive and mixed delirium are commonly seen in cholinergic toxicity, alcohol intoxication or withdrawal, stimulant intoxication, serotonin syndrome, and benzodiazepine withdrawal. In other cases, hypoactive delirium is often due to benzodiazepines, narcotic overdose, or hypnotic intoxication.[36] The mechanism of drug-induced delirium is not well defined. Aging, polypharmacy, and age-related pharmacokinetic or pharmacodynamic changes are thought to contribute to the incidence of drug-induced delirium in the elderly.

Surgery is another common cause of delirium, especially in the elderly. The risk of postoperative delirium is increased in patients with cognitive dysfunction. The most common surgery causing delirium is thoracic surgery including cardiac and noncardiac surgery. Depth of anesthesia during surgery and development of postoperative delirium are thought to be related; however, there is no sufficient evidence.[38] Regional anesthesia might be beneficial in reducing the incidence of postoperative delirium compared with general anesthesia; however, there are relatively few studies supporting this.[38]

Other iatrogenic precipitating factors include environmental factors usually found at a hospital setting: restraints, urinary catheter, multiple procedures, sleep deprivation, or untreated pain.[34]

Pathologic conditions are an important precipitating factor of delirium in the elderly. Especially, lesions of the brain can lead to delirium. Metabolic insult or inflammations are more vulnerable to delirium than vascular damage among them hepatic and

TABLE 13.6 Common Predisposing and Precipitating Factors of Delirium	
Predisposing Factors	**Precipitating Factors**
Old age	Drugs and drug withdrawal Narcotics, benzodiazepine, anticholinergics, methyldopa, nonsteroidal antiinflammatory agents
Male	Electrolyte imbalance
Dementia	Infection/fever
Depression	Sleep deprivation
Immobility	Severe/acute illness
History of falls	Hypoxia
Polypharmacy	Intensive care unit admission
Alcoholism	Emotional stress and pain
Malnutrition	Shock/dehydration

uremic encephalopathies are the most common causes of delirium. Of course, condition decline due to any illness other than the central nervous system could increase the prevalence of delirium. Common predisposing and precipitating factors of delirium are described in Table 13.6.

Diagnosis of Delirium

The Global Attentiveness Rating, Memorial Delirium Assessment Scale (MDAS), Confusion Assessment Method (CAM), Delirium Rating Scale Revised-98 (DRS-R-98), Clinical Assessment of Confusion (CAC), and Delirium Observation Screening Scale are used to diagnose delirium. The most pertinent choice of a tool may depend on the amount of time available and the discipline of the examiner; however, the most widely used and supported tool by sufficient evidence is CAM.[35] It is an instrument based on an algorithm. To diagnose delirium, acute onset of changes and fluctuations in the course of mental status (feature 1) and inattention (feature 2), and either disorganized thinking (feature 3) or altered level of consciousness (feature 4) is required. Anyone who is trained for optimal measure can use CAM, and an instruction manual is available online (http://www.hospitalelderlifeprogram.org/uploads/disclaimers/Short_CAM_Training_Manual_8-29-14.pdf). There are several adapted versions for using in various clinical settings such as the ICU, emergency department, and nursing home.

Before the evaluation of the causes of delirium, the clinician should secure the airway, breathing, and circulation of patients suspected of delirium. After securement, a detailed history including previous cognition, recent symptoms of medical illness, and newly added or dose changes of medication should be evaluated. However, delirious patients often are confused; hence, clinicians usually cannot get sufficient and accurate information from the patient. A detailed interview with caregivers, family, and nursing staff is particularly important. Physical examination and neurologic examination are essential steps to assess delirious patients to find out the causes of delirium. A laboratory test, chest X-ray, and electrocardiogram are necessary to identify any systemic disease, especially infection. If focal neurologic deficit exists, brain imaging including CT, MRI, and lumbar puncture should be obtained. Especially lumbar puncture to patients with head trauma, after neurosurgical procedures, or who are immunocompromised is indispensable even in the absence of cerebral infection signs. If the cause of delirium is not identified after this screening workup, comprehensive and extensive tests should be started. Additional serologic tests such as those for ammonia, thyroid function, morning cortisol, vitamin B12, or autoimmune serologies and more specific sequences of MRI including diffusion-weighted and gadolinium-enhanced MRI may be needed. Electroencephalogram should be applied to anyone who is suspected of nonconvulsive status epilepticus as soon as possible, and this helps to differentiate metabolic encephalopathy.

Treatment of Delirium

The most effective way to treat delirium is to remove the precipitating factors. Although age and preexisting cognitive dysfunction are nonmodifiable, many precipitating factors are iatrogenic that are modifiable. Discontinuation or change in the provoking drugs, natural recovery from surgery, removal of intervenient tools such as catheter and lines might help delirious patients to improve. If the hospital system is available, it is better to orientate the patient frequently: who and where they are and what your role is; provide easily visible clocks, calendars, good lighting, and signage; and facilitate visits from friends and family. Encouraging early mobility under supervision and performing active exercises are another effective nonpharmacologic treatment of delirium.

Current evidence does not support the use of antipsychotics for the prevention or treatment of delirium.[39] Medications are primarily reserved when the symptoms of delirium threaten the patient's own safety or the safety of others or would result in the interruption of essential therapy. Because FDA black box warning indicates increased mortality of patients who were exposed to antipsychotics, clinicians should (1) check ECG for elongated QTc (time between the start of the Q wave and the end of the T wave > 470 ms) before and after starting antipsychotics and (2) monitor the sedated patients for respiratory rate, pulse oximetry, blood pressure, pulse, and temperature, when considering pharmacologic intervention. The common pitfalls in pharmacologic management of delirium include using antipsychotic medications in excessive doses, administering them very late, or overuse of benzodiazepines.[40] If the patient is older than 65 years, haloperidol 0.5–1 mg hourly, maximum 5 mg in 24 h, or haloperidol 0.5–1 mg every 2 h, maximum 5 mg daily is permitted. Patients with a history of dystonia can be given olanzapine 2.5–5 mg orally, maximum 20 mg daily (10 mg in the elderly) other than haloperidol.[41] These drugs can relieve the symptoms of delirium; however, they may increase the duration of delirium. Cholinesterase inhibitors should not be newly prescribed to treat delirium.[38] Benzodiazepines are not recommended for the control of delirium except in the case of nonalcohol withdrawal–related delirium.[42]

Prevention of Delirium

Delirium has been shown to be preventable in up to one-third of the cases in hospitalized elderly patients.[43] The American Geriatrics Society recommends clinical practice guidelines for the prevention of postoperative delirium in the elderly.[38] According to the guidelines, multicomponent nonpharmacologic interventions delivered by an interdisciplinary team and medical evaluation should be administered to at-risk older adults to prevent delirium. Early and pertinent pain management including injection of regional anesthesia should be regulated, and medication with high risk should be avoided. Although there is a study reporting moderate-quality evidence that Bispectral Index (BIS)-guided anesthesia reduces the incidence of delirium compared with BIS-blinded anesthesia or clinical judgment,[33] use of several technologies such as processed electroencephalographic monitors of anesthetic depth during intravenous sedation or general anesthesia has insufficient evidence of efficacy.

CONCLUSION

Depression, dementia, and delirium (3Ds) are highly prevalent in the elderly, with the presence of one condition potentially increasing the risk of developing others. The impact of these conditions on the function and quality of life may surpass the impact of physical impairment. A high index of suspicion and proactive preventive strategies are the keys to reduce the risk for these conditions. Clinicians should be knowledgeable about pharmacologic and nonpharmacologic interventions for these cognitive conditions.

REFERENCES

1. Paykel ES, Priest RG. Recognition and management of depression in general practice: consensus statement. *BMJ.* 1992;305(6863):1198–1202.
2. Eggermont LH, Penninx BW, Jones RN, Leveille SG. Depressive symptoms, chronic pain, and falls in older community-dwelling adults: the MOBILIZE boston study. *J Am Geriatr Soc.* 2012;60(2):230–237.
3. Erlangsen A, Conwell Y. Age-related response to redeemed antidepressants measured by completed suicide in older adults: a nationwide cohort study. *Am J Geriatr Psychiatry.* 2014;22(1):25–33.
4. Zhao KX, Huang CQ, Xiao Q, et al. Age and risk for depression among the elderly: a meta-analysis of the published literature. *CNS Spectr.* 2012;17(3):142–154.
5. Baldwin RC. Is vascular depression a distinct sub-type of depressive disorder? A review of causal evidence. *Int J Geriatr Psychiatry.* 2005;20(1):1–11.
6. Ro J, Park J, Lee J, Jung H. Factors that affect suicidal attempt risk among Korean elderly adults: a path analysis. *J Prev Med Public Health.* 2015;48(1):28–37.
7. Taylor WD. Clinical practice. Depression in the elderly. *N Engl J Med.* 2014;371(13):1228–1236.
8. Cheng ST, Chan AC. A brief version of the geriatric depression scale for the Chinese. *Psychol Assess.* 2004;16(2):182–186.
9. Roose SP, Sackeim HA, Krishnan KR, et al. Antidepressant pharmacotherapy in the treatment of depression in the very old: a randomized, placebo-controlled trial. *Am J Psychiatry.* 2004;161(11):2050–2059.
10. Oslin DW, Ten Have TR, Streim JE, et al. Probing the safety of medications in the frail elderly: evidence from a randomized clinical trial of sertraline and venlafaxine in depressed nursing home residents. *J Clin Psychiatry.* 2003;64(8):875–882.
11. WHO. W. ICD-10 Version:2016. http://apps.who.int/classifications/icd10/browse/2016/en#/V.
12. Simpson JR. DSM-5 and neurocognitive disorders. *J Am Acad Psychiatry Law.* 2014;42(2):159–164.
13. McKhann GM, Knopman DS, Chertkow H, et al. The diagnosis of dementia due to Alzheimer's disease: recommendations from the National Institute on Aging-Alzheimer's Association workgroups on diagnostic guidelines for Alzheimer's disease. *Alzheimers Dement.* 2011;7(3):263–269.
14. Petersen RC, Smith GE, Waring SC, Ivnik RJ, Tangalos EG, Kokmen E. Mild cognitive impairment: clinical characterization and outcome. *Arch Neurol.* 1999;56(3):303–308.
15. DeCarli C. Mild cognitive impairment: prevalence, prognosis, aetiology, and treatment. *Lancet Neurol.* 2003;2(1):15–21.
16. Langa KM, Levine DA. The diagnosis and management of mild cognitive impairment: a clinical review. *JAMA.* 2014;312(23):2551–2561.
17. Eshkoor SA, Hamid TA, Mun CY, Ng CK. Mild cognitive impairment and its management in older people. *Clin Interv Aging.* 2015;10:687–693.
18. Bosch J, Yusuf S, Pogue J, et al. Use of Ramipril in preventing stroke: double blind randomised trial. *BMJ.* 2002;324(7339):699–702.
19. Querfurth HW, LaFerla FM. Alzheimer's disease. *N Engl J Med.* 2010;362(4):329–344.
20. Hirtz D, Thurman DJ, Gwinn-Hardy K, Mohamed M, Chaudhuri AR, Zalutsky R. How common are the "common" neurologic disorders? *Neurology.* 2007;68(5):326–337.
21. Selkoe DJ. Alzheimer's disease: genes, proteins, and therapy. *Physiol Rev.* 2001;81(2):741–766.
22. Mallik A, Drzezga A, Minoshima S. Clinical amyloid imaging. *Semin Nucl Med.* 2017;47(1):31–43.
23. Lee VM, Goedert M, Trojanowski JQ. Neurodegenerative tauopathies. *Annu Rev Neurosci.* 2001;24:1121–1159.
24. McKeith IG, Dickson DW, Lowe J, et al. Diagnosis and management of dementia with lewy bodies: third report of the DLB consortium. *Neurology.* 2005;65(12):1863–1872.
25. Gorelick PB, Scuteri A, Black SE, et al. Vascular contributions to cognitive impairment and dementia: a statement for healthcare professionals from the American Heart Association/American Stroke Association. *Stroke.* 2011;42(9):2672–2713.
26. Zhang Y, Xu Y, Nie H, et al. Prevalence of dementia and major dementia subtypes in the Chinese populations: a meta-analysis of dementia prevalence surveys, 1980–2010. *J Clin Neurosci.* 2012;19(10):1333–1337.
27. Pantoni L. Cerebral small vessel disease: from pathogenesis and clinical characteristics to therapeutic challenges. *Lancet Neurol.* 2010;9(7):689–701.
28. Folstein MF, Folstein SE, McHugh PR. "Mini-mental state". A practical method for grading the cognitive state of patients for the clinician. *J Psychiatr Res.* 1975;12(3):189–198.
29. Markwick A, Zamboni G, de Jager CA. Profiles of cognitive subtest impairment in the montreal cognitive assessment (MoCA) in a research cohort with normal mini-mental state examination (MMSE) scores. *J Clin Exp Neuropsychol.* 2012;34(7):750–757.
30. Knopman DS, DeKosky ST, Cummings JL, et al. Practice parameter: diagnosis of dementia (an evidence-based review). Report of the quality standards subcommittee of the American Academy of Neurology. *Neurology.* 2001;56(9):1143–1153.
31. Rogers SL, Friedhoff LT. The efficacy and safety of donepezil in patients with Alzheimer's disease: results of a US multicentre, randomized, double-blind, placebo-controlled trial. The donepezil study group. *Dementia.* 1996;7(6):293–303.

32. Cacabelos R, Takeda M, Winblad B. The glutamatergic system and neurodegeneration in dementia: preventive strategies in Alzheimer's disease. *Int J Geriatr Psychiatry*. 1999;14(1):3–47.

33. Siddiqi N, Harrison JK, Clegg A, et al. Interventions for preventing delirium in hospitalised non-ICU patients. *Cochrane Database Syst Rev*. 2016;3:CD005563.

34. Douglas VC, Josephson SA. Delirium. *Continuum (Minneap Minn)*. 2010;16(2 Dementia):120–134.

35. Wong CL, Holroyd-Leduc J, Simel DL, Straus SE. Does this patient have delirium?: Value of bedside instruments. *JAMA*. 2010;304(7):779–786.

36. Alagiakrishnan K, Wiens CA. An approach to drug induced delirium in the elderly. *Postgrad Med J*. 2004;80(945): 388–393.

37. Han L, McCusker J, Cole M, Abrahamowicz M, Primeau F, Elie M. Use of medications with anticholinergic effect predicts clinical severity of delirium symptoms in older medical inpatients. *Arch Intern Med*. 2001;161(8):1099–1105.

38. American Geriatrics Society Expert Panel on Postoperative Delirium in Older Adults. American geriatrics society abstracted clinical practice guideline for postoperative delirium in older adults. *J Am Geriatr Soc*. 2015;63(1):142–150.

39. Neufeld KJ, Yue J, Robinson TN, Inouye SK, Needham DM. Antipsychotic medication for prevention and treatment of delirium in hospitalized adults: a systematic review and meta-analysis. *J Am Geriatr Soc*. 2016;64(4):705–714.

40. O'Keeffe ST, Mulkerrin EC, Nayeem K, Varughese M, Pillay I. Use of serial mini-mental state examinations to diagnose and monitor delirium in elderly hospital patients. *J Am Geriatr Soc*. 2005;53(5):867–870.

41. Tropea J, Slee JA, Brand CA, Gray L, Snell T. Clinical practice guidelines for the management of delirium in older people in Australia. *Australas J Ageing*. 2008;27(3): 150–156.

42. Lonergan E, Luxenberg J, Areosa Sastre A. Benzodiazepines for delirium. *Cochrane Database Syst Rev*. 2009;(4):CD006379. https://doi.org/10.1002/14651858. CD006379.

43. Inouye SK, Bogardus Jr ST, Charpentier PA, et al. A multicomponent intervention to prevent delirium in hospitalized older patients. *N Engl J Med*. 1999;340(9):669–676.

CHAPTER 14

Exercise Recommendations for Older Adults for Prevention of Disability

DAVID Z. PRINCE, MD • MATTHEW N. BARTELS, MD, MPH

EPIDEMIOLOGY

As the global population continues to advance in age, the value of maintaining physical function grows in importance from an individual goal to a societal mandate. The "Aging of America" and the "Silver Tsunami" in Asia are compelling epidemiologic evidence that it is essential to maintain the elderly in their homes and communities to reduce healthcare costs.[1] More importantly, this also improves the quality of life for older adults and their families. The number of elderly people globally will steadily increase until approximately 22% of the population will be considered elderly by 2050.[2] One of the most effective ways to maintain independent function in older adults is the initiation of regular conditioning programs specifically designed for older individuals.[3,4] There is already interest in physical activity by highly motivated members of the older population; however, these participants remain at high risk for injury and complications while exercising.[5-7] Expanding physical activity programs for the older adults will expand the benefits of conditioning to a broader segment of the population and one at increased risk for morbidity and disability.

An essential part of this is addressing cardiovascular and cerebrovascular diseases, which continue to increase in the American population as a whole. Simply increasing physical activity in targeted patient populations can reduce many risk factors for both of these highly prevalent disease states,[8] because physical activity is the cornerstone of coordinated efforts to reduce hypertension, hypercholesterolemia, and hyperglycemic states.[9-11]

The aging of the baby boomer population is affecting every aspect of life in the United States, both as consumers of commercial products, consumers of information, and consumers of exercise-related products and activities.[12,13] The increased participation in athletic events for older participants, or "Masters Events," continues to increase to new levels and supports the assertion that there is growing interest and commitment to maintaining physical fitness at the highest possible level even into older years by those seniors interested in maintaining function as they age.[14] At the high end of the functional spectrum, increased enrollment of those older than 50 years in endurance and even ultraendurance events continues to rise.[15,16] Although the media interest generated by centenarian yoga teachers, marathon runners, and cyclists captures the imagination of the general population, this belies the reality that only 49% of the general population meets the Physical Activity Guidelines for aerobic physical activity.[17] In the United States, more than one-third of older adults 65 years and older are obese.[18] In addition, there is an increased rate of obesity in individuals between 65 and 74 years of age compared with those older than 75 years, and the rate of falls may be correlated with a low fitness level and general inactivity.[19] The epidemic of obesity and sedentarism leading to deconditioning, falls, and increased cardiovascular and cerebrovascular disease demands attention and intervention by medical professionals to translate current medical knowledge into actionable plans for patients and health consumers.

Although older individuals benefit greatly from regular conditioning programs, there are also potential complications in cardiovascular and musculoskeletal systems that need to be considered when initiating an exercise program in this population. The rate of osteoarthritis, decreased connective tissue elasticity, and reduced recovery reserve can lead to a higher rate of injury, especially during initiation of a new exercise program or when returning to a previous activity after prolonged interruption.[20,21] Medical professionals, especially physiatrists, are uniquely positioned to offer education, structure, and accountability and provide appropriate rehabilitation services when needed to maintain physical function and safe conditioning for this population.

PHYSIOLOGY OF AGING

To advise, educate, and prescribe exercise appropriately in older adults, it is essential to bear in mind that the physiology of natural aging leads to changes in the

TABLE 14.1
Physiologic Changes of Aging Relevant to Exercise Prescription

Organ System	Changes With Aging	Impact on Exercise Performance	Decrease Per Year
Cardiac[25]	↓ Maximum heart rate ↓ Stroke volume	↓ Peak cardiac output ↑ Risk of ischemia	↓ 1%–2%/year after age 25 years
Pulmonary[26]	↓ Lung capacity ↓ Lung compliance	↓ DL_{CO}	↓ Ventilation: 1%/year after age 30 years ↓ DL_{CO}: 1%/year
Muscle[27]	↑ Fatty infiltration ↑ Fibrous infiltration ↓ Lean body mass	↓ Peak muscle strength ↓ Type 2 fibers ↓ Peak performance ↓ Strength	↓ Muscle strength of 1%–2%/year after age 25 years
Neurologic[28,29]	↓ Coordination ↓ Reaction times	↓ Balance ↓ Coordination ↓ Peak performance	↑ Dementia with aging ↑ Blood flow and cognition with exercise

DL_{CO}, diffusing capacity of the lung for carbon monoxide.

pulmonary, cardiac, musculoskeletal, and vascular systems, among others. Reduced sex hormone levels lead to reduced muscle mass and power generation during exercise. If the patient is interested in achieving the highest level of conditioning possible, an assessment of the maximum exercise capacity can provide a patient specific VO_2max (a measure of the maximum amount of oxygen). Individuals in their 80s have half the peak capacity of individuals in their 20s because of the physiologic decrement of 10% in VO_2max per decade. For example, a 25-year-old sedentary individual who has a VO_2max of 35 mL O_2/kg/min at age 25 years would have a VO_2max of 17.5 mL O_2/kg/min at age 80 years.[22] Scaled to measurements of metabolic equivalents (METs) of energy, this equals a decrement in peak capacity from 10 METs to 5 METs. It is important to keep these general values in mind, especially when an older patient is initiating an exercise program and seeks advice regarding expectations and realistic goal setting. Referring to an MET table can be helpful in educating patients regarding objective measures of energy expenditure.[23] The Duke's Activity Scale Index is a 12-question administered questionnaire that estimates functional capacity and can be used to establish some degree of baseline functional capacity when the gold-standard, maximal exercise testing is not feasible.[24] A more detailed comparison of the physiologic changes with aging is summarized in Table 14.1.

DECONDITIONING AND EXERCISE

Deconditioning is physiologic and anatomic changes in multiple systems induced by physical inactivity that can be reserved through physical activity. Skeletal muscle is the effector of movement and function in the human body. Age-related muscle mass decline or sarcopenia begins in the third decade of life and continues throughout the life cycle.[30] Although deconditioning causes cardiac, vascular, pulmonary, and neurologic impairments, here we focus on the reduction in muscle mass due to inactivity, either acute or chronic, that is seen in deconditioning. Chronic lack of movement, immobility, and an inactive lifestyle (sedentarism) can all contribute to deconditioning. Acute deconditioning (e.g., from hospitalization) superimposed on age-related sarcopenia can lead to a synergistic loss of function and independence in older adults.[31,32] As the population ages, this becomes a phenomenon of greater significance to society. Between 10% and 35% of the American population is considered to be at an increased risk for a physical disability based on reduced skeletal muscle mass, a number that will continue to increase over time. In 2004 the estimated cost to the American healthcare system attributable to sarcopenia was estimated to be more than $18 billion.[33] Sarcopenia is associated with increased disability, frailty, and healthcare costs. Regular exercise can reduce the incidence of sarcopenia with its associated disability and decline in function.[34] The details of deconditioning in other organ systems are described in Chapter 8 of this book.

Exercise as medicine is a new paradigm in healthcare.[35] To this end exercise must be considered and categorized similarly to classes of medications—different types, different mechanisms of action, and different effects on organs and overall function. Aerobic conditioning is the type of exercise most commonly associated with a therapeutic benefit in older populations, partially because of the increasing awareness of cardiac rehabilitation/aerobic conditioning following cardiac events.[36] Progressive resistance training (PRT) or weightlifting is less often associated with the geriatric population, but it has been proved to benefit the elderly, as skeletal muscle responds to training throughout the lifecycle.[37,38] Flexibility training is important and usually a benefit of slow velocity movement-based systems. Balance training should be initiated as far in advance of an anticipated loss of balance as possible. Lastly, postural training is typically overlooked as an exercise modality, but the benefits of lifelong postural alignment are significant and allow all other modalities to have an optimal effect.

PRECONDITIONING ASSESSMENT

Owing to the standing recommendation "check with your doctor before starting any exercise program," many patients consult their primary physician before starting an exercise program, although this usually does not guarantee a thorough preconditioning assessment that incorporates goal setting specifically focused on functional preservation. This admonition also implies that exercise is a hazardous activity in middle-aged and older individuals when the opposite is actually true—sedentarism is a more significant risk than exercise. Perhaps the warning should be altered to: "Check with your doctor before NOT starting an exercise program." Because the greatest risk from a sudden increase in physical activity is the unmasking of occult coronary artery disease in the setting of an acute coronary syndrome, this is usually the sole focus of standard medical evaluation. Maximal exercise testing with or without a cardiology consult can provide scientifically valid risk stratification, but it should be remembered that the solution for coronary artery disease is not inactivity, a common misconception that should be challenged whenever possible. Patients found to be at an increased risk for cardiovascular events should be stabilized and referred to cardiac rehabilitation as the first step to preventing further lifelong disability. Progression of exercise program can be carried out following an introduction to exercise in the monitored setting.

In parallel to cardiovascular risk stratification the physiatrist is uniquely suited to complete an overall functional assessment to determine the patient's ability to perform activities of daily living independently, as well as higher-level tasks that are functional priorities for that individual patient. There are many standardized measurement tools available to assist the busy clinician in the objective evaluation of a patient's conditioning status, including an approximation of predicted METs extrapolated from daily activities and numerous balance assessment tools.[24] The evaluation of muscle power generation and flexibility are best determined by the physiatric physical examination. The same evaluations and tools that are used to inform a physiatric prescription for physical therapy should be used to prescribe exercise activities for older adults (Table 14.2).

EXERCISE PRESCRIPTION

All prescriptive exercise should follow the FITT principle, where the acronym FITT stands for: frequency, intensity, time, and type of exercise.[42] Following a detailed medical examination and thorough functional history, conditioning and functional goals can be identified. **It is essential to tie the exercise prescription to functional goals that hold high personal value for each individual patient**. Physically writing an exercise prescription on a prescription pad, now less common with the advent of electronic prescribing, has been shown to be more effective at modifying patient behavior than verbal instruction alone.[43] The exercise prescription should be rooted in patient interests, and ideally the clinician will review in detail how each recommendation will directly benefit the patient.

Techniques of motivational interviewing may be effective tools in facilitating behavioral change and because of their ease of use can be incorporated into patient discussions.[44,45] An initial assessment regarding patient "stage of change" at the time of office visit will prevent patient and clinician frustrations based on misunderstanding of the motivational state. This includes an assessment of patient interest and motivation to make a change using an analogue scale or "readiness ruler" for scoring. The readiness ruler is simply a 0–10 analog scale going from 0: "Not prepared to change" to 10: "Already changing" (see Fig. 14.1). The patient marks where they feel on the scale from 1–10. Patients whose motivation is 3 or less should be approached again at the next medical visit to determine if they are ready to initiate an exercise program at the next clinical visit.[46] For clinicians or their staff who are interested in incorporating health-coaching techniques and motivational interviewing into their practice, there are numerous resources available throughout the United States. The efficacy of these techniques is promising and currently an area of active investigation.[47,48]

Another possible tool to use to assess readiness to accept exercise is the Exercise Stages of Change Questionaire[49] seen in Box 14.1.

TABLE 14.2
Evaluation Tools for Cardiac and Muscular Capacity

Area of Evaluation	Measurement Tool	Example of Intervention
Exercise capacity	Duke's Activity Scale Index[24]	Exercise prescription with recommended intensity level
Maximal predicted heart rate	Karvonen formula[39] Target HR = (Max HR − Resting HR) × Target training intensity + resting HR Max HR can be measured on exercise test or estimated by the formula Max HR = 220 − age.	Target heart rate zones for warm-up/cool-down and aerobic conditioning Target intensity: • Low: 60%–70% • Moderate: 70%–85% • High: 85%–95%
Blood pressure management	Patient blood pressure log	Recommend optimal blood pressure range for patient during exercise
Balance assessment	Berg balance scale[40]	Prescription of balance training or activity to improve balance, e.g., Tai Chi
Aerobic conditioning	Resting heart rate Maximum heart rate[41]	Frequency and intensity of exercise intervention to achieve aerobic conditioning
Muscle power generation	Manual muscle testing or 1-repetition max testing[42]	Recommend exercise, starting weight and repetitions for Progressive Resistance Training program (PRT), e.g., Weight training.
Flexibility	Range-of-motion testing[42]	Referral to physical therapy for musculotendinous unit restriction. Recommendation of low-velocity home-based stretching program/activity, e.g., Yoga, Tai-Chi

HR, heart rate.

FIG. 14.1 Readiness ruler.

AEROBIC EXERCISE RECOMMENDATIONS

Aerobic conditioning should be the cornerstone of every exercise program designed to prevent disability in older individuals. Aerobic training effectively lowers blood pressure in adults with hypertension and can significantly reduce the risk of future cerebrovascular disease.[50–52] The current recommendation for aerobic conditioning is that all adults should participate in at least 30 min of moderately vigorous aerobic exercise most days of the week or 150 min total exercise per week.[53–58] The most effective aerobic exercise is the type that a patient will actually perform on a regular basis. The most common conceptualization of prescriptive exercise is walking on a treadmill, but this should be challenged, as there may be barriers to access or other limitations that prevent treadmill walking. It

is far more important to teach patients that any activity involving movement that elevates the heart rate can be considered to fulfill the exercise recommendations, including walking, cycling, dance, and other activities. Intensity can be directed with the use of the Borg scale of perceived exertion—a validated scale that has been shown to correlate with heart rate and is applicable in this setting.[59,60]

Guidelines for when to consider a cardiac stress test before initiating an exercise program are well defined by the American College of Sports Medicine and American Heart Association risk stratification screening classification into low, moderate, and high-risk groups. This stratification is based on cardiac risk.[61] Patients who are asymptomatic and have one or less risk factors are low risk; patients with no symptoms and 2 or less risk

BOX 14.1
Exercise Stages of Change Questionnaire

For each statement, please mark yes or no

1. I am currently physically active   ■ Yes   ■ No
   (at least 30 min per week).

2. I intend to become more   ■ Yes   ■ No
   physically active in the next
   6 months.

3. I currently engage in regular   ■ Yes   ■ No
   physical activity.

4. I have been regularly physically   ■ Yes   ■ No
   active for the past 6 months

Exercise Stages of Change—Scoring Key

No to 1, 2, 3, and 4	Precontemplation stage
No to 1, 3, and 4, Yes to 2	Contemplation stage
Yes to 1 and 2, No to 3 and 4	Preparation stage
Yes to 1 and 3, Yes or No to 2, No to 4	Action stage
Yes to 1, 3, and 4, Yes or No to 2	Maintenance stage

From American College of Sports Medicine. *Exercise Is Medicine: Healthcare Providers' Action Guide.* Available at: http://www.exerciseismedicine.org/assets/page_documents/HCP_Action_Guide.pdf; with permission.

factors are moderate risk; and patients with symptoms of known cardiac, pulmonary, or metabolic disease or 3 or more risk factors are high risk. For patients with low risk, no screening or testing is required for moderate or vigorous exercise. For moderate-risk patients, there is no screening for moderate exercise and only a medical examination for high level exercise. For patients who are high risk, there should be a physical examination and exercise test before both moderate and high-level exercise.[61]

THE ROLE OF EXERCISE THERAPY AND PREVENTION OF DISABILITY

Aerobic conditioning has been shown to reduce multiple cardiovascular and cerebrovascular risk factors simultaneously.[61] Improved blood pressure control in hypertensive patients leads to a reduced risk of cardiac events and stroke. Functional independence is affected by energy reserve that directly affects the ability to execute functional activities such as walking and dressing. As an example, we examine exercise in stroke.

Stroke survivors usually have a VO_2max that is 50% peak aerobic power of healthy age-matched controls.[62] Individuals with reduced aerobic capacity gradually reduce their intended activities to match their level of cardiopulmonary reserve, and it has been demonstrated that, although most stroke survivors are able to ambulate, less than 10% achieve normal ambulation parameters.[63] Improving aerobic capacity in stroke survivors will provide the energy store needed to participate in functionally important activities of daily living that require both higher short-term energy expenditure and longer endurance. Currently, stroke survivor conditioning protocols have a goal intensity of 40%–70% of VO_2max. Aerobic conditioning has been shown to improve the energy reserve from 10% to 15% in varied older populations, whether obese, frail, or older than 75 years.[64,65] Clearly, the advantages of aerobic conditioning are significant throughout the lifecycle, but initiating a regular conditioning program before age 75 years yields greater benefits both in terms of the percentage of conditioning achieved and time to accumulate benefit from overall risk reduction of chronic disease.[66]

The most common contributor to disability in older individuals is arthritis.[67] Any intervention shown to improve functional outcomes in patients with arthritis can be considered to be of significant benefit to the general population in preventing disability given the lifetime risk of being affected by arthritis. Exercise therapy has been shown to benefit patients with osteoarthritis of the knee in both pain reduction and increasing physical function.[68] An umbrella review of meta-analyses of randomized controlled trials demonstrated that 85 meta-analyses with 22 different chronic diseases resulted in statistically significant improvements for 126 of 146 (86%) functional capacity outcomes, compared with the control groups.[69] One can extrapolate from this that exercise therapy is a cost-effective way to preserve physical function and prevent disability.

BENEFITS OF SPECIFIC EXERCISE MODALITIES
Progressive Resistance Training

Muscle mass and strength first begins to decline in the third decade of life; however, a more rapid rate of decline at 2% each year starts in the sixth decade and continues into old age.[70] Changes in muscle physiology and overall muscle mass contribute to age-related strength decline that can be attenuated by resistance training. Muscle tissue responds to training even into the ninth decade; however, the presence of comorbidities can reduce the effectiveness of PRT.[71,72] Therefore, it is of greater benefit to begin training as early as possible. As with all exercise therapy, regularity is the key to achieving maximum benefit, and studies have consistently shown benefit from PRT that takes place at least two to three times a week. Consistent PRT has been correlated with numerous functional improvements, including improvement in the timed up-and-go test, timed chair rise, and gait speed.[73,74] Extrapolation to activities of daily living based on these objective tests is reasonable. For example, stair-climbing is often difficult for older adults because of pain from osteoarthritis of the knees. The combination of decreased strength and pain can lead to a fear of falling and an increased time to climb stairs. PRT is a solution that has been demonstrated in numerous studies to reduce time to climb stairs.[75–77] It is important to keep in mind that with resistance training greater intensity is not necessarily better. One can assume that higher-intensity resistance training is more likely to cause injury and potential disability, even if temporary. In one small study there was no significant difference between variable-intensity resistance training and high-intensity training in a group of older adults participating in a 25-week training program.[78] This challenges the assumption that resistance training should be performed at the highest intensity that is considered feasible and safe, a contrast from aerobic conditioning, which has been shown to be of greater benefit at higher intensities.

Resistance training can potentially reduce the risk of disability due to osteoporotic fracture, although there is no clear consensus on what is the most effective type of resistance training to prevent fracture-related disability. Osteoporosis is of significant concern globally, with more than 200 million people estimated to be affected by this disease.[79] Consequently, there has been extensive interest devoted to the study of nonpharmacologic approaches to improve bone mineral density (BMD) through resistance training. Various resistance training programs from two to six times a week in duration, using upper and lower body exercises, has suggested but not definitively proved positive effects on femoral neck and lumbar spinal BMD scores. The lack of statistically significant proof still makes definitive clinical recommendations elusive.[80–84] Numerous training protocols have been investigated in recent trials including resistance only and resistance with high-impact or weight-bearing exercises added in a combined training protocol. Owing to variable training protocols, sample sizes, and inconsistent results, meta-analysis may suggest current recommendations and future directions of research. Zhao et al. completed a meta-analysis of 24 controlled trials pooling data for 1769 healthy postmenopausal women who were not regular exercisers before enrollment in the study. Analysis suggested that a combination resistance training, which included high-impact and weight-bearing exercise, was more effective than PRT alone. In general, females of all ages should be encouraged to incorporate resistance training into their conditioning routines with individual modifications for those at risk for osteoporotic fracture.

Tai Chi

Tai Chi is a gentle system of traditionally standing group exercise that integrates breathing and rhythmic movements to achieve a conditioning effect. As Tai Chi has become a popular intervention to study in medical settings, programs integrating Tai Chi have proliferated to include poststroke rehabilitation, chronic obstructive pulmonary disease (COPD), heart failure, and multiple other medical diseases.[85–87] Tai Chi has been adapted for wheelchair participants to include people with restricted mobility and spinal cord injury.[88] Owing to the lack of reported adverse events and overall safety of Tai Chi, new variations are being developed, including a weighted-vest Tai Chi to improve lower extremity strength and water-based Tai Chi.[89,90] These programs illustrate that proliferation is giving rise to creative applications of this form of therapy. For example, the specific benefits of Tai Chi are seen in the setting of stroke rehabilitation with improved balance, reduced fall rates, and improved quality of life.[91–93] Tai Chi can be adapted to suit the particular health needs of special populations because of lack of adverse effects and an excellent safety profile.

In addition, Tai Chi may benefit older individuals in improving dynamic balance and postural control and reducing fall-related disability. Home- and community-based Tai Chi has been demonstrated to reduce falls compared with a standard physical therapy supervised program of lower extremity strengthening.[87] Efficiency of postural control and specifically control of the center of pressure have also been demonstrated following 6 months of Tai Chi instruction.[94] It is unlikely there are any adverse psychological effects from Tai Chi; however, owing to the heterogeneous nature of medical studies concerning Tai Chi, no definitive conclusion regarding the psychological effects in older adults can be drawn at this time. Still, it is logical to assume that older adults would benefit from a community-based group exercise activity that has demonstrated numerous other benefits. It is reasonable to recommend that patients who are at risk for falling begin a regular Tai Chi practice, as there is evidence to support the assertion that participation in this activity improves balance and reduces the future possibility of falling.

Walking Programs

Walking is arguably the most functional of all conditioning modalities. There are few barriers to beginning a walking program, and there is no financial expenditure required. Self-directed walking programs have been determined to be safe even for participants at high risk for adverse cardiovascular events.[95] Goodrich et al. reported that, in a clinic-coordinated home-based walking program with 274 participants at high risk for cardiovascular events, almost 90% of all reported adverse events were not related to the exercise program. The walking program is safe, and numerous technological aides exist to support participants who are undertaking a walking program. Pedometers, smartphone accelerometers, and GPS-enabled devices are all available to help track, measure, and motivate patients seeking to begin a walking program. Self-directed walking programs are a safe and effective way to increase physical activity levels with low risk of adverse events.

Walking programs should be strongly encouraged by providers throughout the medical community. The US Preventive Services Task Force and the American College of Cardiology/American Heart Association have both concluded that rigorous examination and exercise testing is not required for patients who want to begin an exercise program of moderate intensity as long as the participants are in communication with their physicians.[96,97] As with all interventions that involve a behavioral change, it is important not to use a "one size fits all" approach when it comes to exercise counseling. Patients should be encouraged to tailor their walking programs to suit their own preferences. Adherence is improved when patients can select the type of walking program that they prefer.[98]

Wearable electronic devices can have significant benefits when added to a self-directed walking program. Use of pedometers has been associated with increased physical activity, significant decrease in body mass index, and improved blood pressure control.[99] By downloading an appropriate app, patients can use their cell phones as pedometers to track their steps, turning the phones into pedometers and allowing patients to use the accelerometer that they likely were not aware is part of all smartphones. As goal setting and attainment is critical to achieving lasting behavior modification, pedometers can play an important and economical role. Use of a pedometer allows the assignment of a measurable goal—steps/day. Having a step goal is a predictor of participants' ability to successfully achieve an increased level of physical activity. It is important for participants to keep a step diary in which they record the total number of daily steps. Interventions that use step goals and step diaries have been shown to be more effective at increasing participants' physical activity than those that do not.[100,101] It has also been demonstrated that use of a pedometer can improve glycemic control in type 2 diabetic participants.[102] Better glycemic control reduces future disability from multiple causes.

INJURY PREVENTION IN OLDER ADULTS

Fall in the elderly remain an important cause of morbidity and mortality. Increasing mobility in older adults through exercise prevents falls even while it exposes the individual to a higher-risk environment. Each clinician must determine the risk/benefit ratio for an individual patient whether the proposed activity benefits the patient more than the risk of falling during that activity. Exercise in general can also be delivered in a seating position, reducing fall risk. It is important to help patients maintain a safe exercise routine because exercise-based fall prevention programs can reduce falls and their resultant injuries in older adults.[103,104] The most effective programs in preventing falls incorporate multiple approaches to improve lower extremity strengthening, endurance, and flexibility.

Falls are not the only cause of injury in the older population. At the higher end of the functional spectrum, increasing numbers of older adults participating in physically demanding and competitive sports have increased the rate of sport-related injuries.[105,106] Therefore it is essential that physiatrists understand their important and unique role in preventing injury and repeat injury when evaluating both sedentary individuals who are beginning an exercise program and providing care for the older athlete who is already exercising. Older athletes have been shown to sustain higher rates of lower extremity injuries whether at recreational or elite levels of performance.[107,108] In Sweden the rate of acute Achilles tendon rupture has increased between 2001 and 2012, especially in the older population. The most common lower extremity cause of disability in older populations is due to osteoarthritis of the knees. Prevention of significant disability in an older population can be accomplished by stabilizing the knees as much as possible with exercise to improve balance and quad strength. Early referral to physical therapy when indicated can treat existing pain, improve gait, and prevent injury. Patients should be taught how to incorporate a physical therapy–derived home exercise program into an overall routine of physical activity. Physical therapy maintenance exercises are often ideal warm-up exercises, as they use stabilizing muscles and provide range of motion before the mechanical stress of prolonged exercise.

TABLE 14.3
Exercise Training Modalities to Prevent Disability

Modality	Benefits	Risks	Recommendation
Aerobic conditioning	Improvement in VO$_2$max Reduction in cardio/ cerebrovascular risk factors Improved energy reserve	Acute coronary syndromes	150 min per week of moderate- to high-intensity exercise Target heart rate: 60%–80% of predicted maximum heart rate Physiatric evaluation before starting to screen for MSK conditions
Progressive resistance training	Improved LE strength Reduction in falls Improved bone health	MSK injury	≥2 training sessions per week Progress slowly to prevent injury Demonstrated benefit from high intensity (70%–85% of 1RM) Combined training programs more beneficial for osteoporosis
Tai Chi	Balance, well-being, fall reduction, improved shoulder ROM, reduced systolic blood pressure[109]	No adverse effects reported	Twice a week—1 h minimum per session
Walking	No cost, excellent safety profile	Rare cardiac events, potential hypoglycemia Fall risk	Increase walking distance and progress intensity within level of comfort (RPE 10–15 in 6–20 Borg scale)

1RM, 1 repetition maximum; *LE*, lower extremity; *MSK*, musculoskeletal; *ROM*, range of motion; *RPE*, rate of perceived exertion.

Injuries in older athletes are not restricted to the lower extremities. There is a more than 20% prevalence of full-thickness tears of the rotator cuff in senior athletes, and there was no significant correlation between the severity of pain and degree of tear.[109] This is consistent with previous studies that described full-thickness rotator cuff tears in approximately 25% of individuals older than 60 years. Therefore one must always maintain a high rate of clinical suspicion for either the possibility of a preexisting rotator cuff tear or the potential to create a new tear with a sudden increase in physical activity. A careful history and thorough physical examination with detailed focus on the range of motion of the shoulder should identify patients with shoulder dysfunction who are at risk for rotator cuff impingement or tear. These patients should be sent to physical therapy before participating in any sport that involves stress to the shoulder girdle or rotator cuff. About 4 to 6 weeks of scapular stabilization with incorporation of appropriate exercises into a preexercise warm-up can prevent shoulder complications from arising.

The overall benefits of a regular conditioning program are clear: improved balance, glycemic control, hypertensive control, improved overall endurance, and fall reduction make a compelling case that the most efficient way to prevent disability in the older adult is to undertake a regular conditioning program that incorporates both aerobic and PRT methods. Additional benefits from Tai Chi and walking are worthwhile and complimentary. The prevention of upper and lower extremity injuries when undertaking a new exercise program or when returning to a well-established program can be facilitated by early involvement of the rehabilitation professional and rehabilitation team (Table 14.3).

FUTURE DIRECTIONS

Although the literature is mature regarding the benefits of exercise and the role of exercise in preventing and treating disability, there are new and exciting investigations that can be highlighted as areas of future opportunity and interest. Well-designed investigations of high-velocity PRT or "Power training" should be undertaken in the older population. With aging, the ability to generate lower extremity muscle power is lost more rapidly than muscle strength.[70,110] Improvement in lower extremity power generation has been demonstrated in older adults.[111] If the ability of lower extremity muscles to rapidly generate power can be reliably improved with specialized training, hypothetically fall risk could be reduced even more than has been demonstrated with traditional conditioning programs. Because normal ambulation can be viewed as "controlled falling" through the cumulative effect of a series of small perturbations in balance resulting in successful and safe forward locomotion, power training could have implications for fall prevention programs by improving the ability to generate a corrective force quickly. A caution with power training is the increased potential for soft tissue injury, which should be investigated in the controlled setting of trials under medical supervision.

Smartphones and wearable devices continue to be an exciting area of developing interest to enhance physical conditioning. As the older population continues to adopt smartphone and social media, wearable devices are the next logical iteration of e-fitness. The potential for technology to improve physical function and conditioning is only limited by the creativity of the investigators who choose to explore this area. At the low end of the functional spectrum, home-based conditioning programs and wearables could be used to collect and catalogue physiologic information during home-based therapy.[112-114] This valuable information can also assist providers to assess the effect, progress, and medical necessity of the therapy being provided. In both hospital and outpatient settings, smartphones are being used to relay patient communications, satisfaction, and activity level to care providers.[115-117] Technology that was initially used to bring patient information back to the provider is now facilitating the flow of information from provider to patient as well. Finally, patient education is a fertile area for the development of apps and interactive programs that will allow providers to query, respond to, and send clinically relevant information to patients in real time.

Another area of potential growth in helping older adults be more active is through motion-sensing technology commonly seen in the consumer computer gaming industry. These technologies could be developed as physical therapy coaching programs to monitor and offer form correction either remotely or under indirect supervision. Wearable devices can monitor cardiovascular response to therapy to keep participants within a safe heart-rate range.[118] Lastly, patients can receive instruction, feedback on their sessions, and home exercise programs on their smartphones to reinforce compliance with home exercises and medical follow-up visits.[119]

In conclusion, the knowledge base regarding the benefits of exercise is mature and exercise is being accepted by the general population as an important way to maintain independence and prevent disability throughout the life cycle. As the population ages, there

will be ever increasing demand for physiatrist-led educational initiatives as well as the expertise habilitating older individuals, from athletes at all fitness levels to those with disabilities. The impact of technology on the already existing multibillion-dollar fitness industry will continue to produce novel ways to enhance the motivation, safety, and rehabilitation of older adults as they engage in lifelong fitness regimens. Opportunities are waiting for researchers who ask "how can I prevent disability and rehabilitate injury using emerging technology." The answers to this question will ultimately yield the greatest rewards for patients, researchers, and society as a whole in the quest to prevent disability and preserve function for all older adults.

SUMMARY OF RECOMMENDATIONS

Aerobic exercise is the foundational modality to prevent disease progression and disability.

Moderate-intensity aerobic exercise (40%–60% of predicted heart rate maximum) can be safely used in almost all situations. Higher-intensity training may be appropriate for some patients as well whenever determined to be safe and feasible.

Frequency of training should be a minimum of twice a week, preferably three or more times a week.

Resistance training of variable intensity may be of equal benefit to high-intensity training while potentially reducing the risk of injury.

Adverse events for PRT are not adequately reported, and patient education, "prehab," and close follow-up are recommended in the older adult who is beginning an exercise program.[120]

Presentation of written physical prescriptions for exercise should continue to be given to patients, even in the presence of electronic medical records.

Musculoskeletal optimization before conditioning of any type is recommended.

Longer follow-up studies with functional outcomes are needed regarding the benefits of exercise modalities other than aerobic conditioning.

REFERENCES

1. United Nations. *World Population Aging 2013*. Department of Economic and Social Affairs PD; 2013.
2. UN. World Population Ageing 2007. In: DoEaS, ed. *Affairs*. New York: United Nations; 2007.
3. Gill TM, Beavers DP, Guralnik JM, et al. The effect of intervening hospitalizations on the benefit of structured physical activity in promoting independent mobility among community-living older persons: secondary analysis of a randomized controlled trial. *BMC Med*. 2017;15(1):65.

4. Alexander KP. Walking as a window to risk and resiliency. *Circulation.* 2017;136(7).

5. Kallinen M, Markku A. Aging, physical activity and sports injuries. An overview of common sports injuries in the elderly. *Sports Med.* 1995;20(1):41–52.

6. Chen AL, Mears SC, Hawkins RJ. Orthopaedic care of the aging athlete. *J Am Acad Orthop Surg.* 2005;13(6):407–416.

7. American College of Sports Medicine Position Stand. Exercise and physical activity for older adults. *Med Sci Sports Exerc.* 1998;30(6):992–1008.

8. Benjamin EJ, Blaha MJ, Chiuve SE, et al. Heart disease and stroke statistics-2017 update: a report from the American Heart Association. *Circulation.* 2017;135(10):e146–e603.

9. Myers J. Exercise and cardiovascular health. *Circulation.* 2003;107(1):e2–e5.

10. Stone NJ, Robinson JG, Lichtenstein AH, et al. 2013 ACC/AHA guideline on the treatment of blood cholesterol to reduce atherosclerotic cardiovascular risk in adults: a report of the American College of Cardiology/American Heart Association task force on practice guidelines. *J Am Coll Cardiol.* 2014;63(25, Part B):2889–2934.

11. Hu FB. Globalization of diabetes: the role of diet, lifestyle, and genes. *Diabetes Care.* 2011;34(6):1249–1257.

12. Rice NE, Lang IA, Henley W, Melzer D. Baby boomers nearing retirement: the healthiest generation? *Rejuvenation Res.* 2010;13(1):105–114.

13. Twigg J, Majima S. Consumption and the constitution of age: expenditure patterns on clothing, hair and cosmetics among post-war 'baby boomers'. *J Aging Stud.* 2014;30:23–32.

14. Tayrose GA, Beutel BG, Cardone DA, Sherman OH. The masters athlete: a review of current exercise and treatment recommendations. *Sports Health.* 2015;7(3):270–276.

15. Jokl P, Sethi PM, Cooper AJ. Master's performance in the New York City Marathon 1983–1999. *Br J Sports Med.* 2004;38(4):408–412.

16. Hoffman MD, Ong JC, Wang G. Historical analysis of participation in 161 km ultramarathons in North America. *Int J Hist Sport.* 2010;27(11):1877–1891.

17. Ward BW, Clarke TC, Nugent CN, Schiller JS. Early release of selected estimates based on data from the 2015 National Health Interview Survey. In: *Statistics USDoHaHSCfD-CaPNCfH* 2015.

18. Fakhouri THI, Ogden CL, Carroll MD, Kit BK, Flegal KM. National Health and Nutrition Examination Survey, 2007–2010. In: *Services USDoHH.* Atlanta, GA: National Center for Health Statistics; 2012.

19. Mertz KJ, Lee D, Sui X, Powell KE, Blair SN. Falls among adults: the association of cardiorespiratory fitness and physical activity with walking-related falls. *Am J Prev Med.* 2010;39(1):15–24.

20. Zhang Y, Jordan JM. Epidemiology of osteoarthritis. *Clin Geriatr Med.* 2010;26(3):355–369.

21. Sherratt MJ. Tissue elasticity and the ageing elastic fibre. *Age.* 2009;31(4):305–325.

22. Burtscher M. Exercise limitations by the oxygen delivery and utilization systems in aging and disease: coordinated adaptation and deadaptation of the lung-heart muscle axis – a mini-review. *Gerontology.* 2013;59(4):289–296.

23. Jette M, Sidney K, Blumchen G. Metabolic equivalents (METS) in exercise testing, exercise prescription, and evaluation of functional capacity. *Clin Cardiol.* 1990;13(8):555–565.

24. Hlatky MA, Boineau RE, Higginbotham MB, et al. A brief self-administered questionnaire to determine functional capacity (the Duke activity status index). *Am J Cardiol.* 1989;64(10):651–654.

25. van Empel VP, Kaye DM, Borlaug BA. Effects of healthy aging on the cardiopulmonary hemodynamic response to exercise. *Am J Cardiol.* 2014;114(1):131–135.

26. Sharma G, Goodwin J. Effect of aging on respiratory system physiology and immunology. *Clin Interv Aging.* 2006;1(3):253–260.

27. Ali S, Garcia JM. Sarcopenia, cachexia and aging: diagnosis, mechanisms and therapeutic options – a mini-review. *Gerontology.* 2014;60(4):294–305.

28. Tarumi T, Gonzales MM, Fallow B, et al. Central artery stiffness, neuropsychological function, and cerebral perfusion in sedentary and endurance-trained middle-aged adults. *J Hypertens.* 2013;31(12):2400–2409.

29. Guiney H, Machado L. Benefits of regular aerobic exercise for executive functioning in healthy populations. *Psychon Bull Rev.* 2013;20(1):73–86.

30. Janssen I, Heymsfield SB, Wang ZM, Ross R. Skeletal muscle mass and distribution in 468 men and women aged 18–88 yr. *J Appl Physiol.* 2000;89(1):81–88.

31. Dos Santos L, Cyrino ES, Antunes M, Santos DA, Sardinha LB. Sarcopenia and physical independence in older adults: the independent and synergic role of muscle mass and muscle function. *J Cachexia Sarcopenia Muscle.* 2017;8(2):245–250.

32. Marques EA, Baptista F, Santos DA, Silva AM, Mota J, Sardinha LB. Risk for losing physical independence in older adults: the role of sedentary time, light, and moderate to vigorous physical activity. *Maturitas.* 2014;79(1):91–95.

33. Janssen I, Baumgartner RN, Ross R, Rosenberg IH, Roubenoff R. Skeletal muscle cutpoints associated with elevated physical disability risk in older men and women. *Am J Epidemiol.* 2004;159(4):413–421.

34. Steffl M, Bohannon RW, Sontakova L, Tufano JJ, Shiells K, Holmerova I. Relationship between sarcopenia and physical activity in older people: a systematic review and meta-analysis. *Clin Interv Aging.* 2017;12:835–845.

35. Katz PP, Pate R. Exercise as medicine. *Ann Int Med.* 2016;165(12):880–881.

36. Golwala H, Pandey A, Ju C, et al. Temporal trends and factors associated with cardiac rehabilitation referral among patients hospitalized with heart failure: findings from get with the guidelines-heart failure registry. *J Am Coll Cardiol.* 2015;66(8):917–926.

37. Bechshoft RL, Malmgaard-Clausen NM, Gliese B, et al. Improved skeletal muscle mass and strength after heavy strength training in very old individuals. *Exp Gerontol.* 2017;92:96–105.

38. Churchward-Venne TA, Tieland M, Verdijk LB, et al. There are no nonresponders to resistance-type exercise training in older men and women. *J Am Med Dir Assoc.* 2015;16(5): 400–411.

39. Karvonen MJ, Kentala E, Mustala O. The effects of training on heart rate; a longitudinal study. *Ann Med Exp Biol Fenniae.* 1957;35(3):307–315.

40. Berg KO, Wood-Dauphinee SL, Williams JI, Maki B. Measuring balance in the elderly: validation of an instrument. *Can J Public Health.* 1992;83(suppl 2):S7–S11.

41. Karvonen J, Vuorimaa T. Heart rate and exercise intensity during sports activities. Practical application. *Sports Med.* 1988;5(5):303–311.

42. Pescatello LS, American College of Sports M. *ACSM's Guidelines for Exercise Testing and Prescription.* Philadelphia: Wolters Kluwer/Lippincott Williams & Wilkins Health; 2014.

43. Swinburn BA, Walter LG, Arroll B, Tilyard MW, Russell DG. The green prescription study: a randomized controlled trial of written exercise advice provided by general practitioners. *Am J Public Health.* 1998;88(2):288–291.

44. Rubak S, Sandbaek A, Lauritzen T, Christensen B. Motivational interviewing: a systematic review and meta-analysis. *Br J Gen Pract.* 2005;55(513):305–312.

45. Britt E, Hudson SM, Blampied NM. Motivational interviewing in health settings: a review. *Patient Educ Couns.* 2004;53(2):147–155.

46. Enhancing motivation for change in substance abuse treatment. In: Treatment CfSA, ed. *Treatment Improvement Protocols. TIP Series – Treatment Improvement Protocols.* Rockville MD: Substance Abuse and Mental Health Services Administration; 1999.

47. Huang B, Willard-Grace R, De Vore D, et al. Health coaching to improve self-management and quality of life for low income patients with chronic obstructive pulmonary disease (COPD): protocol for a randomized controlled trial. *BMC Pulm Med.* 2017;17(1):90.

48. Willard-Grace R, Chen EH, Hessler D, et al. Health coaching by medical assistants to improve control of diabetes, hypertension, and hyperlipidemia in low-income patients: a randomized controlled trial. *Ann Fam Med.* 2015;13(2):130–138.

49. http://www.exerciseismedicine.org/assets/page_documents/HCP_Action_Guide.pdf.

50. Johnson BT, MacDonald HV, Bruneau Jr ML, et al. Methodological quality of meta-analyses on the blood pressure response to exercise: a review. *J Hypertens.* 2014;32(4): 706–723.

51. Pescatello LS, MacDonald HV, Ash GI, et al. Assessing the existing professional exercise recommendations for hypertension: a review and recommendations for future research priorities. *Mayo Clin Proc.* 2015;90(6): 801–812.

52. Whelton SP, Chin A, Xin X, He J. Effect of aerobic exercise on blood pressure: a meta-analysis of randomized, controlled trials. *Ann Intern Med.* 2002;136(7):493–503.

53. James PA, Oparil S, Carter BL, et al. 2014 evidence-based guideline for the management of high blood pressure in adults: report from the panel members appointed to the Eighth Joint National Committee (JNC 8). *JAMA.* 2014;311(5):507–520.

54. Eckel RH, Jakicic JM, Ard JD, et al. 2013 AHA/ACC guideline on lifestyle management to reduce cardiovascular risk: a report of the American College of Cardiology/American Heart Association task force on practice guidelines. *J Am Coll Cardiol.* 2014;63(25 Pt B):2960–2984.

55. Chobanian AV, Bakris GL, Black HR, et al. The seventh report of the Joint National Committee on prevention, detection, evaluation, and treatment of high blood pressure: the JNC 7 report. *JAMA.* 2003;289(19):2560–2572.

56. Brook RD, Appel LJ, Rubenfire M, et al. Beyond medications and diet: alternative approaches to lowering blood pressure: a scientific statement from the American Heart Association. *Hypertension (Dallas, Tex: 1979).* 2013;61(6):1360–1383.

57. Pescatello LS, Franklin BA, Fagard R, Farquhar WB, Kelley GA, Ray CA. American College of sports medicine position stand. Exercise and hypertension. *Med Sci Sports Exercise.* 2004;36(3):533–553.

58. Mancia G, Fagard R, Narkiewicz K, et al. 2013 ESH/ESC practice guidelines for the management of arterial hypertension. *Blood Press.* 2014;23(1):3–16.

59. Borg GA. Psychophysical bases of perceived exertion. *Med Sci Sports Exerc.* 1982;14(5):377–381.

60. Nelson ME, Rejeski WJ, Blair SN, et al. Physical activity and public health in older adults: recommendation from the American College of Sports Medicine and the American Heart Association. *Med Sci Sports Exerc.* 2007;39(8):1435–1445.

61. Fletcher GF, Balady G, Blair SN, et al. Statement on exercise: benefits and recommendations for physical activity programs for all Americans. A statement for health professionals by the Committee on Exercise and Cardiac Rehabilitation of the Council on Clinical Cardiology, American Heart Association. *Circulation.* 1996;94(4):857–862.

62. Kelly JO, Kilbreath SL, Davis GM, Zeman B, Raymond J. Cardiorespiratory fitness and walking ability in subacute stroke patients. *Arch Phys Med Rehabil.* 2003;84(12): 1780–1785.

63. Hill K, Ellis P, Bernhardt J, Maggs P, Hull S. Balance and mobility outcomes for stroke patients: a comprehensive audit. *Aust J Physiother.* 1997;43(3):173–180.

64. Ehsani AA, Spina RJ, Peterson LR, et al. Attenuation of cardiovascular adaptations to exercise in frail octogenarians. *J Appl Physiol.* 2003;95(5):1781–1788.

65. Villareal DT, Chode S, Parimi N, et al. Weight loss, exercise, or both and physical function in obese older adults. *N Engl J Med.* 2011;364(13):1218–1229.

66. Kohrt WM, Malley MT, Coggan AR, et al. Effects of gender, age, and fitness level on response of VO$_2$max to training in 60-71 yr olds. *J Appl Physiol.* 1991;71(5):2004-2011.

67. Prevalence of disabilities and associated health conditions among adults-United States, 1999. *MMWR Morb Mortal Wkly Rep.* 2001;50(7):120-125.

68. Nguyen C, Lefevre-Colau MM, Poiraudeau S, Rannou F. Rehabilitation (exercise and strength training) and osteoarthritis: a critical narrative review. *Ann Phys Rehabil Med.* 2016;59(3):190-195.

69. Pasanen T, Tolvanen S, Heinonen A, Kujala UM. Exercise therapy for functional capacity in chronic diseases: an overview of meta-analyses of randomised controlled trials. *Br J Sports Med.* 2017;51(20):1459-1465.

70. Hughes VA, Frontera WR, Roubenoff R, Evans WJ, Singh MA. Longitudinal changes in body composition in older men and women: role of body weight change and physical activity. *Am J Clin Nutr.* 2002;76(2):473-481.

71. Aguirre LE, Villareal DT. Physical exercise as therapy for frailty. *Nestle Nutr Inst Workshop Ser.* 2015;83:83-92.

72. Fiatarone MA, O'Neill EF, Ryan ND, et al. Exercise training and nutritional supplementation for physical frailty in very elderly people. *N Engl J Med.* 1994;330(25):1769-1775.

73. de Vreede PL, van Meeteren NL, Samson MM, Wittink HM, Duursma SA, Verhaar HJ. The effect of functional tasks exercise and resistance exercise on health-related quality of life and physical activity. A randomised controlled trial. *Gerontology.* 2007;53(1):12-20.

74. Kalapotharakos VI, Michalopoulos M, Tokmakidis SP, Godolias G, Gourgoulis V. Effects of a heavy and a moderate resistance training on functional performance in older adults. *J Strength Cond Res.* 2005;19(3):652-657.

75. Suetta C, Magnusson SP, Rosted A, et al. Resistance training in the early postoperative phase reduces hospitalization and leads to muscle hypertrophy in elderly hip surgery patients - a controlled, randomized study. *J Am Geriatr Soc.* 2004;52(12):2016-2022.

76. Ouellette MM, LeBrasseur NK, Bean JF, et al. High-intensity resistance training improves muscle strength, self-reported function, and disability in long-term stroke survivors. *Stroke.* 2004;35(6):1404-1409.

77. Kongsgaard M, Backer V, Jorgensen K, Kjaer M, Beyer N. Heavy resistance training increases muscle size, strength and physical function in elderly male COPD-patients - a pilot study. *Respir Med.* 2004;98(10):1000-1007.

78. Hunter GR, Wetzstein CJ, McLafferty Jr CL, Zuckerman PA, Landers KA, Bamman MM. High-resistance versus variable-resistance training in older adults. *Med Sci Sports Exerc.* 2001;33(10):1759-1764.

79. Reginster JY, Burlet N. Osteoporosis: a still increasing prevalence. *Bone.* 2006;38(2 suppl 1):S4-S9.

80. Bocalini DS, Serra AJ, dos Santos L, Murad N, Levy RF. Strength training preserves the bone mineral density of postmenopausal women without hormone replacement therapy. *J Aging Health.* 2009;21(3):519-527.

81. Kerr D, Ackland T, Maslen B, Morton A, Prince R. Resistance training over 2 years increases bone mass in calcium-replete postmenopausal women. *J Bone Miner Res.* 2001;16(1):175-181.

82. Maddalozzo GF, Widrick JJ, Cardinal BJ, Winters-Stone KM, Hoffman MA, Snow CM. The effects of hormone replacement therapy and resistance training on spine bone mineral density in early postmenopausal women. *Bone.* 2007;40(5):1244-1251.

83. Nelson ME, Fiatarone MA, Morganti CM, Trice I, Greenberg RA, Evans WJ. Effects of high-intensity strength training on multiple risk factors for osteoporotic fractures. A randomized controlled trial. *JAMA.* 1994;272(24):1909-1914.

84. Pruitt LA, Taaffe DR, Marcus R. Effects of a one-year high-intensity versus low-intensity resistance training program on bone mineral density in older women. *J Bone Miner Res.* 1995;10(11):1788-1795.

85. Caminiti G, Volterrani M, Marazzi G, et al. Tai Chi enhances the effects of endurance training in the rehabilitation of elderly patients with chronic heart failure. *Rehabil Res Pract.* 2011;2011:761958.

86. Ngai SP, Jones AY, Tam WW. Tai Chi for chronic obstructive pulmonary disease (COPD). *Cochrane Database Syst Rev.* 2016;(6):Cd009953.

87. Hwang HF, Chen SJ, Lee-Hsieh J, Chien DK, Chen CY, Lin MR. Effects of home-based Tai Chi and lower extremity training and self-practice on falls and functional outcomes in older fallers from the emergency department-a randomized controlled trial. *J Am Geriatr Soc.* 2016;64(3):518-525.

88. Wang YT, Li Z, Yang Y, et al. Effects of wheelchair Tai Chi on physical and mental health among elderly with disability. *Res Sports Med (Print).* 2016;24(3):157-170.

89. Su Z, Zhao J, Wang N, Chen Y, Guo Y, Tian Y. Effects of weighted Tai Chi on leg strength of older adults. *J Am Geriatr Soc.* 2015;63(10):2208-2210.

90. Macias-Hernandez SI, Vazquez-Torres L, Morones-Alba JD, et al. Water-based Tai Chi: theoretical benefits in musculoskeletal diseases. Current evidence. *J Exerc Rehabil.* 2015;11(3):120-124.

91. Kim H, Kim YL, Lee SM. Effects of therapeutic Tai Chi on balance, gait, and quality of life in chronic stroke patients. *Int J Rehabil Res.* 2015;38(2):156-161.

92. Au-Yeung SS, Hui-Chan CW, Tang JC. Short-form Tai Chi improves standing balance of people with chronic stroke. *Neurorehabil Neural Repair.* 2009;23(5):515-522.

93. Taylor-Piliae RE, Hoke TM, Hepworth JT, Latt LD, Najafi B, Coull BM. Effect of Tai Chi on physical function, fall rates and quality of life among older stroke survivors. *Arch Phys Med Rehabil.* 2014;95(5):816-824.

94. Zhou J, Chang S, Cong Y, et al. Effects of 24 weeks of Tai Chi exercise on postural control among elderly women. *Res Sports Med (Print).* 2015;23(3):302-314.

95. Goodrich DE, Larkin AR, Lowery JC, Holleman RG, Richardson CR. Adverse events among high-risk participants in a home-based walking study: a descriptive study. *Int J Behav Nutr Phys Act.* 2007;4:20.

96. Gibbons RJ, Balady GJ, Bricker JT, et al. ACC/AHA 2002 guideline update for exercise testing: summary article. A report of the American College of Cardiology/American Heart Association task force on practice guidelines (Committee to update the 1997 exercise testing guidelines). *J Am Coll Cardiol.* 2002;40(8):1531–1540.

97. Fowler-Brown A, Pignone M, Pletcher M, Tice JA, Sutton SF, Lohr KN. Exercise tolerance testing to screen for coronary heart disease: a systematic review for the technical support for the U.S. Preventive Services Task Force. *Ann Intern Med.* 2004;140(7):W9–W24.

98. Loew L, Brosseau L, Kenny GP, et al. An evidence-based walking program among older people with knee osteoarthritis: the PEP (participant exercise preference) pilot randomized controlled trial. *Clin Rheumatol.* 2017;36(7):1607–1616.

99. Bravata DM, Smith-Spangler C, Sundaram V, et al. Using pedometers to increase physical activity and improve health: a systematic review. *JAMA.* 2007;298(19):2296–2304.

100. Izawa KP, Watanabe S, Omiya K, et al. Effect of the self-monitoring approach on exercise maintenance during cardiac rehabilitation: a randomized, controlled trial. *Am J Phys Med Rehabil.* 2005;84(5):313–321.

101. Ransdell LB, Robertson L, Ornes L, Moyer-Mileur L. Generations exercising together to improve fitness (GET FIT): a pilot study designed to increase physical activity and improve health-related fitness in three generations of women. *Women Health.* 2004;40(3):77–94.

102. Shenoy S, Guglani R, Sandhu JS. Effectiveness of an aerobic walking program using heart rate monitor and pedometer on the parameters of diabetes control in Asian Indians with type 2 diabetes. *Prim Care Diabetes.* 2010;4(1):41–45.

103. El-Khoury F, Cassou B, Charles MA, Dargent-Molina P. The effect of fall prevention exercise programmes on fall induced injuries in community dwelling older adults: systematic review and meta-analysis of randomised controlled trials. *BMJ.* 2013;347:f6234.

104. Lord SR, Ward JA, Williams P, Strudwick M. The effect of a 12-month exercise trial on balance, strength, and falls in older women: a randomized controlled trial. *J Am Geriatr Soc.* 1995;43(11):1198–1206.

105. Kannus P, Niemi S, Sievanen H, Parkkari J. Fall-induced wounds and lacerations in older Finns between 1970 and 2014. *Aging Clin Exp Res.* 2017. https://doi-org.elibrary.einstein.yu.edu/10.1007/s40520-017-0753-4.

106. Ng N, Soderman K, Norberg M, Ohman A. Increasing physical activity, but persisting social gaps among middle-aged people: trends in Northern Sweden from 1990 to 2007. *Glob Health Action.* 2011;4:6347.

107. Svensson K, Alricsson M, Karneback G, Magounakis T, Werner S. Muscle injuries of the lower extremity: a comparison between young and old male elite soccer players. *Knee Surg Sports Traumatol Arthrosc.* 2016;24(7):2293–2299.

108. Ostermann RC, Hofbauer M, Tiefenbock TM, et al. Injury severity in ice skating: an epidemiologic analysis using a standardised injury classification system. *Int Orthop.* 2015;39(1):119–124.

109. McMahon PJ, Prasad A, Francis KA. What is the prevalence of senior-athlete rotator cuff injuries and are they associated with pain and dysfunction? *Clin Orthop Relat Res.* 2014;472(8):2427–2432.

110. Bean JF, Kiely DK, Herman S, et al. The relationship between leg power and physical performance in mobility-limited older people. *J Am Geriatr Soc.* 2002;50(3):461–467.

111. Caserotti P, Aagaard P, Larsen JB, Puggaard L. Explosive heavy-resistance training in old and very old adults: changes in rapid muscle force, strength and power. *Scand J Med Sci Sports.* 2008;18(6):773–782.

112. Garabelli P, Stavrakis S, Po S. Smartphone-based arrhythmia monitoring. *Curr Opin Cardiol.* 2017;32(1):53–57.

113. Lin F, Wang AS, Zhuang Y, Tomita MR, Xu WY. Smart insole: a wearable sensor device for unobtrusive gait monitoring in daily life. *IEEE Trans Ind Inf.* 2016;12(6):2281–2291.

114. Ongvisatepaiboon K, Vanijja V, Chignell M, Mekhora K, Chan JH. Smartphone-based audio-biofeedback system for shoulder joint tele-rehabilitation. *J Med Imaging Health Inf.* 2016;6(4):1127–1134.

115. Perry TT, Marshall A, Berlinski A, et al. Smartphone-based vs paper-based asthma action plans for adolescents. *Ann Allergy Asthma Immunol.* 2017;118(3):298–303.

116. Strickler JC, Lopiano KK. Satisfaction data collected by e-mail and smartphone for emergency department patients how do responders compare with nonresponders? *J Nurs Adm.* 2016;46(11):592–598.

117. Lee W, Evans A, Williams DR. Validation of a smartphone application measuring motor function in Parkinson's disease. *J Parkinsons Dis.* 2016;6(2):371–382.

118. Skobel E, Knackstedt C, Martinez-Romero A, et al. Internet-based training of coronary artery patients: the heart cycle trial. *Heart Vessels.* 2017;32(4):408–418.

119. Matera G, Boonyasirikool C, Saggini R, Pozzi A, Pegoli L. The new smartphone application for wrist rehabilitation. *J Hand Surg Asian Pac Vol.* 2016;21(1):2–7.

120. Liu CJ, Latham NK. Progressive resistance strength training for improving physical function in older adults. *Cochrane Database Syst Rev.* 2009;(3):CD002759.

FURTHER READING

1. Chiang CE, Wang TD, Ueng KC, et al. 2015 guidelines of the taiwan society of cardiology and the taiwan hypertension society for the management of hypertension. *J Chin Med Assoc.* 2015;78(1):1–47.

CHAPTER 15

Spine Disorders in Older Adults

ADELE MERON, MD • VENU AKUTHOTA, MD

INTRODUCTION

Back pain is one of the most common presenting complaints to physicians and a leading cause of disability in patients of all ages. Disorders of the spine have a considerable burden on both the quality of life of affected patients and the healthcare economy. Although it was previously suggested that back pain was an ailment of the working-age patient, more recent studies have shown that severe back pain increases with age. Spine disorders affect both the hospitalized and ambulatory communities and appear to affect the geriatric population to a greater extent. The global point prevalence of symptomatic low-back pain has been estimated to reach 10%, with both prevalence and disease impact increasing with age.[1] Low back pain has been cited as the highest burden of disability globally. In 2010 patients older than 65 years made up 17% of the US population and 48% of hospital discharges for low back disorders for an estimated 350,000 hospitalizations for low back pain in patients over 65 years in 2010.[2] The aging population will contribute significantly to the burden of spine disorders on the healthcare economy in both hospital admissions and ambulatory pain management. Analysis of the Medicare database estimated that Medicare beneficiaries used 4.8 million interventional spine procedures in 2011, which represented a 228% increase since 2000.[3] Rehabilitation physicians practice in a variety of settings from inpatient acute and subacute rehabilitation facilities, inpatient consult services, and skilled nursing facilities to outpatient rehabilitation clinics and spine centers, all of which have the responsibility of caring for older adult patients with spine disorders. The multidisciplinary nature of a rehabilitation team provides an ideal model for treating spine disorders. Care should be longitudinal, with a sharp focus on optimizing function and realistic goal setting. Understanding spine disorders that affect the aging population is essential for all members of the rehabilitation team.

SPINE STRUCTURE AND FUNCTION

The spine is a complex modular structure composed of alternating bony and fibrocartilage elements that provides protection of neurologic structures and support to the trunk while allowing movement in multiple planes. In all, 33 vertebrae make up the spine, including 7 cervical, 12 thoracic, 5 lumbar, 5 sacral, and 4 coccygeal. At each level, excluding the unique atlas and axis, the cylindrical bony vertebral body forms the anterior weight-bearing component of the spine. Paired pedicles and lamina form an arch and convalesce posteriorly to form the spinous process. From the arch emanate the superior and inferior articular processes that articulate to form the zygapophysial joints, which connect adjacent vertebrae and prevent anteroposterior translation and twisting of the vertebrae. The vertebral body's connection to the posterior bony elements by the pedicles forms the ring-shaped vertebral foramen, which houses the spinal cord and surrounding cerebrospinal fluid. The vertebral body comprises a shell of cortical bone encasing a form of transverse and vertical trabeculae promoting dynamic load bearing while minimizing mass. The intervertebral disc is a strong but deformable ring of fibrocartilage surrounding a gelatinous central nucleus pulposus, the purpose of which is to transmit force between vertebrae while allowing the rocking movement that permits flexion, extension, and lateral bending of the spine. The segmental motion at each level is limited owing to the shape of the articular and spinous processes and by the splinting of the rib cage at the thoracic level. Although the combination of bony elements and intervertebral disks provides stability and protection of neurologic structures, while allowing segmental movement, the actions of the powerful flexor and extensor muscle groups augment motion, stability, and position control of the spine from axis to sacrum. As these structures age, they lose their ability to perform these essential functions (Fig. 15.1A–C).

AGING

At birth the entire spine is kyphotic and remains so until the erect postures of sitting and upright walking are initiated. At this point, the cervical and lumbar spines become lordotic. Over the first year of life, the sacral and coccygeal vertebrae fuse to form a single wedge-shaped base. Each component of the spine

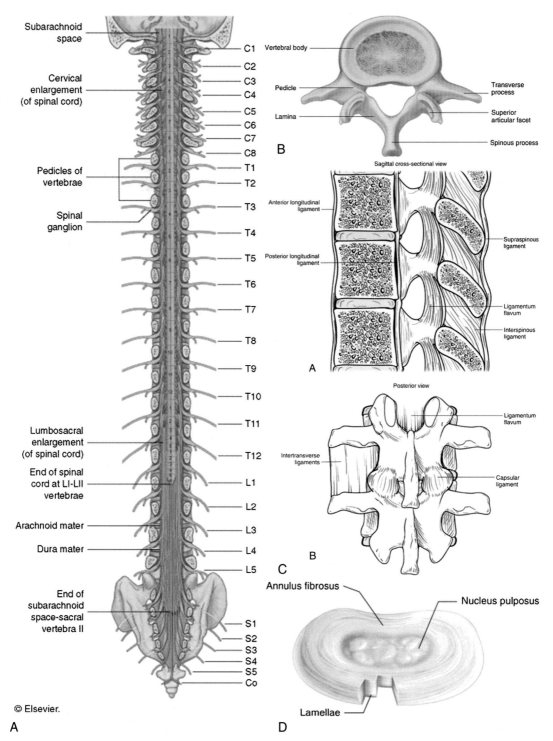

FIG. 15.1 **(A–D)** Spinal anatomy. (**(A)** © Elsevier. Drake, et al. *Gray's Anatomy for Students*. www.studentconsult.com. Reproduced with permission. **(B)** From Lawry GV, Hall H, Ammendolia C, et al. The spine. In: Lawry GV, Kreder HJ, Hawker GA, et al., eds. *Fam's Musculoskeletal Examination and Joint Injection Techniques*. 2nd ed. Philadelphia: Mosby, Inc.; 2010; with permission. **(C)** From Moulton AW. Clinically relevant spinal anatomy. In: Errico TJ, Lonner BS, Moulton AW, eds. *Surgical Management of Spinal Deformities*. 1st ed. Philadelphia: Saunders; 2009; with permission. **(D)** From Arakal RG, Mani M, Ramachandran R. Applied anatomy of the normal and aging spine. In: Yue JJ, Guyer RD, Johnson JP, et al., eds. *The Comprehensive Treatment of the Aging Spine*. Philadelphia: Saunders; 2011; with permission.)

undergoes degenerative changes over time, contributing to a cycle that alters the biomechanical properties of the spine, leading to a new environment that contributes to further degenerative changes. Degenerative processes of the individual tissues vary, but all share the basic principles of initial biochemical changes leading to microstructural and then macrostructural failure.

IS DEGENERATIVE DISC DISEASE A DISEASE?

Although the aging process is subject to various genetic and external factors, overall the process is fairly uniform. Thus the definition of a normal spine structure varies by age. In the absence of painful processes or functional limitations, it may be misleading to describe these changes as a disease process rather than simply the typical process of aging.

INTERVERTEBRAL DISC

The basic structure of the intervertebral disc includes the central nucleus pulposus surrounded by the peripheral annulus fibrosus (Fig. 15.1D). Although the disc is distinctly different at the center and at the periphery, the area where the two components merge is not a discrete line but a gradual merging of the two structures, which share common components but are differentiated by their relative concentrations. In young adults, the nucleus pulposus is a semifluid mass of mucoid substance composed of 70%–90% water (although this varies with age). The dry weight of the nucleus is approximately 65% proteoglycans and 15%–20% collagen with rare chondrocytes interspersed within the matrix. The biomechanical properties are similar to that of a fluid-filled balloon that stretches and deforms with compression. In contrast, the annulus fibrosus is 60%–70% water, with a dry content of 50%–60% collagen and 20% proteoglycans, primarily in the aggregated form. In the transition from outer annulus to inner nucleus the proteoglycan content increases as the collagen content decreases. The annulus consists of highly ordered layers of lamellae arranged in concentric rings. The hydrostatic pressure in the nucleus is contained by the surrounding annulus, allowing the distribution of force over the entire surface of the adjacent vertebral body. Maintaining the proteoglycan and collagen content requires metabolically active chondrocytes and fibroblasts, which require oxygen, glucose, and other substrates. As the disc lacks a robust blood supply to provide these nutrients, they are generally delivered by

diffusion. The balance of anabolic and catabolic activities of the cells is critical to maintaining the health and structure of the disc.[4]

Biochemical changes within the disc are central to the changes that occur with age. The balance between synthesis and degradation of matrix breaks down, leading to alterations in relative proportions of water, proteoglycans, and collagen. Biochemical processes within the disc begin changing at birth as the blood supply to the disc diminishes and the cells adapt to anaerobic metabolism over the first decade of life. Cell content also changes with age as the proportion of cells that exhibit necrosis goes from 2% in infancy to 50% in young adults and 80% in the elderly. The proteoglycan content and size decrease with age. Within the nucleus pulposus, the proteoglycan content decreases from 65% in early adult life to 30% at age 60 years. In contrast, the collagen content in the nucleus and annulus both *increase* with age, whereas elastin decreases. The water content in the disc also decreases from 88% at birth to 65%–72% at age 75 years.[4] In summary, the discs become drier, more fibrous, and less elastic, making them more resistant to deformation and less able to regain their shape after deformation occurs. A drier nucleus pulposus with decreased hydrostatic pressure can no longer transmit and disperse weight, and thus the annulus fibrosus bears a larger proportion of the weight with age. With chronic weight bearing on the annulus, over time microcracks develop and provide the foundation for larger concentric fissures and radial tears to develop with continued load bearing. These mechanical changes can lead to diffuse bulging of the disc even without a discrete herniation of nucleus material through the annular ring. In addition, owing to the arrangement of the lamellae, the posterior and posterolateral segments of the annulus are susceptible to thinning and can serve as a weak point for overt herniation of the nucleus pulposus. Although loss of disc height is frequently cited as a sign of age-related pathology in the spine, studies have shown this may not be the case. In the absence of alternate pathologic deterioration, the intervertebral discs actually increase in size, both in the anteroposterior dimension and in height.[4]

VERTEBRAL BODY AND ENDPLATE

The vertebral body is designed for longitudinal load bearing. The external cortical shell is augmented with internal vertical trabeculae that are able to sustain great longitudinal loads and horizontal trabeculae that prevent bowing of the vertical trabeculae. The horizontal trabeculae also transmit tension horizontally, increasing the resilience of the structure. With age, vertebral bodies exhibit a decrease in bone density and strength as a result of the change in structural composition of the enclosed trabeculae. The strength and weight-bearing capacity of the vertebral body rely on the horizontal trabecular bracing of the vertical trabeculae. The cortical shell typically provides only 15% of the load-bearing capacity of the vertebral body. Over time, there is a relative loss of the horizontal trabeculae, decreasing the load-bearing capacity of the central surface of the vertebral body and forcing the cortical bone to support a greater proportion of the applied load.

The vertebral endplate lies at the interface between the vertebral body and intervertebral disc and is formed by layers of subchondral bone and cartilage of approximately equal thickness. The function of the endplate is to distribute force over the surface of the vertebral body as well as provide a connection between the fibrous disc and the vertebral bone. The endplate is permeable enough to allow water and solutes to pass through to supply nutrients to the disc; however, it is dense enough to prevent extrusion of the disc material. Endplate thickness is variable, with increased thickness at the periphery, which has been shown to correlate with endplate strength. Disc properties also appear to influence the endplate structure. A connection has been shown between the proteoglycan content of the disc and the thickness of the underlying endplate, suggesting that the previously described age-related loss of proteoglycan content of the disc may contribute to changes in the endplate. Given the importance of load distribution on maintaining the structural integrity of the spinal elements, as the endplate undergoes degradation, further structural changes in the vertebral body are initiated. Concurrently, the vertebral body loses bone density, causing a two-hit model of degradation of the vertebral body from both internal and external factors. Biomechanical studies have shown the endplate to be the weakest component of the vertebral body under repetitive loading conditions.[5] Weakened endplates and vertebral bodies predispose the spine to a variety of structural failures, including endplate fractures, vertebral body fractures, and Schmorl nodes, all of which are discussed later in this chapter.

FACET JOINTS

The facet joints are diarthrodial, synovial joints that add to the stability of the spine in flexion and extension, limit axial rotation, and partially contribute to weight bearing (Fig. 15.2). They are composed of subchondral bone covered by hyaline cartilage. It has been

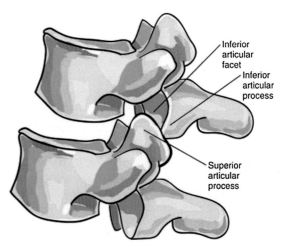

FIG. 15.2 Applied anatomy of the thoracic and lumbar spine. (From Waldman SD. Functional anatomy of the lumbar spine. In: Waldman SD, ed. *Physical Diagnosis of Pain*. 3rd ed. St. Louis: Elsevier, Inc.; 2016; with permission.)

shown that facet degeneration follows disc degeneration.[6] Loss of disc height and segmental instability lead to increased load on the facets and increased joint subluxation. The process of facet degeneration is similar to that of other diarthrodial joints. The process consists of erosion of the hyaline cartilage, hypertrophy of the synovial membrane, sclerosis of subchondral bone, and formation of osteophytes. This begins a cycle of remodeling that contributes to decreased mobility of the joint. Facets are innervated, and their degeneration may cause its own painful syndrome. In addition, facet hypertrophy can lead to a cascade of structural changes, including nerve root impingement, central stenosis, or spondylolisthesis.

MUSCLES AND LIGAMENTS

In addition to providing a significant contribution to the mobility and stability of the spinal column, muscles and ligaments have a proprioceptive role. Receptors in these structures stimulate muscle contraction throughout the spine and core to provide stability and balance, support complex movements, and protect from movements that would cause excessive stress on the spine. Ligaments are composed of a high concentration of collagen and serve a relatively minor stabilizing function to the spine, whereas their elastic components allow for some movement and flexibility. For example, the ligamentum flavum, which connects adjacent lamina, has a higher concentration of elastin than most spinal ligaments (80% elastin and 20% collagen)[7] to allow for stretch during flexion and return to rest during neutral and extension. Longitudinal ligaments have a higher collagen concentration and provide resistance to flexion (posterior longitudinal ligament) and extension (anterior longitudinal ligament). As ligaments age, they exhibit both biochemical and structural changes. The elastin concentration increases, decreasing their stabilizing capacity. The ligamentum flavum can undergo hypertrophy, which can contribute to central stenosis.

Core muscles stabilize and mobilize the spine. Muscle fibers degenerate over time and are replaced by adipose. Tendinous attachments degenerate in a similar mechanism to ligaments and osteophytes form at their attachment sites, decreasing their contractile forces.

SPINE CONDITIONS AFFECTING OLDER ADULTS
Osteoporosis and Vertebral Fractures
Normal bone metabolism

Osteoporosis, put simply, is an imbalance of bone homeostasis whereby bone resorption outweighs bone deposition. The primary risk factor for the development of osteoporosis is age. Bone homeostasis is under the control of both intrinsic and extrinsic factors that affect the relative concentrations and activities of osteoblasts (bone-forming cells) and osteoclasts (bone-reabsorbing cells). As described earlier, the vertebral body is mostly trabecular bone, a porous scaffold of interlocking vertical and horizontal supports. A thin exterior of cortical bone surrounds the cancellous central core. Both cortical and cancellous bones are composed of extracellular matrix with varying degrees of mineralization. Osteoid, the nonmineralized component of bone, is made up of collagenous and noncollagenous proteins and is secreted by osteoblasts. The mineralized part of bone is made up of calcium hydroxyapatite, and the mineralization depends on the amounts of calcium and phosphate ions. The strength of mineralized bone increases with increasing concentrations of calcium. Formation and mineralization of osteoid are initiated by osteoblasts with input from parathyroid hormone (PTH) and 1,25-dihydroxyvitamin D. Osteoclast differentiation activity is also mediated by PTH and 1,25-dihydroxyvitamin D, although not through direct binding but through interaction with osteoblasts. Receptor activator of nuclear factor kappa-B (RANK) ligand is an essential mediator of osteoclast differentiation.

The architecture of bone has metabolic consequence and thus influences the susceptibility to osteoporosis. Cancellous (trabecular) bone is more porous and thus

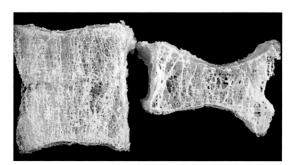

FIG. 15.3 Osteoporotic vertebral body (right) shortened by compression fractures compared with a normal vertebral body (left). Note that the osteoporotic vertebra has a characteristic loss of horizontal trabeculae and thickened vertical trabeculae. (From Kumar V, Abbas AK, Aster JC. Bones, joints, and soft tissue tumors. In: Kumar V, Abbas AK, Aster JC, eds. *Robbins Basic Pathology*. 10th ed. Philadelphia: Elsevier; 2018; with permission.)

more vascular than cortical bone, making cancellous bone more susceptible to the metabolic alterations that lead to osteoporosis.

Risk factors

Clinically, osteoporosis is diagnosed by dual-energy X-ray absorbometry (DEXA) scan with lumbar spine measurements that are 2.5 standard deviations below the average value for a 30-year-old gender-matched individual (t-score < 2.5). Osteoporotic compression fractures occur when the bone density reaches a level where the loads imposed by daily activity exceed the strength of the vertebral body. Vertebral compression fractures are the hallmark of osteoporosis and occur more commonly in the early stages of osteoporosis than any other type of fracture.[8]

Vertebral compression fractures (Fig. 15.3) are predictors of morbidity and mortality, social isolation, and overall quality of life,[9] and thus, identification of risk factors for fracture is of paramount importance. Low bone mass is a clear predictor of osteoporotic vertebral fractures, so it is important to be able to identify all associated risk factors. Peak bone mass is achieved in the second or third decade of life, followed by a slow progressive decrease. Although loss of bone mass is a common cause of osteoporosis, it is important to note that it is not the only cause. Failure to reach peak bone mass can lead to the development of osteoporosis without the acceleration of bone loss later in life. Thus chronic disease during childhood and adolescence is an identifiable risk factor for low bone mass later in life. Female gender is a risk factor for bone loss. Men lose bone at a rate of 0.3% per year. Women lose bone at a rate of 0.5% per year; however, following meno-pause this rate accelerates significantly, up to 5%–6% per year in the first five menopausal years.[10] Other risk factors for low bone mass include estrogen deficiency, low body mass index (BMI), smoking, family history of osteoporosis, and history of prior fracture.[8] Inadequate calcium intake is a risk factor for developing low bone mass. Elderly patients may have a decreased overall food intake or financial constraints that lead to poor calcium intake. In addition, once osteoporosis has manifested, anterior vertebral body compression fractures, leading to thoracic kyphosis, can promote early satiety,[11] creating a self-perpetuating cycle of poor bone health. Decreases in physical activity that often accompany aging also lead to decreased bone mass. Again, a self-perpetuating cycle beginning with decreased activity levels, which result in a decrease in bone mass, leads to vertebral compression fractures that further limit physical activity.

Although low bone mass is a significant predictor of fractures, research indicates that a propensity for falls is another important risk factor for fracture. Fracture risk has been associated with a history of falls, poor vision, environmental hazards, cognitive deficits, slow gait speed, and decreased quadriceps strength. Fall prevention is paramount in the prevention of vertebral fractures.

Secondary osteoporosis is the result of a primary medical condition or medication that leads to decreased bone mass and increased risk of fracture. In women, secondary osteoporosis is most commonly caused by hypoestrogenemia, glucocorticoid use, thyroid hormone excess, and anticonvulsant use. In men, the most common causes are hypogonadism, use of glucocorticoids, and alcoholism.

Diagnosis

Both asymptomatic and symptomatic fractures are predictors of increased morbidity and mortality. Studies have shown that only 25% of vertebral fractures are clinically recognized. This is in part due to not only the lack of presenting symptoms but also the rarity of fracture in relation to the prevalence of back pain. Less than 1% of back pain is related to fracture, so fracture is often not evaluated for in the absence of trauma.[12] Once a vertebral fracture is suspected, or it is determined that screening is warranted based on risk factors, lateral radiographs of the spine should be obtained to evaluate for fracture. There is a lack of standardization for diagnosing and grading vertebral fractures, as vertebral deformity does not always represent a fracture. Fractures commonly occur in a wedge shape

with anterior compression or a biconcave shape with a central depression. There are proposed methods for quantitative and semiquantitative methods for fracture assessment. As there remains a lack of consensus, it was recommended by the US National Osteoporosis Foundation's Working Group on Vertebral Fractures that radiographic assessments should be performed by a radiologist or trained clinician who has specific expertise in the radiology of osteoporosis.[13]

Prevention

Calcium intake is critical for maintaining bone mass, and the recommended intake is not regularly achieved. The recommended intake in adolescence is 1300 mg/day, and it is estimated that 25% of boys and 10% of girls meet this recommendation. For older adults the recommended calcium intake is 1000–1500 mg/day, and 50%–60% of adults are meeting this recommendation. Vitamin D is essential for calcium absorption, and 400–600 IU/day is recommended for adults.

Physical activity throughout life is critical for building bone mass and avoiding vertebral compression fractures. Studies have shown physical activity in childhood and adolescence contributes to higher peak bone mass.[8] There are less data available on the effects of physical activity on bone mass later in life; however, there are strong recommendations for a multicomponent exercise program that includes balance and resistance training in older adults and particularly those who have sustained osteoporotic vertebral fractures[14] for fracture prevention and to maintain functionality. Kyphotic posture is associated with vertebral fractures and can contribute to balance deficits and an increased risk of falls. Accordingly, a supervised exercise program with a physical therapist is recommended.

Screening recommendations have been outlined by the National Osteoporosis Foundation as a means of fracture prevention. Recommendations include screening for all women over the age of 65 years and men over the age of 70 years. Screening can be performed by DEXA of the hip and lumbar spine or calcaneal quantitative ultrasound imaging.[15] Adults under the screening age may also require screening based on the aforementioned risk factors. The FRAX tool (Fracture Risk Assessment tool, World Health Organization Collaborating Centre for Metabolic Bone Diseases, Sheffield, United Kingdom; www.shef.ac.uk/FRAX) has been developed to determine a 10-year fracture risk based on easily obtainable clinical information, such as age, BMI, parental fracture history, tobacco use, and alcohol use.

In addition, there are recommendations for screening specifically for vertebral fractures. Despite a proportion of them being asymptomatic, vertebral fractures are diagnostic of osteoporosis, increase the risk of subsequent fractures, and are an indication for initiating treatment for osteoporosis. Indications for screening imaging to assess for vertebral fractures include women older than 70 years and men older than 80 years with T score < –1.0, women 65–69 years and men 70–79 years with T score < –1.5, and post-menopausal women and men older than 50 years with a low trauma fracture in adulthood, historical height loss of more than 4 cm, prospective height loss of more than 2 cm, or recent or ongoing glucocorticoid treatment.[16]

Management

The National Osteoporosis Foundation recommends initiating pharmacologic treatment for patients with hip or vertebral fractures, those with osteoporosis diagnosed by DEXA (T score < –2.5), postmenopausal women and men over 50 years with a diagnosis of osteopenia by DEXA (T score between –1.0 and –2.5), and those with a 10-year hip fracture probability of >3% or a 10-year major osteoporosis-related fracture probability >20% based on the absolute fracture risk model (FRAX).[16] Current US Food and Drug Administration–approved pharmacologic options include bisphosphonates, calcitonin, estrogen agonist/antagonists, PTH-134, and RANK ligand inhibitor. The selection of the appropriate pharmacologic treatment for osteoporosis depends on efficacy, tolerability, and safety profile and should be a joint decision between patient and clinician.

Facet Arthropathy

Although there is clear evidence of degenerative changes in the facet joints, the role of the facet joint in the etiology of low back pain remains controversial. There is a debate surrounding the prevalence, effectiveness of imaging and clinical testing in diagnosis, and treatment of suspected facet-mediated pain. The prevalence of facet-mediated back pain has been reported between 15% and 52%, with some studies showing a greater prevalence in the elderly[17] (Fig. 15.4).

Pathogenesis

As described earlier, facet joints are synovial joints that form the posterior articulation between adjacent vertebrae. With age and the degeneration of the intervertebral disc, load is transferred to the facet joints. In healthy structures, the facet bears between 3% and 25% of the load, whereas degenerative joints can bear up to 47%.[18] Based on imaging studies, degenerative changes

within the facet joints start at age 30 years and progress until they are nearly ubiquitous by the age of 60 years.

Although there is clear evidence that intervertebral disc degeneration incites degenerative changes in the facet joints, the reverse is also true. Motion abnormalities in the facet joints can lead to enhanced degeneration of the intervertebral disc. Orientation of the joints determines which actions of spinal motion they resist. The L4-5 facet joints are most coronally oriented (about 70 degrees from the sagittal plane), which makes them more protective against flexion and shearing. Conversely, the L2-3 and L3-4 joints are more sagittally oriented (less than 40 degrees from the sagittal plane), which makes them more resistant to axial rotation. The orientation of facet joints also changes with age. With age, facet joints at all levels become more sagittally oriented. Orientation changes can differentially affect the facet joints at the same level, a phenomenon known as tropism.

Degenerative changes that can develop include bony erosions, subchondral sclerosis, osteophyte formation, bony hypertrophy, and synovial cysts. Although these changes are well documented and easily identifiable by standard imaging, the correlation between visual degenerative changes and pain is less clear. To be a pain generator a structure must have a nerve supply. Each facet joint is dually innervated by the posterior primary rami of the levels at the facet joint and one level above. For example, the C5-6 facet joint is innervated by the C5 and C6 medial branches and the L4-5 facet joint is innervated by the L3 and L4 medial branches, relative to the fact that there is a C8 nerve but no C8 vertebrae. The medial branches also innervate the multifidi, interspinous muscles, and the ligament and periosteum of the neural arch.[18]

Clinical presentation

Diagnosis of facet-mediated pain may be the most controversial aspect of this condition. Multiple signs and symptoms have been proposed as predictors or diagnostic criteria for facet-mediated pain; however, there has been little success in their validation. Suggested clinical symptoms include age over 65 years, unilateral or bilateral low back pain in the absence of radicular features, pain not associated with cough or sneeze, and low back pain with groin or thigh pain. Symptoms proposed to be associated with facet-mediated pain include pain with extension, rotation, and lateral flexion that is relieved by flexion and tenderness to palpation over the transverse processes or facet joints.[19] None of these features, however, has been able to predict the response to local anesthetic block of the medial branches. Likewise,

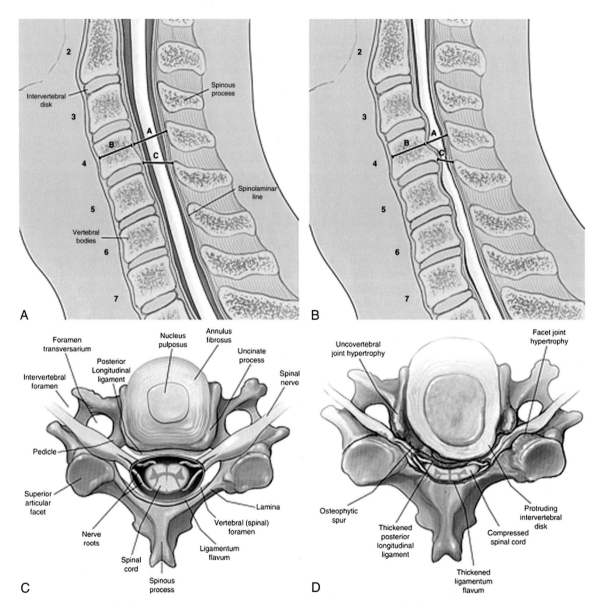

FIG. 15.4 **(A, C)** Midsagittal and axial views of the normal cervical spine. **(B, D)** Midsagittal and axial views of cervical spinal stenosis result from a combination of a congenitally narrow cervical spinal canal and superimposed cervical spondylosis. **(A)** The anteroposterior spinal canal diameter. **(B)** The vertebral body diameter. **(C)** The narrowest spinal canal opening as measured by the distance between the most posterior aspect of a vertebral body, including its osteophytic spur, and the nearest point on the spinolaminar line formed by the junction of the lamina and spinous process. (From Tracy JA, Bartleson JD. Cervical spondylotic myelopathy. *Neurologist*. 2010;16(3):176–187; with permission.)

radiologic studies have failed to show consistent correlation with clinical symptoms.

Localization of pain to a particular joint is similarly challenging. Patient-reported pain maps have been unable to identify consistent referral patterns. There was more consistency with provoked pain via electrical stimulation of the medial branches; however, these did not match patterns provoked with intraarticular facet injection.[20]

Diagnosis

Because of the lack of specificity of clinical signs and symptoms of facet-mediated pain, there are very narrow diagnostic criteria recommended. Facet-mediated pain should be diagnosed by radiologically guided, comparative, or placebo-controlled intraarticular facet injections or medial branch blocks. Comparative blocks are important for the diagnosis owing to a high false-positive rate for a single diagnostic block using lidocaine, reported at up to 40%.[18] As diagnosis requires multiple interventional procedures and the natural history of axial back pain is generally favorable, definitive diagnosis of acute and subacute axial back pain that is suspected to be facet mediated may not be necessary before initiating treatment. Only in the case of pain refractory to conservative measures are interventional diagnostic and therapeutic procedures necessary.

Management

Treatment of facet-mediated pain should consist of a multimodal approach, including medications, physical therapy, procedural interventions, and, in some cases, psychotherapy. Medications can include nonsteroidal antiinflammatory drugs (NSAIDs) and acetaminophen. No specific physical therapy program has been shown to specifically affect facet-mediated pain; however, yoga and tailored exercise program have both been shown to be generally helpful in axial low back pain.[21] The effect of intraarticular steroid injection is under debate. Multiple studies have evaluated the effect of intraarticular steroid, and the results are mixed. Overall, it appears that a subset of patients with facet-mediated pain, particularly those with inflammatory changes, could have intermediate-term pain relief from intraarticular injections.[21] This is based on studies using imaging to detect inflammatory changes, including single-photon emission computed tomography and radionuclide bone scintigraphy; imaging modalities are not routinely used in spine diagnostics.

Radiofrequency denervation is a widely studied treatment for facet-mediated pain that also has conflicting evidence. In this technique, a needle is guided fluoroscopically to the medial branches that supply the affected joint (or in the case of L5, the dorsal ramus is the target). Radiofrequency energy is conducted directly onto the nerve to ablate the nerve supply to the joint via a controlled burn. Some studies have shown a success rate as high as 80% for sustained relief, whereas others have shown much lower rates of success.[21] Inconsistencies stem from varying methods for patient selection; for example, not all studies used comparative or placebo-controlled blocks for patient selection. The most stringent inclusion criteria was used by Dreyfuss, who enrolled only patients who had 80% pain relief following a medial branch block using 0.5 mL of 2% lidocaine and 80% pain relief for greater than 2 h following a medial branch block using 0.5 mL of 0.5% bupivacaine.[22] Of these patients who met these criteria, 87% obtained at least 60% pain relief for 12 months and 60% achieved at least 90% pain relief. In addition to these stringent criteria, Dreyfuss further optimized these procedures by using 16-gauge electrodes and assessing the denervation of the multifidus muscles using electromyography to evaluate the success of the procedure. In combination, these results suggest that radiofrequency denervation can be highly effective if patient selection is optimized.

Cervical Myelopathy

Degenerative cervical myelopathy is a nontraumatic spinal cord injury caused by age-related changes to the axial cervical spine resulting in spinal cord compression. The clinical syndrome is characterized by gait imbalance, hand dysfunction, and loss of sphincter control. This condition has a significant impact on the function and quality of life and is among the most common indications for surgery among older adults. Degenerative cervical myelopathy is the leading cause of spine dysfunction in adults globally, and the annual incidence is estimated at 41 million per year in North America.[23] The pathogenesis of degenerative cervical myelopathy involves age-related progressive changes to a variety of spinal structures, including facet joints, intervertebral discs, or vertebral bodies; hypertrophy or ossifications of the ligamentum flavum or the posterior longitudinal ligament; progressive cervical kyphosis; or any combination of these processes.

Pathogenesis

The process is thought to occur by a cascade of events starting with disc degeneration. Owing to anatomic differences, the degenerative process in the cervical spine is slightly different than that in the lumbar spine. Discs degenerate similarly with alterations in the proteoglycan and collagen contents, resulting in loss of disc height and increased stress on joints. In the cervical spine, uncovertebral joints (joints of Luschka) lie on the lateral aspect of the vertebral body where a superior projection, the uncinate process, articulates with the undersurface of the cephalad vertebral body (Fig. 15.5). As disc height decreases, the load-bearing responsibilities get transferred to the uncovertebral joints, which in turn gradually flatten. This transfers load to the

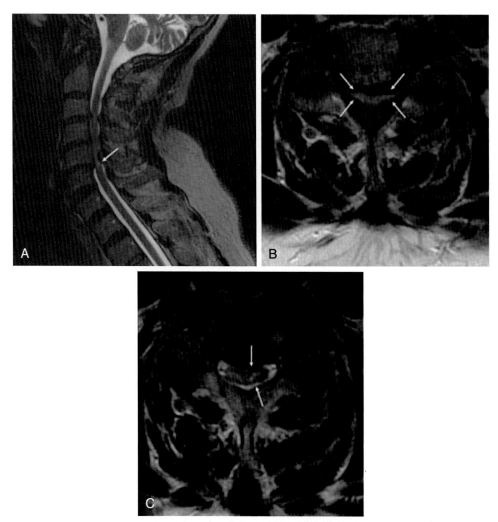

FIG. 15.5 Magnetic resonance imaging of the cervical spine. **(A)** Sagittal T2-weighted image of a 74-year-old woman with multilevel cervical spinal stenosis worse at C5-6, more than C4-5, more than C3-4. There is very little spinal fluid in front of or in back of the spinal cord at these levels. There is increased T2 signal intensity within the spinal cord just below the C5-6 interspace level (*arrow*). **(B)** Axial T2-weighted image at the level of maximal stenosis and spinal cord deformity (C5-6 interspace). The spinal cord is deformed and thinned (*banana-shaped*) by a bulging disk and osteophytic spurring anteriorly and the laminae and ligamenta flava posteriorly (*arrows*). **(C)** Axial T2-weighted image at a level between the interspaces below the area of maximal stenosis showing T2 signal hyperintensity (*arrows*). (From Toledano M, Bartleson JD. Cervical spondylotic myelopathy. *Neurol Clin*. 2013;31(1):293; with permission.)

vertebral endplates. Osteophytes form to improve the load-bearing capacity of the endplates and to stabilize the abnormal motion created by the degeneration. Osteophytes encroach on the central canal, creating anterior central stenosis. Posteriorly, the loss of cervical lordosis in combination with the loss of disc height causes the ligamentum flavum to stiffen and buckle, encroaching on the central canal. Other degenerative changes that can contribute to central stenosis include spondylolisthesis, disc herniation, and ossification of the posterior longitudinal ligament[23] (Fig. 15.6).

In addition to the static factors listed before, dynamic factors contribute to central stenosis that leads to spinal cord compression. Neck flexion causes

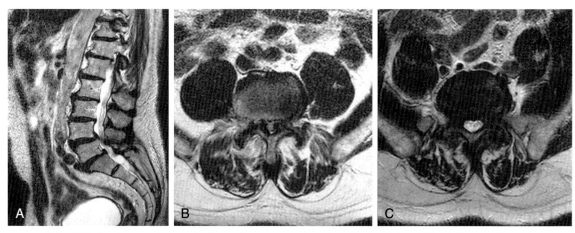

FIG. 15.6 Lumbar canal stenosis. Magnetic resonance imaging. **(A)** Sagittal and **(B)** axial images through L4-5 and **(C)** axial images through L5-S1, showing spinal stenosis at L4-5. (From Perkin GD, Miller DC, Lane RJM, et al. Spinal disorders. In: Perkin GD, Miller DC, Lane RJM, et al., eds. *Atlas of Clinical Neurology*. 3rd ed. Philadelphia: Saunders; 2011; with permission.)

the anterior osteophytes to encroach further into the central canal. Neck extension allows increased laxity in the ligamentum flavum, and the cord can be pinched between the vertebral body and the buckled ligament or the lamina posteriorly.

Biochemical changes within the cord contribute to disruption of normal neurologic signaling. Both vascular and neuroinflammatory changes have been demonstrated in in vivo and in vitro studies. Chronic compression of the cord leads to chronic ischemia induced by microvascular and macrovascular changes that cause an overall decrease in spinal cord perfusion. The result is hypoxic conditions, a decreased number of blood vessels, and reduced blood flow throughout the axonal pathways, including the corticospinal tract. Hypoxic conditions in the cellular milieu lead to ionic imbalance in the neuron and excitotoxic glutamate release, increasing the boundaries of the local injury.[24] Levels C5 through C7 have been shown to be the most susceptible to vascular insult and thus are the most common levels for myelopathic changes.

In addition, studies have shown increased permeability of the blood-spinal cord barrier with chronic compression, leading to edema within the cord, neuroinflammatory changes, and neuronal breakdown. The combination of neuroinflammation and hypoxic conditions leads to cellular apoptosis in the corticospinal tracts.[24] Overall the ischemia, neuroinflammation, demyelination, and neuronal apoptosis lead to abnormal signaling in the spinal cord and the clinical condition associated with degenerative cervical myelopathy.

Clinical presentation

Symptoms of degenerative cervical myelopathy are related to the degree of compression of the various spinal cord tracts. The clinical syndrome ranges from mild difficulties with hand function and mild balance deficits to incontinence and complete paralysis. There are several studies that have shown a surprising prevalence of cervical spine imaging findings in asymptomatic populations. In a study of asymptomatic patients aged 60–65 years, 90% of men and 75% of women had degenerative changes on lateral cervical spine radiograph.[25] Another study of asymptomatic patients aged 20–79 years found significant disc bulging in 87% of patients, evidence of cord compression in 5.3%, high-intensity signal lesions in 2.3%, and flattening of the cord in 3.1%.[26] This highlights the difficulty of correlating imaging findings with clinical symptoms.

As progression of symptoms is often slow, patients may not be able to identify them without specific provocation. Accordingly, a thorough history and physical examination are essential for early diagnosis. History should include difficulty with fine motor tasks, including buttoning, using a smartphone or keyboard, or changes in handwriting. Upper extremity paresthesias and Lhermitte sign are also reported. An early common finding in degenerative cervical myelopathy is the necessity of handrail use when negotiating stairs, which a patient is unlikely to volunteer unless asked by a clinician. Bladder dysfunction, a commonly queried red flag symptom, is a late finding of cervical myelopathy and would suggest advanced disease rather than being used as an early screening question.

Physical examination should include an examination of the cervical spine, including range of motion. Upper extremity function testing should include examination for intrinsic muscle wasting and strength, and sensory examination should include all testable myotomes and dermatomes. Tone examination of the upper and lower extremities may reveal spasticity in a myelopathic patient. Reflex examination should be performed in the upper and lower extremities, as hyperreflexia is a common finding. Hoffman sign is commonly associated with cervical myelopathy, although it has been shown to have a relatively low sensitivity (58%) in clinical studies. There is some evidence that the application of a dorsiflexion force to the distal interphalangeal increased sensitivity to 77%. This is at the cost of specificity, which decreases from 97% to 77% when comparing dorsiflexion force with volar flexion force.[27] Clonus may be present, as well as upgoing plantar responses. Gait examination should include tandem gait and heel and toe walking, assessing for losses of balance and a wide-based, unstable gait pattern.

The natural history of cervical myelopathy is variable and difficult to predict, despite multiple attempts to identify risk factors for disease progression. Being able to predict clinical deterioration would allow clinicians to pursue surgical intervention earlier in patients who were likely to decline. A classic study by Clarke and Robinson in 1956 retrospectively evaluated patients with cervical myelopathy and described distinct patterns of disease progression.[28] They found that 5% had rapid onset of symptoms followed by long periods of remission, 20% had slow and gradual decline in function, and 75% had a stepwise decline in function. However, more recent studies have shown a more variable disease course. Factors that have been suggested or shown in individual studies to predict clinical deterioration include increased neck range of motion, female sex, longer duration of symptoms, worse functional status at presentation, and circumferential cord compression on magnetic resonance imaging (MRI); however, follow-up studies have failed to consistently reproduce these risk factors.

Imaging assessment

Imaging typically starts with radiographs to assess for disc space narrowing, facet arthrosis, osteophyte formation, degree of cervical kyphosis, and presence of ossification of the posterior longitudinal ligament. Flexion-extension films should be included to assess for dynamic instability of any spondylolisthesis or

hypermobility at any segment. MRI provides a more detailed view of the soft tissues and spinal cord and can assess for disc herniations, facet hypertrophy, thickness and position of the ligamentum flavum, and diameter and shape of the spinal canal and spinal cord. It can also identify hyperintense T2 signal within the cord representative of edema or myelomalacia. Absolute stenosis has been defined as a sagittal canal diameter less than 10 mm and relative stenosis as less than 13 mm. However, these absolute numbers should be interpreted with caution, as they are subject to genetic variation and body size.

As described earlier, MRI is able to detect subtle cord compression and signal intensity abnormalities that correspond with variable clinical presentation. There is an overlap in MRI findings between myelopathic and nonmyelopathic cord compression, resulting in a "clinical-radiological mismatch." Prevalence of nonmyelopathic cervical cord compression has been found to be as high as 59% with an increase in age, from 32% in the fifth decade of life to 67% in the eighth.[29]

Management

Controversy exists over the efficacy and timing of surgical intervention for degenerative cervical myelopathy. There have been several attempts to compare surgical decompression with nonoperative treatment; however, there remains a paucity of randomized controlled trials (RCTs) evaluating the subject. These studies typically use the Japanese Orthopedic Association (JOA) score, a patient-oriented outcome measure to grade the severity of cervical myelopathy. The largest RCT compared operative and nonoperative treatment in patients with mild cervical myelopathy and found no significant differences in the mean JOA change score or 10-min walk score between the two groups at 10 years. There were significant differences in outcomes favoring the nonoperative group at 3 years. There was no standardization of conservative care in this study, but treatments included intermittent use of a collar, antiinflammatories, avoidance of high-risk activities, and intermittent bed rest.[30] Other studies comparing operative and nonoperative treatment, as well as many operative studies, have shown improvement in neurologic symptoms following surgical intervention.

A large body of the literature has evaluated outcomes of surgical intervention for cervical myelopathy. Multiple large-scale studies have demonstrated improvement in functional outcomes in patients who underwent surgical decompression for cervical myelopathy.[31,32] These studies have demonstrated greater improvement in patients with higher severity at presentation, suggesting that surgery is most beneficial for those with moderate to severe disease. There is evidence that all patients with symptomatic cervical myelopathy, from mild to severe, show clinically significant functional and quality of life improvement among a variety of populations and surgical approaches.[24] The most common surgical complication across all approaches is postoperative neck pain/discomfort.

Efficacy studies of nonoperative management have shown minimal clinical improvement. Those studies that did show clinically significant improvement with nonoperative care included patients with soft disc herniations and dynamic myelopathy,[33] suggesting this subpopulation may benefit from a trial of conservative care. The rate of conversion to surgical intervention after a trial of conservative treatment ranges from 23% to 54%.[24]

An area of controversy exists over how to manage patients with nonmyelopathic cervical cord compression or ossification of the posterior longitudinal ligament. Studies have sought to determine both the rate of progression to symptomatic myelopathy and risk factors for progression. Patients with asymptomatic cord compression or canal narrowing advanced to symptomatic myelopathy at rates of 8% at 12 months and 23% at 44 months. Based on the lack of evidence for prophylactic surgery in this group and variable rates of progression, it would not be prudent to recommend immediate surgical intervention in all of these patients but to instead counsel patients on the risks and signs and symptoms of disease progression and provide close follow-up with serial neurologic examinations.

Lumbar Spinal Stenosis

Lumbar spinal stenosis is ubiquitous among older adults and is the most common indication for surgery in those older than 65 years. The prevalence of lumbar stenosis is estimated to increase 60% by the year 2025.[2] Degenerative lumbar stenosis is defined by the North American Spine Society as "diminished space available for the neural and vascular elements in the lumbar spine secondary to degenerative changes in the spinal canal."[34] If compression of the neural structures does not occur, the canal is referred to as narrowed but not stenotic. Stenosis can almost always be attributed to three structures: a bulging intervertebral disc, a thickened ligamentum flavum, and hypertrophied facet joints. These degenerative changes are extremely common but not always symptomatic, leading again to a clinical-radiologic mismatch.

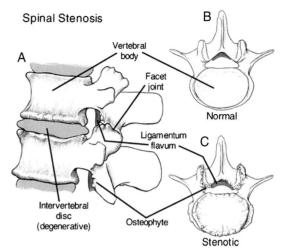

FIG. 15.7 Spinal stenosis pathology. (From Goodman CC, Kelly Snyder TE. Screening the head, neck, and back. In: Goodman CC, Kelly Snyder TE, eds. *Differential Diagnosis for Physical Therapists: Screening for Referral.* 5th ed. St. Louis: Saunders; 2013; with permission.)

Pathogenesis

As with cervical myelopathy, degenerative lumbar stenosis begins with the degenerative cascade, starting with the intervertebral disc (Fig. 15.7). As the disc ages and collagen and proteoglycan contents shift, the disc loses its ability to bear load. The disc itself can encroach on the central canal owing to shortening and widening. Consequently, as weight shifts to the facet joints, and eventually overloads their load-bearing capacity, joint hypertrophy and osteophyte formation ensue. This leads to further encroachment on the central canal. The ligamentum flavum further invades the central canal as disc height decreases. In addition, mechanical stresses induce changes in the tissue structure of the ligamentum flavum, leading to fibrosis and hypertrophy.

Lateral, or neuroforaminal, stenosis is defined as the entrapment of a nerve root, dorsal root ganglion, or spinal nerve as it exits the spinal column. Degenerative lateral stenosis can occur from facet hypertrophy or disc herniation. The superior and inferior borders of the foramen are made up of the superior and inferior pedicles, and this space can be constricted by disc height loss. The foramen can be narrowed laterally by the development of spondylolisthesis. In the case of lateral stenosis, symptoms are more often unilateral radicular pain, radiating in a dermatomal pattern, and weakness in a specific myotomal distribution.

Canal narrowing caused by a combination of the aforementioned mechanisms leads to radiographic, and sometimes clinical, lumbar stenosis. However, not all individuals with radiologic evidence of canal stenosis experience symptomatic stenosis. Studies have found disc degeneration, facet joint arthritis, or osteophytes in 90%–100% of patients older than 64 years at autopsy,[35] and stenosis has been identified in 80% of patients over 70 years. As described earlier with cervical stenosis, there is poor correlation between spine imaging and symptom presentation. Studies have shown that up to 21% of asymptomatic adults over the age of 60 years have radiologic evidence of lumbar stenosis. Therefore there must be other factors that contribute to symptom development in the presence of canal stenosis in addition to neural element compression. Compression on the thecal sac has been shown to alter capillary flow and electrophysiologic balance. Neural pressure also leads to intraneural venous congestion and decreased solute transport.[36] These microscopic and macroscopic changes to the neural environment contribute to an inflammatory response that likely contributes to neuron signaling and the development of symptoms. Although this mechanistic explanation does not differentiate between people who become symptomatic and those who do not, it does open up another avenue for genetic variation to play a role in response to mechanical compression.

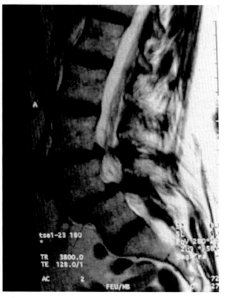

FIG. 15.8 Spinal stenosis decompression. (From von Strempel A. Cosmic: dynamic stabilization of the degenerated lumbar spine. In: Yue JJ, Bertagnoli R, McAfee PC, et al., eds. *Motion Preservation Surgery of the Spine Advanced Techniques and Controversies*. Philadelphia: Saunders; 2008; with permission.)

Clinical presentation

The clinical presentation of lumbar stenosis is a variable combination of gluteal pain or leg pain and fatigue with or without low back pain. The classic presentation includes neurogenic claudication characterized by pain, burning, cramping, heaviness, weakness, and numbness in the lower extremities that is exacerbated with lumbar extension or standing upright and relieved with forward flexion or sitting. Symptoms are typically gradually progressive, and rapid neurologic decline from mild to moderate lumbar stenosis alone is rare.[37]

As multiple diseases can occur concurrently in the elderly population, it is important to consider the differential diagnosis of leg pain and fatigue when evaluating for lumbar stenosis. The greatest mimicker of neurogenic claudication is vascular claudication due to intermittent ischemia to the lower extremities. Patients with advanced neurogenic claudication are unable to descend stairs or may do so backward to avoid the necessary lumbar extension, whereas patients with vascular claudication have more difficulty with ascending stairs owing to the increased cardiovascular demand. The physical examination when evaluating for lumbar stenosis in the elderly begins with observation. Observe seated and ambulatory posture for forward flexion and avoidance of extension. Motor and sensory evaluation of the lower extremities is essential to evaluate for dermatomal or myotomal distribution of symptoms. Moreover, a vascular examination should be performed to distinguish neurogenic from vascular claudication. In the elderly population, the two entities may occur concurrently. It is important to attempt to attribute symptoms specifically to either vascular or neurogenic causes, particularly when surgery is being considered.

Imaging assessment

Radiographic assessment begins with plain radiographs to assess the bony elements of the spine and their relationship to canal size. Flexion-extension views should be obtained if dynamic spondylolisthesis is suspected. MRI provides more detailed imaging of the soft tissue and neural structures. Axial images reveal the level of stenosis of the central canal and presence of lateral recess stenosis. Compression of neural elements can be identified, as well as the offending compressive structures. In cases in which MRI is unobtainable or unclear, CT myelography can be used to visualize the cause, localization, and impact of the stenosis.

Management

The goal of treatment for patients with lumbar stenosis should be to improve function and minimize discomfort (Fig. 15.8). Nonsurgical management should be considered in elderly patients with multiple comorbidities who may not be candidates for, or not desire, surgical intervention. However, absolute age should never be a contraindication to surgery. Goals of therapy should be discussed with the patient before proceeding with a treatment plan. Conservative management consists of medications, physical therapy, injections, and functional support. NSAIDs can be effective in the short term, although they need to be used with caution in the elderly population owing to bleeding, gastrointestinal, renal, and cardiovascular risks.[38] Physical therapy has not been shown to be effective as a stand-alone therapy but can augment other therapies and improve pain and function. Physical therapy program should focus on abdominal flexion exercises and core strength to maintain strength and range of motion and improve global functioning. Physical therapists are also able to provide ambulation and balance training and assess when assistive devices are necessary.

The role for epidural steroid injections in lumbar spinal stenosis remains unclear; however, an RCT demonstrated that epidural steroid injections with both lidocaine alone and glucocorticoid with lidocaine provided clinically significant improvements in pain and function after 6 weeks, although there was no difference in the two groups.[39] This suggests a role for epidural steroid injections for short-term benefit in elderly patients with lumbar stenosis who may prefer a conservative treatment approach.

Surgical intervention is recommended for patients with moderate to severe lumbar stenosis and for those patients who have failed conservative treatments. Studies have shown that after 3–6 months of unsuccessful conservative treatment, surgical intervention was more effective than continued conservative treatment.[40] There is a conception among providers that earlier surgical intervention is always better in the case of lumbar stenosis. However, this condition rarely exhibits rapid progression, and studies have shown that a trial of conservative treatment, particularly in mild to moderate cases, can be advised, and those who fail conservative treatment to go on to surgery still have good outcomes.[41] Overall, operative treatment for lumbar stenosis shows favorable outcomes in pain, disability, and quality of life. Even in the elderly population, mortality rates are low. A study of over 30,000 patients over 65 years who underwent decompression for lumbar stenosis showed mortality rates of 0.3% for decompression alone and 0.6% for decompression and fusion.[42] Importantly, complications in elderly patients have not been shown to be substantially different compared with a younger population. Nevertheless, it remains important to identify patients who will most benefit from surgery and those with a lower risk of harm. Factors predicting poor surgical outcome include radiologic findings not concordant with patient symptoms, diabetes, obesity, female gender, litigation, prior lumbar surgery, and concomitant presence of spondylolisthesis or scoliosis.[42,43] Although none of these factors is strictly prohibitive and surgery remains a safe option overall, these risks should be carefully considered and discussed with patients when making treatment decisions.

Sarcopenia

Sarcopenia is characterized by a global, progressive loss of muscle mass, quality, and strength that is associated with disability and poor quality of life. Loss of muscle mass occurs at 1% per year after the age of 30 years and then accelerates to a 10%–15% per decade after the age of 70 years.[44] Starting at age 50 years, there is a decline in leg strength of 10%–15% per decade until this accelerates to 25%–40% per decade after age 70 years. A decrease in both muscle fiber number and fiber size is seen. Sarcopenia is considered primary if it is age related and secondary if it is activity related, disease related, or nutrition related. Owing to the varying definitions of sarcopenia, prevalence rates vary across studies from 3% to 36% in older adults in the community. In ambulatory and inpatient rehabilitation facilities the prevalence of sarcopenia increases to 40% and 50%, respectively. In post–hip fracture community-dwelling patients, prevalence has been seen as high as 71%. Not surprisingly, loss of muscle mass and strength is associated with disability, falls, fractures, functional decline, decreased quality of life, and increased mortality.[45] Despite the clear impact on functionality, there are no standardized methods for screening for sarcopenia nor is it regularly assessed, even in rehabilitation clinics or inpatient units. Some proposed methods for assessing sarcopenia include grip strength, calf circumference, and relative appendicular skeletal muscle mass. Both DEXA and bioimpedance electric analyzers can be used to evaluate muscle mass.

Pathogenesis

The mechanism of sarcopenia is also not fully understood. Type I muscle fibers are most active during activities of daily living (ADLs), and type II fibers are recruited for higher-intensity activity. There is greater relative loss of type II fibers with aging, likely due in part to the decrease in higher-intensity activities.[44] Muscle fiber activity is also decreased with decreases in actin-myosin bridging and single fiber force. At a cellular level, there is a disproportionate decrease in

TABLE 15.1
Physical Activity Recommendations for Older Adults With Sarcopenia

Type	Frequency	Intensity	Time
Aerobic training			
• Vigorous intensity	3 days/week	70%–80% of max	20 min/day
• Moderate intensity	5 days/week	50%–60% of max	30 min/day
Resistance training	2 days/week	Slow to moderate lifting velocity at 60%–80% max	8–10 exercises 1–3 sets 8–12 repetitions
Power training	2 days/week	High lifting velocity at 30%–60% max	8–10 exercises 1–3 sets 6–10 repetitions

Adapted from Iolascon G, Di Pietro G, Gimigliano F, et al. Physical exercise and sarcopenia in older people: position paper of the Italian Society of Orthopaedics and Medicine (OrtoMed). *Clin Cases Miner Bone Metab*. 2014;11(3):220; with permission.

skeletal muscle protein synthesis and increase in protein breakdown.

Management

Treatment interventions for sarcopenia should focus on a combination of nutritional and physical rehabilitation goals. Protein status is directly linked to muscle mass and function and should be optimized in rehabilitation patients. Aerobic exercise is recommended to improve metabolic control, reduce oxidative stress, and enhance exercise capacity. Resistance training (performing the concentric and eccentric contraction of the muscle group over 2–3 s) is well established as a safe, effective, and feasible technique to increase strength in older adults. Studies have shown that a structured resistance training program (22 weeks, 3 days per week) was able to overcome age-related changes in muscle mass and limb strength. However, although resistance training increases strength, multiple studies have shown minimal effect on functional measures, such as walking speed and timed up and go tests.[46] Regardless, resistance training programs should be started early with progressively increasing loads to optimize results. Muscular power is the product of force and speed and has been shown to decline at a faster rate than muscle strength alone. Muscle power is required for many ADLs and instrumental ADLs, including carrying groceries and laundry, climbing stairs, and rising from sitting. Fast-velocity resistance training (performing the eccentric phase of muscle contraction over 2 s) has been shown to increase muscle power. This type of training can be particularly useful for combating sarcopenia, as it recruits type II fibers that are disproportionately reduced with aging.[44] As with classic resistance

training, in patients with sarcopenia, fast-velocity resistance training should be initiated early and proceed with increasing loads to maximize effect (Table 15.1).

CONCLUSIONS

Rehabilitation physicians are in a unique position to provide comprehensive interdisciplinary spine care to the elderly population. Given the multiple settings in which physiatrists practice, it is crucial for all rehabilitation physicians to understand the full breadth of spine conditions that can affect the elderly and their unique characteristics and treatment considerations compared with the general population.

REFERENCES

1. Hoy D, et al. The global burden of low back pain: estimates from the Global Burden of Disease 2010 study. *Ann Rheum Dis*. 2014;73(6):968–974.
2. Waldrop R, et al. The burden of spinal disorders in the elderly. *Neurosurgery*. 2015;77(suppl 4):S46–S50.
3. Manchikanti L, et al. Utilization of interventional techniques in managing chronic pain in the Medicare population: analysis of growth patterns from 2000 to 2011. *Pain Physician*. 2012;15(6):E969–E982.
4. Bogduk N. *Clinical and Radiological Anatomy of the Lumbar Spine*. 5th ed. Churchill Livingstone; 2012:272.
5. Hansson TH, Keller TS, Spengler DM. Mechanical behavior of the human lumbar spine. II. Fatigue strength during dynamic compressive loading. *J Orthop Res*. 1987;5(4):479–487.
6. Fujiwara A, et al. The relationship between disc degeneration, facet joint osteoarthritis, and stability of the degenerative lumbar spine. *J Spinal Disord*. 2000;13(5):444–450.

7. Yahia H, Drouin G, Newman N. Structure-function relationship of human spinal ligaments. *Z Mikrosk Anat Forsch*. 1990;104(1):33–45.
8. Nih Consensus Development Panel on Osteoporosis Prevention, Diagnosis and Therapy. Osteoporosis prevention, diagnosis, and therapy. *JAMA*. 2001;285(6):785–795.
9. van der Jagt-Willems HC, et al. Mortality and incident vertebral fractures after 3 years of follow-up among geriatric patients. *Osteoporos Int*. 2013;24(5):1713–1719.
10. Riggs BL, Melton 3rd LJ. The prevention and treatment of osteoporosis. *N Engl J Med*. 1992;327(9):620–627.
11. Leidig-Bruckner G, et al. Clinical grading of spinal osteoporosis: quality of life components and spinal deformity in women with chronic low back pain and women with vertebral osteoporosis. *J Bone Miner Res*. 1997;12(4):663–675.
12. Grigoryan M, et al. Recognizing and reporting osteoporotic vertebral fractures. *Eur Spine J*. 2003;12(suppl 2):S104–S112.
13. Kiel D. Assessing vertebral fractures. National Osteoporosis Foundation Working Group on vertebral fractures. *J Bone Miner Res*. 1995;10(4):518–523.
14. Giangregorio LM, et al. Too fit to fracture: exercise recommendations for individuals with osteoporosis or osteoporotic vertebral fracture. *Osteoporos Int*. 2014;25(3):821–835.
15. Force USPST. Screening for osteoporosis: U.S. preventive services task force recommendation statement. *Ann Intern Med*. 2011;154(5):356–364.
16. Cosman F, et al. Clinician's guide to prevention and treatment of osteoporosis. *Osteoporos Int*. 2014;25(10):2359–2381.
17. Manchikanti L, et al. Role of facet joints in chronic low back pain in the elderly: a controlled comparative prevalence study. *Pain Pract*. 2001;1(4):332–337.
18. Saravanakumar K, Harvey A. Lumbar zygapophyseal (facet) joint pain. *Rev Pain*. 2008;2(1):8–13.
19. Laslett M, et al. Zygapophysial joint blocks in chronic low back pain: a test of Revel's model as a screening test. *BMC Musculoskelet Disord*. 2004;5:43.
20. Windsor RE, et al. Electrical stimulation induced lumbar medial branch referral patterns. *Pain Physician*. 2002;5(4):347–353.
21. Cohen SP, Raja SN. Pathogenesis, diagnosis, and treatment of lumbar zygapophysial (facet) joint pain. *Anesthesiology*. 2007;106(3):591–614.
22. Dreyfuss P, et al. Efficacy and validity of radiofrequency neurotomy for chronic lumbar zygapophysial joint pain. *Spine (Phila Pa 1976)*. 2000;25(10):1270–1277.
23. Tetreault L, et al. Degenerative cervical myelopathy: a spectrum of related disorders affecting the aging spine. *Neurosurgery*. 2015;77(suppl 1):S51–S67.
24. Wilson JR, et al. State of the art in degenerative cervical myelopathy: an update on current clinical evidence. *Neurosurgery*. 2017;80(3S):S33–S45.
25. Boden SD, et al. Abnormal magnetic-resonance scans of the cervical spine in asymptomatic subjects. A prospective investigation. *J Bone Joint Surg Am*. 1990;72(8):1178–1184.
26. Nakashima H, et al. Abnormal findings on magnetic resonance images of the cervical spines in 1211 asymptomatic subjects. *Spine (Phila Pa 1976)*. 2015;40(6):392–398.
27. Lebl DR, et al. Cervical spondylotic myelopathy: pathophysiology, clinical presentation, and treatment. *HSS J*. 2011;7(2):170–178.
28. Clarke E, Robinson PK. Cervical myelopathy: a complication of cervical spondylosis. *Brain*. 1956;79(3):483–510.
29. Kovalova I, et al. Prevalence and imaging characteristics of nonmyelopathic and myelopathic spondylotic cervical cord compression. *Spine (Phila Pa 1976)*. 2016;41(24):1908–1916.
30. Kadanka Z, et al. Approaches to spondylotic cervical myelopathy: conservative versus surgical results in a 3-year follow-up study. *Spine (Phila Pa 1976)*. 2002;27(20):2205–2210. Discussion 2210-1.
31. Fehlings MG, et al. Efficacy and safety of surgical decompression in patients with cervical spondylotic myelopathy: results of the AOSpine North America prospective multi-center study. *J Bone Joint Surg Am*. 2013;95(18):1651–1658.
32. Fehlings MG, et al. A global perspective on the outcomes of surgical decompression in patients with cervical spondylotic myelopathy: results from the prospective multi-center AOSpine international study on 479 patients. *Spine (Phila Pa 1976)*. 2015;40(17):1322–1328.
33. Matsumoto M, et al. Relationships between outcomes of conservative treatment and magnetic resonance imaging findings in patients with mild cervical myelopathy caused by soft disc herniations. *Spine (Phila Pa 1976)*. 2001;26(14):1592–1598.
34. Kreiner DS, et al. An evidence-based clinical guideline for the diagnosis and treatment of degenerative lumbar spinal stenosis (update). *Spine J*. 2013;13(7):734–743.
35. Miller JA, Schmatz C, Schultz AB. Lumbar disc degeneration: correlation with age, sex, and spine level in 600 autopsy specimens. *Spine (Phila Pa 1976)*. 1988;13(2):173–178.
36. Lee JY, et al. Lumbar spinal stenosis. *Instr Course Lect*. 2013;62:383–396.
37. Watters 3rd WC, et al. Degenerative lumbar spinal stenosis: an evidence-based clinical guideline for the diagnosis and treatment of degenerative lumbar spinal stenosis. *Spine J*. 2008;8(2):305–310.
38. Issack PS, et al. Degenerative lumbar spinal stenosis: evaluation and management. *J Am Acad Orthop Surg*. 2012;20(8):527–535.
39. Friedly JL, et al. A randomized trial of epidural glucocorticoid injections for spinal stenosis. *N Engl J Med*. 2014;371(1):11–21.
40. Kovacs FM, Urrutia G, Alarcon JD. Surgery versus conservative treatment for symptomatic lumbar spinal stenosis: a systematic review of randomized controlled trials. *Spine (Phila Pa 1976)*. 2011;36(20):E1335–E1351.
41. Amundsen T, et al. Lumbar spinal stenosis: conservative or surgical management?: A prospective 10-year study. *Spine (Phila Pa 1976)*. 2000;25(11):1424–1435. Discussion 1435-6.

42. Shamji MF, et al. Management of degenerative lumbar spinal stenosis in the elderly. *Neurosurgery*. 2015;77(suppl 1):S68–S74.

43. Aalto TJ, et al. Preoperative predictors for postoperative clinical outcome in lumbar spinal stenosis: systematic review. *Spine (Phila Pa 1976)*. 2006;31(18):E648–E663.

44. Iolascon G, et al. Physical exercise and sarcopenia in older people: position paper of the Italian Society of Orthopaedics and Medicine (OrtoMed). *Clin Cases Miner Bone Metab*. 2014;11(3):215–221.

45. Sanchez-Rodriguez D, et al. Prevalence of malnutrition and sarcopenia in a post-acute care geriatric unit: applying the new ESPEN definition and EWGSOP criteria. *Clin Nutr*. 2017;36(5):1339–1344.

46. Latham NK, et al. Systematic review of progressive resistance strength training in older adults. *J Gerontol A Biol Sci Med Sci*. 2004;59(1):48–61.

CHAPTER 16

Assistive Technologies for Geriatric Population

MOOYEON OH-PARK, MD • JEAN H. OH, PHD

INTRODUCTION

All older adults wish to stay independent and enjoy a life of high quality and meaning. Since 1980s, many assistive technologies (ATs) have emerged to provide innovative and effective ways to help seniors be independent and reduce the burden for caregivers. The roles of these technologies are often complementary to traditional healthcare services for enhancing mobility of older adults, reducing hospitalizations, and improving their social participation. Healthcare providers should be knowledgeable on the role of ATs for the specific needs of older adults including the pros and cons of ATs, target population, barriers to implement AT, and how to overcome those barriers. This chapter will review the need of ATs for the care of older adults, different categories of currently available ATs and their effectiveness, and future development and research.

CATEGORIES AND TARGET AREAS OF ASSISTIVE TECHNOLOGIES IN THE CARE OF OLDER ADULTS

ATs are defined as "any item, piece of equipment, product system, whether acquired commercially off the shelf, modified, or customized, that is used to increase, maintain, or improve functional capabilities of individuals with cognitive, physical or communication disabilities." This definition was first described in the Technology-Related Assistance to Individuals with Disabilities Act of 1988 and revised excluding surgically implanted devices in the Individuals with Disabilities Education Act of 2004.[1]

Categories of ATs are as follows:
- Information and communication technology (ICT) (e.g., using computers and the Internet)
- Robotics (examples of research area are shown in Fig. 16.1)
- Telemedicine
- Sensor technology

- Medication management applications
- Video games (e.g., exergames)

Among the categories of ATs, in recent years robotics technology has received increased public and research attention. Research areas in robotics geared toward ATs include mechanical prosthetic designs[2] and cognitive-level artificial intelligence (AI).[3] Whereas mechanical engineering approaches seek solutions to develop physical devices or platforms, the works in cognitive-level AI are centered around software solutions to support cognitive capabilities such as perception and language understanding. For example, Fig. 16.1 illustrates examples of conversational robots that can interact and communicate with humans using natural language. To develop robots that can work in close proximity to humans as in assistive robots, research is being conducted focusing on soft robotics techniques that can be safe around humans; this work on inflated robots[4] inspired a robot caregiver character called Baymax in a Disney movie. Following a similar principle, soft sensor technologies focus on developing new types of sensors[5] that are lightweight, breathable, and flexible.[5] The notion of shared autonomy has been developed to facilitate a new robot control paradigm wherein human users still feel that they have the full control, while the robot's autonomy assists this control in a subtle way.[6] In the end-user interface, speech-based interfaces are becoming viable solutions owing to the availability of high-end microphones and speech processing systems such as Amazon Echo and the recent successes of machine learning and natural language processing.

There are several areas targeted by ATs to maximize the independence and quality of life of older adults. The main target area of ATs that has been researched is chronic disease management via telehealth and medication management, because of their immediate relevance to the health of older adults. The ATs used for these two areas have shown evidence of clear benefits and a high degree of acceptability for older adults.

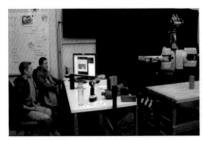
"Robot which can follow instructions of picking up green block"

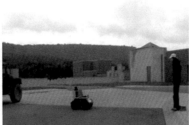
"Robot which can follow the instruction of navigate outdoors"

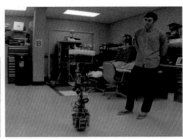
"Robot which can follow the instructions of inspection of environment and reporting to a person"

FIG. 16.1 Robotics applications being developed for the care of older adults.

However, the role of ATs has been increasingly studied in other areas including falls, social isolation, loneliness, well-being, and caregiver burden. Various forms of ATs may be applied to address the specific need of older adults.

Targeted Areas in Aging Care by ATs[7] are as follows:

- Access to general health information
- Chronic disease management
- Medication optimization
- Fall prevention and management
- Social isolation, loneliness, and well-being
- Mobility (physical dependence)
- Caregiver burden
- Other (e.g., dementia, depression)

Accessing and Retrieving Health Information

ICT (e.g., the Internet), which is used to retrieve health information, is the least expensive form of AT. In the United States, the number of Internet users older than 65 years has grown from 4.2 million in 2002 to 19 million in 2012, with a growth rate of 16% per year in contrast to 3% among those aged 30–49 years.[8] A similar trend has also been noted in the United Kingdom, with a 9% increase per year in the number of Internet users aged 65–74 years compared with a 1% increase for the 35–44 age-group. Web designers and engineers have put a great effort into enhancing the usability of the Web by older adults (e.g., readability and clickability). Health information is reported to be one of the main reasons older adults use the Internet (e.g., searching for information about medications prescribed, in addition to hobbies, news, finance, shopping, and socialization).[8,9]

The vast majority of older adults use search engines such as Google and Yahoo to access and retrieve health information, whereas only 17% of this user group visited sites recommended by healthcare professionals.[10] In this study, 70%–82% of participants thought that the information helped only "a little" or "did not help" them to improve self-care skills or to find new resources for exercise, diet, or support programs. In terms of the reliability of information from the Web, only 7% rated this information as extremely reliable. These findings highlight the need for health professionals' guidance in navigating the Internet and finding accurate and helpful information about health issues among older adults.

Among older adults, there are some barriers and potential risks of using the Internet. For those who are not familiar with the ICT, education specifically tailored to older adults is needed. There are a number of organizations and websites available to older adults that provide training to use the computer and the Internet (e.g., skillful senior, SeniorNet, or Microsoft accessibility). These sites generally educate not only on how to use the computer, but also on proper ergonomics for avoiding the development of pain and fatigue. Internet use can be time-consuming and may, in fact, be habit-forming to some individuals, potentially encouraging a sedentary lifestyle. Healthcare providers need to advise older adults about these aspects of Internet use.

Management of Chronic Diseases by Telemedicine and "e-Health"

As the older population dramatically increases worldwide, the prevalence of chronic diseases and physical and/or cognitive disability has increased accordingly. As reported by the Milken Institute, 78% of the healthcare cost in the United States can be attributed to chronic diseases.[11] Older adults tend to prefer living in their own homes; however, difficulties in the management of chronic medical conditions or limited mobility may threaten their independent living. Optimal management of chronic diseases requires frequent monitoring of the patient's status, to prevent exacerbation of these conditions and associated hospital

TABLE 16.1
Examples of Chronic Disease Management by Telemedicine

Disease	Intervention	Outcomes
Chronic heart failure[14]	Home-based telemanagement with one-lead trace to a receiving station with 24/7 healthcare provider access	19% decrease in hospital readmissions due to heart failure Mean costs for hospital readmission were lowered by 35% compared with control group
Diabetes mellitus[15]	Web-enabled computer with modem connection to an existing telephone line. Home telemedicine unit has camera, home glucose meter, blood pressure cuff, access to patient's own clinical data, and communication with nurses	Superior control of diabetes mellitus (HbA1c), systolic blood pressure, and lipid profile No difference in mortality rate between the telemedicine group versus control group
Amyotrophic lateral sclerosis[16]	Ventilator parameters were monitored via modem device connected to the ventilator	Significantly lower rate of readmission and emergency department visits, lowering costs by 50%
Chronic obstructive pulmonary disease[17]	Web phone with a touch-screen monitor. Daily input of data by patient; and the system automatically interacts with the patient and provides advice tailored to changes in their conditions	Increased patient and family satisfaction but no cost reduction

admissions or emergency department visits. The term "e-health" describes a range of the ICT that are used to provide healthcare.[12,13] This term encompasses (but is not limited to) Internet or computer-based technologies, telemedicine (monitoring and management), and electronic health records.[12,13] Telemedicine monitoring the status of the patient at home has shown positive effects on the management of various diseases (Table 16.1) and helps patients avoid unnecessary hospitalizations and visits to the emergency department. The existence of cost savings from using telemedicine as compared with standard care is debatable because of the high implementation cost of hardware and software.[18]

The key aspect of chronic disease management is self-management and behavioral change toward healthy habits. There are many Internet-based educational and self-management interventions that support patients to change the health-related behaviors.[12] The four core interactive design features of Internet-based health behavior interventions are as follows[12]:

- Social context and support: facilitate perceptions of humanlike interaction and social support
- Contact with intervention: provide direct or mediated contact with intervention or individuals responsible for the intervention
- Tailoring and targeting: provide optimally relevant information matched to individual users (tailoring) and groups of users (targeting)

- Self-management: Goal setting and action planning[19] and monitoring health behavior

The programs that have incorporated these features show superior effectiveness in terms of changing the behavior of users (examples of the programs are in Table 16.1). A brief report of 21 older adults showed that this agent was acceptable and resulted in significant increase in physical activity in older adults as compared with the control group.[20]

Medication Optimization

Medication optimization refers to a wide variety of technologies designed to help manage medication reconciliation, adherence, and monitoring.[21] Medication optimization technologies are particularly applicable for older adults, because 87% of older adults take prescription medications.[22] On average, an older adult is prescribed between four and five medications. In addition to prescription medications, 37.9% of older adults take over-the-counter medications, and 63.7% use dietary supplements.[22] The number of medications increases dramatically to an average of 14 medications among older adults discharged from acute hospital care to skilled nursing facilities.[23] Poor adherence to medication is reported as a worldwide problem of striking magnitude.[24] In the United States, for example, only 51% of those diagnosed to have hypertension adhere to their prescribed medication regimen.[25] In a survey done by the American Association of Retired Persons

(AARP), more than three-quarters of caregivers indicated that they were interested in technologies that can help with medication refills, delivery, and adherence.[26] A recent systematic review showed that interventions for improving adherence are not very effective, calling for innovations to assist patients to take medications as prescribed.[27]

There are various ATs available for this problem, ranging in form from very simple to highly sophisticated. A technology can potentially provide one or more functions of the five steps of the medication-use process: (1) assess, (2) prescribe, (3) dispense, (4) administer, and (5) monitor.[21] Assessing and prescribing are the steps delivered by healthcare providers, and medications can be reconciled during this time. Personal health records and medication list software are often used during this process. Dispensing and administration encompass the patients' process of adherence and are potentially the most challenging to address. This process is understood as a series of steps described in Table 16.2.[28]

ATs are available for the steps of fill/education, remind, dispense, report, and adjust. Some technologies are under development for detecting ingestion and metabolizing of medications, including Magne-Trace and Xhale's SMART. The MagneTrace necklace can record exactly when magnetized pills pass through a patient's esophagus and send the information to a smartphone or a computer. Xhale's SMART system is designed to verify whether patients have taken the right dose of breath-based medications. A recent survey about medication dispensing devices showed that more than 90% of older adults reported high ease of use and reliability.[29] Almost all older adults in the study reported that the medication dispenser helped them manage their medications, although initially many were not comfortable with the machine.

Improving Social Isolation, Loneliness, and Well-being

Social isolation among older adults is estimated to be up to 24%, as compared with 7% of the general population, and its prevalence increases with the increasing age.[30] This is a growing concern in this population due to decreasing financial and social resources, functional limitations, death of family members, changes in family structures, and the technically advancing modern society.[31] Social isolation and loneliness are known risk factors for physical and mental deterioration among older adults, including cardiovascular diseases (e.g., coronary artery disease), depression, substance abuse, self-neglecting behavior, and increased mortality and suicide.[30,31] It has been reported that the health risks

TABLE 16.2 The Role of Technology in Medication Adherence	
Steps of Medication Adherence	**Function of Technology**
Education	A drug information app giving information about the drug, instructions on how to take it, potential drug interactions, etc.
Remind	A device or app reminding patients to take medication on time
Dispense	A device that can automatically dispense by day with a locking mechanism to avoid double dosing
Ingest	A device that detects whether the patient took his/her medication
Metabolize	A device that detects whether the patient metabolized his/her medication
Report	A logging function can be added to the dispensing device, which logs the date and time of medication taken and automatically sends the data to the healthcare provider
Adjust	Automatic medication adjustment based on the adherence Assisting healthcare provider

Adapted from Center for Technology and Aging. *Technologies to Help Older Adults Maintain Independence. Advancing Technology Adoption.* Available at: http://www.techandaging.org/briefingpaper.pdf; with permission.

associated with isolation and loneliness are equivalent to the detrimental effects of smoking and obesity.[32]

There are two types of technological interventions that have been introduced to overcome social isolation and loneliness for older adults: ICT and robot technologies. ICT intends to provide easy and affordable communication and activities for older adults and comes in textual, audio, and/or visual forms.[30] In pilot studies, communication programs (e.g., smartphones, iPads, emailing, videoconferencing via Skype, and online chat rooms) and entertainment technology applications (e.g., Wii, TV gaming system, a virtual pet companion) have shown positive effects on alleviating loneliness.

The potential benefits of using ICT are as follows[30]:

- Intergenerational communication: ICT allows older adults to adjust to their younger family members, including their grandchildren, enhancing both the quantity and quality of their intergenerational communication
- Gaining social inclusion and support
- Engaging in activities of interest (connecting with the outside world, e.g., via videoblogging)
- Boosting self-confidence ("feeling young," "becoming one of the modern generation," "overcome challenges," "help others online")

The role of ICT in reducing loneliness, however, still needs further investigation to better define social isolation/loneliness and the type, duration, and intensity of the intervention ICT. A recent systematic review revealed a high attrition rate of older adults in ICT studies, although some older adults can benefit from ICT and will use it consistently after training. Many factors including living setting, cultural barriers, level of interest in and motivation for ICT, level of cognition and education, vision health, and ability to use the computer (e.g., using a mouse) are to be considered in determining the suitability of ICT for the elderly.

Robotics technologies have been used to reduce loneliness and promote well-being among older adults. Such social robots are designed to provide assistance, guidance, education, and entertainment to older adults.[33] For instance, robot therapy—using robots in place of the animals in animal-assisted therapy—has been tried. A seal-type robot named Paro was developed in long-term care facilities in several countries. This type of robot has specific features to stimulate people's experiences of animals and to bring out their feelings when they are interacting with animals.[33] It has been reported that the use of interactive robots in care facilities improved the mood, stress level, and loneliness of older adults and reduced the burnout of nursing staff.[33,34] The price of these robots and ethical debates concerning the use of robots remain for further discussion.[35]

More recently, with steep progress being made in the field of machine learning and AI in general, the idea of robotic assistants/companions is becoming more plausible than ever. Affordable speech interface systems such as Amazon Echo/Alexa or Google Home have brought the possibility of older adults having an interactive, conversational, caregiving robot. Techniques for language comprehension and dialoging have been developed for indoor and outdoor navigation problems, but for such technologies to be transferred to the companion/caregiving domain, there are several new challenges to be addressed, including safety and trust issues, as well as the mobility and perception challenges of physical robotic platforms.

Falls and Physical Functioning

The fall rate in acute care hospital settings can be as high as 9.1 falls per 1000 patient days, and the rate in a long-term care facility can be twice that number. Bedside rails and restraints have been traditionally used to reduce falls, although their use is less frequent in recent years because of their ineffectiveness and even potential harmfulness to patients. As an alternative, sensor technology–based alarm systems (e.g., bed-exit) have been used to alert the nursing staff and other caregivers that a patient is attempting to leave the bed unassisted and to facilitate an immediate response to the patient's need. Because a pressure sensor is embedded under the sheet, mattress, or chair seat, nuisance false alarms are not uncommon. A recent systematic review showed that false (nuisance) alarms account for about 16% of all alarms, which is too high, possibly causing staff desensitization to alarms, as well as being intrusive to patients and their family.[36] Dual sensor alarms using both pressure sensors and infrared beam detectors seem to detect a patient's true attempt to get out of bed with a higher accuracy as compared with a single pressure sensor–based alarm.[37] Even with dual sensor alarm systems, the significant rate of false alarms still remains an issue. Although one report found a reduction of up to 77% in fall-related injuries using sensor-based technologies, overall the evidence is inconsistent as to whether these technologies can prevent falls.[38]

Alarm systems monitoring patient movement in bed and wheelchairs are widely used in long-term-care facilities and endorsed by the Joint Commission on Accreditation of Healthcare Organizations.[39] Incorporating user opinions in developing and introducing alarm systems is an essential aspect of successful implementation of these technologies. Nursing staff report positive perceptions about the usefulness of alarm systems. However, receiving a sufficient amount of training on the use of alarm technologies is necessary for the staff to experience their full benefits. Bressler reported on a downside of using alarm systems in which systematically planned removal of alarm systems led to a reduced number of falls and a calmer environment for the patients and staff. This report emphasized that staff members began to become more attuned to the need of patients once they ceased to rely on alarms.[36] An alarm is not a substitute for staff, and thus adequate staff availability is necessary when residents wish to leave their beds.[37]

For community living settings, an unobtrusive, in-home sensor system that continuously monitors older adults for assessment of fall risk and detects falls has been developed.[40] This sensor system consists of a pulse-Doppler radar, a Microsoft Kinect, and two web cameras as a part of a more complete sensor network. The results of a pilot study showed a fall detection rate of 98% and a strong correlation between in-home gait velocity and gold standard fall risk measures.[40] Measuring in-home gait speed may provide a more accurate and precise picture of the physical function of older adults; however, the installment of such equipment and associated costs remain as limitations.[41]

Exercise-based video games, also known as exergame technologies, have been used to improve physical function and prevent falls.[42–45] Traditional exercise interventions demonstrate a benefit in reducing fall risk. However, adherence to exercise programs has been a great challenge for many older adults. Exergames were developed to improve adherence to exercise via engaging in recreation, performance feedback, and social connectivity via competition.[42] Older fallers tend to make a stepping error during a perturbed situation. They often take a step in the wrong direction, take too short a step, or step too slowly.[46] Schoene et al. investigated the effectiveness of a stepping exergame to improve the stepping ability of older adults. This study showed that a stepping exergame improved stepping reaction time and physical functional scores, reducing the risk of fall in older adults.[42] However, as per a recent systematic review of the use of virtual reality (e.g., Wii balance board, Mario & Sonic on Olympic Games, Nintendo video sports games), there is still no substantial evidence that exergame use facilitates improvements in physical functioning among older adults, either as a complement or an alternative to other types of interventions.[45]

Mobility Assistance

The main interest of mobility research in ATs has been an integration of the capabilities of the user and the AT via improving the AT mechanics, the user-technology physical interface, and sharing of control between the user and the technology.[47]

Power wheelchairs

In addition to traditionally joystick-operated power wheelchairs, a collaborative wheelchair assistant was developed for those who are not able to use the standard power wheelchair but have sufficient sensory abilities to detect when stopping is necessary. A collaborative wheelchair assistant guides the user on a known pathway, and the user only needs to focus on obstacle avoidance and speed control without thinking about path-planning or navigation.[48]

Wearable devices

Wearable robotic exoskeletons have been studied for gait training in spinal cord injury or stroke populations. For individuals with lower motor neuron disease (e.g., poliomyelitis), innovative knee-ankle-foot orthosis can assist people with leg weakness to achieve normal joint kinematics during walking. An interesting point for wearable devices for mobility is whether using ATs leads to a therapeutic effect. This combined assistive-therapeutic model for AT has been demonstrated for foot drop stimulators, in which long-term use of a foot drop stimulator improves the ability of a person to walk and may strengthen corticospinal connection.[49]

Assisting Caregiving

Millions of people are providing care for their loved ones by providing emotional support, help in daily activities, aid in household chores, and medical management. An estimated 43.5 million adults in the United States have served as unpaid family caregivers.[50] On average, caregivers spend 20.4 h per week providing care. More than 50% of caregivers are aged 50 years or older, with 10% being ≥75 years of age. Although caregiving has essential value for keeping older adults in their homes and avoiding institutionalization, it can be stressful and burdensome. There have been behavioral and psychologic interventions to reduce caregivers' stress. Although these interventions may help caregivers' stress, they do not reduce the actual work of caregiving. Technology-based interventions, however, can reduce the burden on caregivers by assisting in caregiving activities (e.g., monitoring of care recipient, medication adherence), as can be seen in Fig. 16.2.

One of the advantages that ATs can realize is persistent care (i.e., 24/7 monitoring) and attention, which is required for patients with advanced cognitive impairment. In the case of mild cognitive impairment patients, a conversational companion system can help patients to participate in socially engaging activities that are central in preventing cognitive decline. Technologies for intelligent dialoging systems are still in their early stages, and thus further investigation is needed to study the effects of such systems.

Based on a report from the AARP, 57% of caregivers used technology at least once a week in at least one way

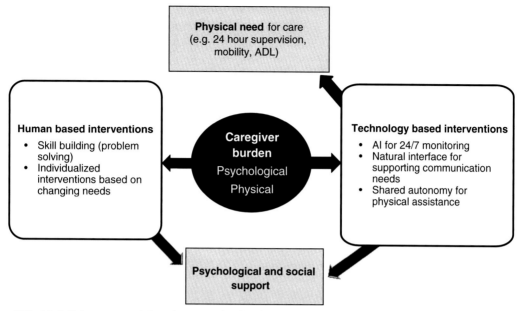

FIG. 16.2 Future approach to reduce caregiver burden using technology. *ADL*, activities of daily living; *AI*, artificial intelligence.

to assist with their caregiving duties.[26] The common uses for ATs were electronic scheduling, organizing, and medication refill and delivery. More than three-quarters of caregivers expressed that they were interested in technology that helps them check on or monitor a loved one, although monitoring technology is currently used by only 10% of caregivers.[26,51] The barriers to adopting ATs include lack of awareness, cost, perceptions that it may not be helpful, and lack of time to learn new technologies. The following are the greatest interest of caregivers for the possible role of AT.

- Prescription refill and pickup
- Making and supervising medical appointments
- Assessing health needs and conditions
- Ensuring home safety
- Monitoring medication adherence
- Checking and monitoring care recipient
- Managing stress and emotional challenges of caregivers

FUTURE DIRECTIONS IN THE DEVELOPMENT AND ADOPTION OF ASSISTIVE TECHNOLOGY IN THE CARE OF OLDER ADULTS

Technology use will rise with time across healthcare settings and patients' homes. Many older adults are interested in using technology for management of their health conditions and to maximize their independence. Among caregivers, lack of awareness was the most frequently reported barrier to adopting ATs.[26] Older patients and their family need to be educated by "tech-health" coaches who are not only knowledgeable about the quality of various ATs and their applications for health conditions, but also understand the social situations of patients. Healthcare providers caring for older adults need to be familiar with ATs currently available for patients to make appropriate recommendations to meet the specific needs of individual patients. Costs of ATs remain another main barrier to the dissemination of ATs. Two-thirds of patients and their family reported that they had to pay for ATs, and efforts with insurance payers should be made for coverage of the costs of AT working.

There are technical challenges as well. The components used in ATs need to be durable, light, and small. The control interfaces must be intuitive and user-friendly. For robotic devices, software algorithms may not be mature enough to produce a natural motion. Involvement of the end user throughout the development process is essential to come up with truly transformative ATs that can enhance the lives of the older adults.

REFERENCES

1. Individuals with Disability Education Act (IDEA). https://legcounsel.house.gov/Comps/Individuals%20With%20Disabilities%20Education%20Act.pdf.
2. Thatte L, Geryer H. Towards local reflexive control of a powered transfemoral prosthesis for robust amputee push and trip recovery. In: *IEEE/RSJ International Conference on Intelligent Robots and Systems*. 2014:2069–2074.
3. Oh J, Suppe A, Duvallet F, et al. Toward mobile robots reasoning like humans. In: *Proc. of AAAI Conference on Artificial Intelligence (AAAI)*. 2015.
4. Sanan S, Moidel JB, Atkeson CG. Robots with inflatable links. In: *Proc. of IEEE/RSJ International Conference on Intelligent Robots and Systems (IROS)*.
5. Chossat JB, Yiwei T, Duchaine V, Park YL. Wearable soft artificial skin for hand motion detection with embedded microfluidic strain sensing. In: *2015 IEEE International Conference on Robotics and Automation (ICRA)*. 2015:2568–2573.
6. Mulling K, Venkatraman A, Valois J-S, et al. Autonomy infused teleoperation with application to BCI manipulation. In: *Proc. of Robotics: Science and Systems (R: SS)*. 2015.
7. Khosravi P, Ghapanchi AH. Investigating the effectiveness of technologies applied to assist seniors: a systematic literature review. *Int J Med Inf*. 2016;85(1):17–26.
8. Nielsen J. *Seniors as Web Users*; 2013. http://www.nngroup.com/articles/usability-for-senior-citizens/.
9. Morrell RW, Mayhorn CB, Bennett J. A survey of World Wide Web use in middle-aged and older adults. *Hum Factors*. 2000;42(2):175–182.
10. Gatto SL, Tak SH. Computer, internet, and e-mail use among older adults: benefits and barriers. *Educ Gerontol*. 2008;34:800–811.
11. DeVol R, Bedroussian A. *An Unhealthy America: The Economic Burden of Chronic Disease*. Milken Institute; 2007.
12. Morrison LG, Yardley L, Powell J, Michie S. What design features are used in effective e-healthy interventions? A review using techniques from critical interpretive synthesis. *Telemed e-Health*. 2012;18(2):137–144.
13. Eng TR. *The Ehealth Landscape: A Terrain Map of Emerging Information and Communication Technologies in Health and Health Care*. Princieton, NJ: The Robert Wood Johnson Foundation; 2001.
14. Giordano A, Scalvini S, Zanelli E, et al. Multicenter randomised trial on home-based telemanagement to prevent hospital readmission of patients with chronic heart failure. *Int J Cardiol*. 2009;131(2):192–199.
15. Shea S, Weinstock RS, Teresi JA, et al. A randomized trial comparing telemedicine case management with usual care in older, ethnically diverse, medically underserved patients with diabetes mellitus: 5 year results of the IDEATel study. *J Am Med Inf Assoc*. 2009;16(4):446–456.
16. Pinto A, Almeida JP, Pinto S, Pereira J, Oliveira AG, de Carvalho M. Home telemonitoring of non-invasive ventilation decreases healthcare utilisation in a prospective controlled trial of patients with amyotrophic lateral sclerosis. *J Neurol Neurosurg Psychiatry*. 2010;81(11):1238–1242.

17. Sicotte C, Pare G, Morin S, Potvin J, Moreault MP. Effects of home telemonitoring to support improved care for chronic obstructive pulmonary diseases. *Telemed J e-health*. 2011;17(2):95–103.
18. Palmas W, Shea S, Starren J, et al. Medicare payments, healthcare service use, and telemedicine implementation costs in a randomized trial comparing telemedicine case management with usual care in medically underserved participants with diabetes mellitus (IDEATel). *J Am Med Inf Assoc*. 2010;17(2):196–202.
19. Webb TL, Joseph J, Yardley L, Michie S. Using the internet to promote health behavior change: a systematic review and meta-analysis of the impact of theoretical basis, use of behavior change techniques, and mode of delivery on efficacy. *J Med Internet Res*. 2010;12(1):e4.
20. Bickmore T. 'It's just like you talk to a friend' relational agents for older adults. *Interact Comput*. 2005;17(6):711–735.
21. *Technologies for Optimizing Medication Use in Older Adults*. Position paper. Center for Technology and Aging; 2011. http://www.techandaging.org/MedOpPositionPaper.pdf.
22. Qato DM, Wilder J, Schumm LP, Gillet V, Alexander GC. Changes in prescription and over-the-counter medication and dietary supplement use among older adults in the United States, 2005 vs 2011. *JAMA Intern Med*. 2016;176(4):473–482.
23. Saraf AA, Petersen AW, Simmons SF, et al. Medications associated with geriatric syndromes and their prevalence in older hospitalized adults discharged to skilled nursing facilities. *J Hosp Med*. 2016;11(10):694–700.
24. Sabaté E. *Adherence to Long-Term Therapies: Policies for Action*; 2001. http://www.who.int/chp/knowledge/publications/adherencerep.pdf.
25. Critical overview of antihypertensive therapies: what is preventing us from getting there? Based on a presentation by Mark A. Munger, PharmD. *Am J Manag Care*. 2000;6(4 suppl):S211–S221.
26. *Caregivers & Technology: What They Want and Need*. AARP; 2016. http://www.aarp.org/content/dam/aarp/home-and-family/personal-technology/2016/04/Caregivers-and-Technology-AARP.pdf.
27. Haynes RB, McDonald H, Garg AX, Montague P. Interventions for helping patients to follow prescriptions for medications. *Cochrane Database Syst Rev*. 2002;(2):Cd000011.
28. *Technologies to Help Older Adults Maintain Independence. Adavancing Technology Adoption*. Center for Technology and Aging; 2009. http://www.techandaging.org/briefingpaper.pdf.
29. Reeder B, Demiris G, Marek KD. Older adults' satisfaction with a medication dispensing device in home care. *Inf Health Soc Care*. 2013;38(3):211–222.
30. Chen YR, Schulz PJ. The effect of information communication technology interventions on reducing social isolation in the elderly: a systematic review. *J Med Internet Res*. 2016;18(1):e18.

31. Courtin E, Knapp M. Social isolation, loneliness and health in old age: a scoping review. *Health Soc Care Community*. 2017;25(3):799–812.

32. Holt-Lunstad J, Smith TB, Layton JB. Social relationships and mortality risk: a meta-analytic review. *PLoS Med*. 2010;7(7):e1000316.

33. Shibata T, Wada K. Robot therapy: a new approach for mental healthcare of the elderly – a mini-review. *Gerontology*. 2011;57(4):378–386.

34. Kanamori M, Suzuki M, Tanaka M. Maintenance and improvement of quality of life among elderly patients using a pet-type robot. *Jpn J Geriatr*. 2002;39:214–218.

35. Tergesen A, Inada M. It's not a stuffed animal, it's a $6,000 medical device. Paro the Robo-seam aims to comfort elderly, but is it ethical? *Wall Str J*. 2010. https://www.wsj.com/articles/SB10001424052748704463504575301051844937276.

36. Bressler K, Redfern RE, Brown M. Elimination of position-change alarms in an Alzheimer's and dementia long-term care facility. *Am J Alzheimers Dis Other Demen*. 2011;26(8):599–605.

37. Capezuti E, Brush BL, Lane S, Rabinowitz HU, Secic M. Bed-exit alarm effectiveness. *Arch Gerontol Geriatr*. 2009;49(1):27–31.

38. Kosse NM, Brands K, Bauer JM, Hortobagyi T, Lamoth CJ. Sensor technologies aiming at fall prevention in institutionalized old adults: a synthesis of current knowledge. *Int J Med Inf*. 2013;82(9):743–752.

39. JCAHO (Joint Commission on the Accreditation of Healthcare Organizations). *Sentinel Event Alert Issue 14: Fatal Falls: Lessons for the Future*; 2000. Available at: https://www.jointcommission.org/sentinel_event.aspx.

40. Rantz M, Skubic M, Abbott C, et al. Automated in-home fall risk assessment and detection sensor system for elders. *Gerontologist*. 2015;55(suppl 1):S78–S87.

41. Stone E, Skubic M, Rantz M, Abbott C, Miller S. Average in-home gait speed: investigation of a new metric for mobility and fall risk assessment of elders. *Gait Posture*. 2015;41(1):57–62.

42. Schoene D, Lord SR, Delbaere K, Severino C, Davies TA, Smith ST. A randomized controlled pilot study of home-based step training in older people using videogame technology. *PLoS One*. 2013;8(3):e57734.

43. Donath L, Rossler R, Faude O. Effects of virtual reality training (exergaming) compared to alternative exercise training and passive control on standing balance and functional mobility in healthy community-dwelling seniors: a meta-analytical review. *Sports Med*. 2016;46(9):1293–1309.

44. Laufer Y, Dar G, Kodesh E. Does a Wii-based exercise program enhance balance control of independently functioning older adults? A systematic review. *Clin Interv Aging*. 2014;9:1803–1813.

45. Molina KI, Ricci NA, de Moraes SA, Perracini MR. Virtual reality using games for improving physical functioning in older adults: a systematic review. *J Neuroeng Rehabil*. 2014;11:156.

46. Maki BE, McIlroy WE. Control of rapid limb movements for balance recovery: age-related changes and implications for fall prevention. *Age Ageing*. 2006;35(suppl 2):ii12–ii18.

47. Cowan RE, Fregly BJ, Boninger ML, Chan L, Rodgers MM, Reinkensmeyer DJ. Recent trends in assistive technology for mobility. *J Neuroeng Rehabil*. 2012;9:20.

48. Zeng Q, Burdet E, Teo CL. Evaluation of a collaborative wheelchair system in cerebral palsy and traumatic brain injury users. *Neurorehabil Neural Repair*. 2009;23(5):494–504.

49. Everaert DG, Thompson AK, Chong SL, Stein RB. Does functional electrical stimulation for foot drop strengthen corticospinal connections? *Neurorehabil Neural Repair*. 2010;24(2):168–177.

50. *Caregiving in the U.S. National Alliance for Caregiving AARP*. http://www.aarp.org/content/dam/aarp/ppi/2015/caregiving-in-the-united-states-2015-report-revised.pdf.

51. *e-Connected Family Caregiver: Bringing Caregiving into the 21st Century*. National Alliance for Caregiving; 2011.

Index

Note: 'Page numbers followed by "f" indicate figures, "t" indicate tables and "b" indicate boxes.'

Printed in the United States
By Bookmasters